"Phil's backyard Camino is a ritual space where ┌ the clarity of desire slowly merge through the s┐ praying. This is embodied prayer—body and so┐ medium of the deeper wisdom of the heart. . . . Ph┐ ....us with our own; we find we are not alone. Perhaps that is what the world most needs now."

—PAUL JANOWIAK, SJ,
Jesuit School of Theology of Santa Clara University

"As his rehabilitation physician, I witnessed Phil face his stage-four cancer, haltingly at first, then with growing kindness and confidence. Befriending his disease, Phil walks a transformational path that guides him beyond death and into spirit, joy, and wisdom. This work is a gentle cartography of the soul, an intimate portrait of one man's courageous journey with important lessons for each of us."

—DAVID S. ZUCKER, MD,
Swedish Cancer Institute

"Phil created a Camino in his backyard and a global neighborhood in his blog. In this neighborhood, there is a 'tapas table' where everyone is welcome to have a seat and rest; a place for hearts, souls, and minds to open and where meaningful, healing conversations flow. This book is an open window to that 'tapas table' . . . an invitation for us all to join . . . no matter where we are."

—CRIS MILHER,
Universidad de Buenos Aires

"Faith, hope, and love. In a time when so many are looking for things to be hopeful for, we have a book that restores our faith. In ourselves, in humanity. Phil harnesses the power of love by walking. Walk with him in this healing journey. You'll be glad you did."

—JOHN CONWAY,
veteran, farmer, pilgrim

"Phil, in this book, shows himself to be a wise, kind, and humorous guide. He's just the person you want as a traveling companion on the Camino de Santiago or the Camino of Life."

—JESSIKA SATORI,
author of *Come to My Dinner Party: The Odes*

"Phil tells his story, encouraging the reader to reflect upon and make the most of their real life. Central is his understanding of and commitment to true healing which leads to well-being with a charming and memorable style. I have enjoyed sharing this story with family and friends."

—RON ANGERT,
hospitalero in training, Camino de Santiago

"When Phil walked the Camino de Santiago, he received a new set of eyes. He's now able to see things that have always been there that he'd never seen before. In these pages, we learn that Phil's story is the story of each of us. It's all about our new set of eyes."

—TOM HALL, CSP
commander, chaplain corps, US Navy, Retired

"Phil Volker was a remarkable human being with an authentic human story that only he can tell. Ultimately, I believe it's about resiliency and courage in the face of adversity. *Walking in the Mud* can inspire a sense of resilience among all of us—regardless of our own medical and life circumstances."

—ARASH ASHER, MD,
Cedars-Sinai Cancer Center

Through the act of walking the Camino de Santiago (on a pathway carved out through his own backyard), Phil learns to stop fighting to cure his cancer and embraces physical, emotional, and spiritual healing. . . . With a great gift for musing and finding grace in the present, he invites us to join him: to not just show up for life but to partake. Join us on the pilgrimage. Savor the walk. It'll do your heart good."

—TERRY HERSHEY,
author of *Stand Still: Finding Balance When the World Turns Upside Down*

Walking in the Mud

The Diary of a DIY Camino

PHIL VOLKER

Edited by KATHRYN BARUSH
with REBECCA GRAVES

Foreword by DAVID S. ZUCKER, MD
Afterword by ANNIE O'NEIL

RESOURCE *Publications* · Eugene, Oregon

Resource Publications
An Imprint of Wipf and Stock Publishers
199 W. 8th Ave., Suite 3
Eugene, OR 97401

www.wipfandstock.com

PAPERBACK ISBN: 978-1-6667-1953-6
HARDCOVER ISBN: 978-1-6667-1954-3
EBOOK ISBN: 978-1-6667-1955-0

MAY 23, 2022 1:44 PM

Contents

A Note from the Editor

THIS BOOK IS AN EDITED version of Phil Volker's daily blog (caminoheads.com) which, as Phil pointed out to me, amounts to more than twice the length of *Don Quixote*. It is also a pilgrimage in and of itself, for the reader and for Phil, telling the story of what he called his "three C's"—overlapping and intertwined journeys with Camino, Catholicism, and Cancer. It is part memoir, part spiritual autobiography, and part *Old Farmer's Almanac* (in fact, you'll encounter a fourth "C"—the corn crop Phil tends and labors over each year). Trimming it down to a book-length manuscript was a labor of love for me. It took over two years, and Phil oversaw the entire process. When we were close to the end (and as Phil neared the end of his earthly pilgrimage) we had weekly meetings about his vision.

Why a book? Well, not everyone is a blog reader - although the online, live version of his diary amassed a community of daily readers and commenters that Phil affectionately referred to as "the neighborhood." Our hope is that this book can be carried in a backpack or to be brought along to chemo treatments, where Phil (with his gentle narration, folk wisdom, and humor) will be a welcome companion. In fact, you will read about when he and a friend accompanied each other to treatments and brought fancy tablecloths, battery-operated candles, wine glasses, and snacks. It was this DIY spirit that led Phil to transform spaces including a backyard in the Pacific Northwest.

I met Phil through Annie O'Neil, producer and director of *Phil's Camino* (which was, at that time, still in its infancy). We were chatting over a glass of wine and tapas at the College of William and Mary Symposium for Pilgrimage Studies. She asked what I do, and I described my academic work which, at the time, was a book about people who go on pilgrimage and create an artwork, space, or built environment to engender the experience for others. Her mouth dropped open and she said, "you gotta meet my friend Phil!" The rest is history. Annie invited me to put on my art history hat and give some notes on an early cut of the film. Shortly afterward, I flew out to Vashon to meet Phil and interview him for my book. He was always a little bemused that I called him a "land artist" and would say, "Catalina, I have a trail where I paint with mud." His backyard Camino became the case study for the first chapter in my book, *Imaging Pilgrimage: Art as Embodied Experience* (Bloomsbury, 2021). At some stage, I was transcribing interviews from Phil and it occurred to me that someone should write his biography. After chatting to him, I actually had a brief go of it but nothing conveyed his spirit like his own writing, so we had the idea to distill the blog into an autobiography.

There are too many people to thank and you will meet them throughout Phil's blog. I do want to especially acknowledge a few people who contributed a great deal of time and energy to the project: David Zucker, MD, PhD, FAAPMR (codename DZ), Cris Milher and Karen Kelly for their judicious comments on early drafts, Cynthia Barush and Mary Reilly for helping to extract the blog text into a document, Jen Huntley for her help wrapping up the manuscript, Annie O'Neil for being a catalyst for so many good things, and Dana Illo and Catherine Johnson for their support of Phil through his life and as we hashed out this project. I am also grateful to Phil's family: Rebecca Graves, Wiley and Henna Volker, and Tesia and Ramon Elani, for their patience, permissions, and contributions.

The biggest debt is to Rebecca Graves. As a novelist, a former school teacher, and Phil's wife of 45 years, she was the *only* person who could copyedit the blog with sensitivity to Phil's quirks, eccentricities in spelling, and coined words and phrases. I am so grateful to her for plowing ahead with the editing, even after Phil left us for the heavenly Santiago de Compostela in October of 2021. By that point, he had walked the equivalent of five Caminos (from Saint Jean Pied de Port to Santiago de Compostela—2500 miles, about the distance from Vashon WA to New York City). It was our duty to bring the project to fruition, and we have done so on what would have been his birthday, as well as the anniversary of the beginning of his first backyard Camino walk in 2013. We hope that you enjoy the journey as much as we have.

KATHRYN "CATALINA" BARUSH
Berkeley, CA
Winter Solstice (and Phil's birthday) December 21, 2021

Foreword

THE DAZZLING BRILLIANCE OF this work sneaks up on the reader, as Phil Volker, in his unassuming daily accounts, weaves a narrative that maps his journey through the medical and spiritual worlds into the far reaches of faith. He plies together his experiences and insights of living and dying with cancer into a powerfully coherent vision of healing and well-being. Through befriending his cancer, Phil threads the eye of fear's needle and is graciously received into spirit's ineffability. And, through the power invested in him by Spirit, he grows into a faith that transcends his own person and reaches outward into the heart of each of us who had the privilege of knowing him. Phil's story is as personal as it is universal—personal because it is uniquely his, universal because one day each of us will of necessity heed death's obligatory bidding. But how do we negotiate this, the ultimate challenge of human existence? In this remarkable work, Phil Volker leaves recognizable signposts, a kind of code that reminds us that we never, ever must walk this path alone.

Phil began blogging about his life with cancer 2 years after he was first diagnosed and 1 year after the cancer recurred. Derived from his blog, this book documents Phil's creative genius of visioning his cancer rehabilitation exercise program as a spiritual pilgrimage. Pilgrimage implies much more than just exercise. It is a mind, body, spirit endeavor that, when whole-heartedly embodied, promises transformation. Phil describes to us in accessible and unpretentious language the miraculous evolution of his journey. But there is a story that precedes by 2 years this one: Phil's initial diagnosis and awakening to his own mortality. As his rehabilitation physician, I witnessed this prelude to what is so beautifully articulated in this book. This introduction is meant to fill in the gap between diagnosis and blog by bringing you into one physician's experience of watching the development of Phil's remarkable human transformation.

It's only fitting here that I follow Phil in kind with a few excerpts from my "blog" (my clinic notes) early in my decade-long journey with Phil. I first met Phil in April 2012, fully 2 years before he started the blog from which this book is derived, and well before any thought of the Camino. He came to my clinic as a newly diagnosed patient, "pretty beat up", about halfway through his first course of chemotherapy. Increasingly fatigued under the physiologic rigors of chemotherapy with yet many weeks left, he was unable to walk more than about 100 yards without fatiguing. Following our first clinic visit, Phil committed himself to gaining strength and stamina during chemotherapy. I introduced rehabilitation strategies to him, including gradually progressive exercise as well as helped him build skills in adapting energy expenditure and physical activity to the inevitable fatigue that comes with chemotherapy. He returned a week later having taken on board my recommendations as well as acknowledging the understandable disease and treatment-related anxiety he that he was experiencing.

04/19/12

Phil has initiated a conditioning program consisting of slowly walking three quarters of a mile in 20 minutes every other day alternating with use of an elliptical trainer for 10 minutes. He is monitoring exercise intensity to avoid pushing beyond his current physiologic limits. We reviewed the patient's fatigue management program focusing on energy conservation and aerobic conditioning. We discussed Phil's exercise log and how to utilize this tool to minimize cyclic fatigue during treatment as well as the distress he was experiencing as a result of his cancer and its impact on his function, manifest as anxiety.

Over the next weeks, Phil progressively increased his physical activity. He chose to begin rebuilding his stamina and strength through regular walking and learning to pace his activity to manage his limited energy reserves. We were joined in the training program by Michelle Edelman, PT, a member of my cancer rehabilitation medicine team. While I used my specialized medical skills to focus his rehabilitative care, Michelle used her specialized physical therapy skills to help guide his developing training program. Phil learned that more is *not* better while on treatment, rather, "slow and steady wins the race." He learned that working hard was listening to his body, not pushing the body to its physical limits and exhaustion.

When Phil returned about a month later, it was clear that he had taken to heart Michelle and my recommendations. Both his fatigue and participation in daily activities had improved. He'd also progressed his aerobic conditioning program, now 20 minutes 6 days a week. His gains were all the more remarkable because he was only three quarters of the way through chemotherapy with 6 weeks left. At this point in treatment, most patients are more debilitated, not more fit.

05/14/12

Today Phil's wife, Rebecca, was here for the entire visit. We discussed "chemo brain" and its manifestations, and how to manage it. We also reviewed the patient's conditioning exercise program, reviewing its purpose in managing treatment-related fatigue. We changed some aspects of his program, in particular focusing on exercising earlier in the day. We reviewed the patient's chemotherapy-related side effects. Fortunately to date these have not been problematic. A relaxation training session with our biofeedback therapist had been helpful for his anxiety. Overall, Phil is doing extremely well with his chemotherapy and concurrent cancer rehabilitation. We also discussed the importance of adherence to balance home program exercises.

Phil disappeared from our clinic for about a year, only to return with the unanticipated recurrence of his cancer and resumption of chemotherapy. Nonetheless, he had continued to build his training program, now at least 4 hours a day of walking, carpentry, and ranch work. Anxiety was still present, waking him early in the morning. He was experiencing some balance issues.

11/11/13

We discussed Phil's rehabilitation management skills, focusing on sleep, energy conservation and moderate intensity conditioning exercise. The goal is to combine exercise, energy conservation and good sleep to minimize fluctuations in fatigue across each day and across each cycle of chemotherapy and, more, so that the whole system is synced and ready for action. We discussed the reasons why chemotherapy can impair balance, and the 3 systems that are responsible for keeping a person steady on their feet: vision, inner ear, and proprioception (the body's ability to sense its orientation in space). I encouraged Phil to resume physical therapy to help increase muscle strength and rehabbing the body's balance system.

Then, the big turnaround! Phil converted to Catholicism and, along the way, hatched the idea (more aptly, perhaps, it hatched him) of his own backyard pilgrimage, integrating his cancer rehabilitation program with the inspiration of "the Godfather of do-it-yourselfers, Eratosthenes", his love of "walking and praying the rosary in the weather" and Martin Sheen's *The Way*. Brilliant! His training moved more deeply into his mind and heart, fortified by his increasing ease in negotiating the ebb and flow of his energy reserves. Despite the background of physiologic instability, Phil's presence radiated emotional and spiritual stability. And such joy! Remarkable to witness. At that visit, I became as much a coach and counselor as a physician.

12/10/13

DISCUSSION: We discussed Phil's plan to set up a trekking course on his ranch on Vashon Island as the next best thing to walking "El Camino de Santiago" in Spain. There are several things to consider here. First is that with continued chemotherapy, fatigue tends to become cumulative. To progress the duration of conditioning exercise sessions during treatment, the training needs to be monitored very closely. What we are aiming for is maintaining moderate aerobic intensity across fatigue fluctuations of each treatment cycle. If you are, for example, more fatigued early in each cycle, you will find yourself walking slower and less far in the same amount of time, but still at moderate intensity. You are giving your body the training stimulus it needs to progressively build fitness even while at lower levels of capacity. The correct "dose" of exercise is the goal, not how far or how fast you are walking.

We reviewed the overtraining syndrome, which means physical activity pushed beyond the body's ability to restore and continue to build fitness. This can easily happen with exercise or daily activity. We discussed its 3 components: physical (outstripping body energy resources), behavioral (acting on the belief that "more is better") and emotional (aiming to maintain one's pre-cancer sense of identity and role). So tempting, but ultimately a training error! I emphasized the importance of his cultivating "physiologic stewardship" to meet the long-term goal of maintaining or building fitness. Practicing energy conservation and a well-thought-out conditioning exercise program can help avoid "burning out"—overtraining.

True to form, Phil continued to progress his training program. When he returned a month later:

01/07/14

We discussed the outstanding training progress Phil has made over the past month. I think this is largely due to his strong commitment to developing fitness with the goal of the long trek in Spain. We reviewed in detail his current program and discussed progression. I noted that when he resumes construction work that he may need to modify his program. I am confident he'll be able to do this successfully because he has excellent energy conservation skills. We also discussed the general pattern of long-term cancer treatment which involves chemotherapy and frequent scans to assess disease status.

By March, Phil was training 2 and a half hours a day. He was sleeping well and optimistic. Yet we did not yet know whether his disease would be stable enough for the month long "chemotherapy holiday" and pilgrimage to Spain. No problem! Phil remained undaunted.

03/20/14

Today we reviewed the continued progress Phil has made in his training program. His current volume of aerobic conditioning exercise is 900 minutes/week compared to the national minimal recommendation of 150 minutes/week. His fatigue has actually improved since his last visit. There is, as expected, a cyclic characteristic. He is managing this well.

We also discussed the impact that his "stewardship" of his healthy cells has had on the existential issues of living with cancer. The recognition that "mortality applies to me" has helped propel Phil into vivid awareness of what is important in his life, moment-to-moment and day-to-day. This includes appreciation of cycles of nature, friendship, and exploration of spiritual and religious domains of human existence. This is consistent with what is in the medical and psychological literature is called "posttraumatic growth" or "benefit finding."

Phil's cyclic, cumulative rhythms of fatigue were inevitable with his chemotherapy cocktail, but he had learned to roll with it, not push against it. He was learning to dance with the changing physiologic environment he now inhabited. Armed with this awareness (and unparalleled motivation), Phil became an active participant in his treatment. He paced himself well, progressively increasing his cardiorespiratory fitness, balance, and strength. With the energy uplift that rewarded him, he turned towards the furthest reaches of his spiritual heart and discovered inspired coherence in living with his cancer and its future uncertainty.

What Phil calls the "3 C's"—Cancer, Catholicism and Camino—is his code name for the reliable compass that navigated him through his unpredictable future. Perhaps Catholicism should be first in the list, because it became his North Star, with Mother Mary "the font of comfort, and [his] learning how to open [himself] to that, to her." But Cancer *is* first. Why? Because it "was the spark that started the whole thing ablaze," the "jarring announcement" that shook Phil awake to the one life he had. Cancer's herald of early death was also the death of great expectations. And here is where Camino fits in because the death of expectations is one of its lessons. Not surprisingly, his anxiety and sleep problems faded away.

Still, more progress in his training program:

05/15/14

Today we reviewed Phil's continuing progress in his rehabilitation program. Spain and El Camino de Santiago remains in his sight. He is consistently training 3 hours, 6 days a week carrying his backpack on his backyard Camino. His fitness and activity tolerance are remarkable given the fact that he has been on palliative chemotherapy since recurrence in July 2013. His fatigue is minimal in this context. I expect that he will be able to do well in Spain on his pilgrimage. We continued our discussion of the existential and spiritual issues that have informed Phil's relationship to his illness. We still don't know if his disease will be stable enough to head to Spain.

By July, Phil was training 3 hours a day while carrying his backpack. And, to our great delight, Phil's CT scan confirmed that his disease was stable. Phil's pilgrimage to Spain was now a reality! El Camino de Santiago was on the horizon. One more chemotherapy treatment and then on the plane 2 days later to face the Pyrenees, just when fatigue from chemotherapy would be at its peak. Phil, take it from here!

DAVID S. ZUCKER, MD, PHD, FAAPMR
Attending Physician
Cancer Rehabilitation Medicine Services
Swedish Cancer Institute
Seattle, WA

The Bio of Phil Volker

MY LAST EIGHT YEARS have been dominated by my cancer diagnosis, my conversion to Catholicism and my walking the pilgrimage trail the Camino de Santiago in Spain—my Three C's. Of course, none of this would have been possible without the love and support of my wife Rebecca and our family. Nor would it have been possible without the continuing care and treatment given me at Swedish Cancer Institute, Seattle, through physicians Philip Gold, MD and David Zucker, MD, PhD, FAAPMR. Nor would it have been possible without the continuing support of Teleios Bible Study, my parish and the Archdiocese of Seattle.

This is my story in short: In 2011 I was diagnosed with colon cancer. I was operated on at Swedish Medical Center, Seattle to remove the tumor, a short section of my large intestine and associated lymph nodes. That was basically successful although some cancer evidence was found in those nodes. Therefore, I started on chemotherapy to minimize the possibility of spreading and that lasted for six months and was brutal.

Then there was some good news—I had a year off! But then a periodic scan revealed that the cancer had spread to my liver and lungs. That upped my stage two cancer to stage four. That started chemo treatments for a solid year which, remarkably, I was able to deal with better. Part of the reason that I was able to do so is that my oncologist replaced one of the standard drugs in the cocktail with a newer one that seemed a better fit.

As part of my Cancer Rehabilitation, I developed a trail here on our property to be an exercise program. One day years ago here on Vashon Island I had opened up a used book, turned to a random page, and was treated to the story of Eratosthenes. He was a Greek, the head librarian at the famous library in Alexandria, Egypt and most importantly he was a poet who wondered. Somehow he envisioned a way to measure the circumference of the earth from his little corner of the Mediterranean Sea using a well and a stick in the ground separated by a 500-mile distance and a geometric principle. Oh, and the sun. He used a shadow from the sun on Summer Solstice. He calculated this circumference to be 25,000 miles, amazingly close to the actual 24,000 for his time (200 BC). This is mind-boggling! For me, this guy was the Grand Godfather of do-it-yourselfers - how can someone pull off this kind of a caper with things at hand in his own backyard? It got me thinking, what else can come out of one's backyard?

Walking and being in the outdoors appealed to me as I was already out praying my rosary daily in the weather. At some point in all this I had seen Martin Sheen's *The Way* and was taken with the idea of it, this pilgrimage thing. The idea that I could somehow do a pilgrimage right here where I was, in the condition that I was in, gelled for me. It could be said that it was a fantasy, a myth but whatever it was it proved incredibly helpful and vital for my overall health and well-being. It was part medical, part athletic, part historical, part religious, part spiritual and I would learn that it would connect me to a whole new world.

In February 2014 we saw *Walking the Camino—Six Ways to Santiago,* the feature length documentary where we were introduced to Annie O'Neil, my future cohort. Rebecca and Annie started communicating through Facebook and Annie came to visit us and walk Phil's Camino in March of that same year.

At this time I was very weak from rounds of chemotherapy and was tentatively walking my camino, never expecting to go to Spain to do the real thing. Remarkably Annie was at this time working on her book *The Everyday Camino With Annie* in which she was giving readers a glimpse of the magic of walking the Camino from wherever they might be physically. So artistically we were working on some of the same ideas. And that was the magic that occurred between us, and the genesis of the documentary, *Phil's Camino.*

So through a series of small miracles the film got started and my pilgrimage to Spain looked like it would happen "for real." It was a marvelous time and it taught us a lot about each other and about ourselves. With much help from numerous sources the film progressed and came to be, premiering in the spring of 2015. And now the years have started to pass and the film has gathered momentum. It is a joy to be associated with it as it continues to educate and inspire. Sometimes just being us becomes noteworthy.

PHIL VOLKER
Raven Ranch, Vashon Island
Summer, 2020

Part I

We're on Shore!

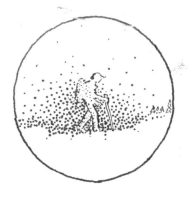

May 21, 2014 / Saint James Again

Caminoheads—it was hard fought and tough on the treasury but we are on the shore and moving inland rapidly. Bullets, beans and bandages will be coming in behind us. So glad that we had so many friends egging us on to get this blog established. We will have fun! We will keep each other inspired! All that and more. That's all the writing for one day.

SJA (St. James Again), Phil.

May 23, 2014 / A Little Story

OK, day three and we are going non-linear. Just wanted to post a little story about stuff, as in material things. A dear friend brought the topic up and I thought that I would jump on it before it got away. And this is walking related!

Several years ago I started teaching a class on survival for the State of Washington to students that were purchasing their first hunting license. As part of the process of my learning about the topic I read every account that I could find. One that sticks out in my mind was one called "The Longest Walk." This is by a Polish officer in WWII who was captured by the Russians and sent to Siberia to one of their famous gulags. Grim is not the word for it. So, he gets it in his head to escape by getting a group together and heading south in the winter (or is it always winter?). He winds up walking all the way to India. I forget how long it takes him but what I remember is that he slept for two months in a hospital there after arriving. And not everyone made it.

But the point is that they did it with practically no stuff. They decided not to carry weapons. They had no shoes or belts. Scraps of furs on the feet and held their pants up with one hand. And somewhere along the "trail" one of the troops found a roll of wire. The roll was such that he put it over his head and carried it the rest of the way. Trading stock he figured. So, they are walking and at some point they are befriended by a man who lives alone in a cave. He takes them in and feeds them for two or three days. And his only possession is a cast iron pot that he fed them out of. It used to have a bail handle, like a bucket, but it was missing. Hard to picture handling a heavy pot over an open fire with no handle. So, wire man gets out one of the only things that they possess and fashions a handle for pot man. And this is one of the best things that ever happens to pot man and maybe to both of them.

In our lives today we are overwhelmed really with stuff. We have to fend it off and manage it and deal with it to such an extent that it takes up valuable time. Can we streamline our gear and start having a "better" experience? Walking the Camino and living out of a small backpack would be a good learning experience for us. What is really important? He who dies with the most toys wins? Or is the point something else?

May 28, 2014 / Backyard Camino

Phase two walking is to try and duplicate the French Camino as much as possible. Phase one was for me and my original needs and capabilities and that has been satisfied. Now we are interested in testing and breaking in gear, team building and increasing our daily mileage.

May 31, 2014 / A Tale of Two Journeys

I got my hiking boots on early today and am ready for whatever. Roy is here in one hour to pick me up and take us to our weekly Bible class. All kinds of stuff happening today and winding up teaching an archery class to kids from the Zen Center this evening. Keeping busy is good medicine.

I got to hold two of our children yesterday, one a son and one a grandson. The grandson is working on being three weeks old and the son is twenty-five (years). Osian is the new grandboy and he has caused all sorts of excitement around here. Two grandmoms on the hover right now. Osian is a Gaelic name meaning little deer or dear, not quite sure at the moment. Wiley is our rough and tumble son who is off on another adventure and our goodbye included a chance for me to hold him.

Wiley is off to join some of his buddies who are hiking the Pacific Crest Trail (PCT). They started at the Mexican border and are set on getting to Canada. Wiley is flying out today to meet them somewhere around Bakersfield, CA. So far they have been doing twenty miles a day. Rough and tumble they are. So, we wish them all the luck and give them our prayers.

And Osian, he is not quite walking yet but showing great promise! He is eight pounds now. He was born with lots of hair.

So, I got to hold the future which is humbling. All the good and the bad to come will be influenced by these guys and their peers. Have we taught them well? Are we teaching them well?

June 3, 2014 / Cheap Thrills

Janis Joplin, of course! Though what I am thinking of are a few things that have happened along the Camino lately. But first I am going to show you my numbers from yesterday which I want to get in place as part of the reporting while on the trip. This will include the number of miles/kilometers covered, steps on pedometer and other metrics.

June 2nd—6 miles on the Vashon Meseta (Old Mill Rd), 13910 steps for all day.

So, Kelly and I were walking what we started calling Kelly's Hills two days ago. This could also be called the Vashon Pyrenees. Vashon is basically, geologically speaking, a pile of glacial till. Close up till is rounded stones worn smooth by the movement and pressure of the ice. The last ice left Vashon in its present form, give or take some erosion. In some areas the surface of the island is fairly flat but in some it is fairly steep going to 300 some feet in elevation above the salt water. We were climbing these undulating piles that form part of the present landscape. Anyway, the day was getting warmer and we were breaking a sweat and were taking off another layer of clothing when we both realized that we had the zip off pants on and that we could get to shorts pretty darn quick. This was a first!

Of course, normally this would be/should be a small thing that would not merit recording but the Camino is beyond normal, right? Realizing that small changes can bring big results in comfort and performance is big and worth paying attention to. Walking with shorts was such a joy just for the immediate freedom and to celebrate that the darn winter was finally gone! A Cheap Thrill for sure.

Also, out on the Vashon Meseta I was really able to stretch out and get in cruisin' mode. This was something that I learned about on the cross-country team in high school. It's about economy. To eliminate movement that is counterproductive is a good thing. Two types of bad movement are bobbing up and down and side to side motion. Also, length of stride comes into play.

Anyway, I get a sensation at the point of max economy, cruisin' speed, when my contact with the earth becomes very light. I am not beating on it with my boots or my sticks. All energy is focused on going forward. It is overdrive gear. It is akin to skipping a flat stone on the water. I got there finally yesterday and it was a real big breakthrough to be back there! Again, maybe a small thing in some ways of thinking but huge in the "here and now" of the Camino. Truly a Cheap Thrill!

June 4, 2014 / Inner Camino

Yesterday's Stats: 5 miles on Kelly's Hills with 20040 steps for all day.

Yesterday was a banner day. Kelly blew us all out of the water, the guy is all heart! To start I had a record day with breaking twenty thousand steps. But Kelly was off with

Rick to walk in the early morning and then with me in the late morning, non-stop. So, he had twelve miles and 27370 steps before noon! No slouch, that Kelly.

What is this Inner Camino, anyway? Doesn't sound like the usual fun and games. Why does it come up in regard to this one walk? Why not just walk, drink wine and call it good?

I guess what I am struggling with is my inability to talk about the Inner Camino as an idea in itself in any substantial way but I'll give it a shot. Well to start, it is generally the inner spiritual journey that we are all on anyway. We are in different places along it but we are definitely all on it somewhere. Most of the time we are too busy and distracted to see it, much less work on it.

But I know that the Camino offers a great venue to do this in if this is what we want to do. It is all set up and going now for over a thousand years to be a sort of spiritual boot camp. A rough and ready experience that works us over for the good!

Look at me pontificating on this thing that I haven't experienced yet. Or have I? Not in Spain anyway. I have over 500 miles in already on Camino de Vashon, remember, and have been worked over by the best of them: Saint James, Sister Joyce and Annie O'Neil to mention a few.

Eight thirty! Oh, I have to go. That animal Kelly will be here momentarily and will be pumped to walk! Spiritual boot camp, up, up and away!

June 5, 2014 / Mushroom Wavelength

Yesterday's stats—walked with Kelly here at Phil's and did 4 miles, pedometer reading I failed to record but was approximately 14000.

OK, I have 20 minutes before Kelly is waiting for me to walk this morning. I need the Mission Impossible music! Just a little story to start. When I was in art school and afterward, I was always on the lookout—gathering and to some extent hoarding materials for future projects. This was time consuming and took away from the here and now of actually creating stuff. Then at some point I began to realize that materials were really all over the place. Everywhere all the time. People were throwing stuff away that were just perfect material. This realization was very freeing.

OK, two stories. Here in the Pacific NW it is the perfect place for the gathering of mushrooms in the wild or not so wild. People know of certain spots where they grow usually, given the right rain and warmth. So off you go to find them. But there is also just walking through the woods and fields looking for certain species that you want to find. You're walking and walking and looking and looking. And after what seems like too long a time you find one. Hurray! And then, of course, you start finding more and more. But you are never quite sure that it wasn't you that was the weak link in the process and that if you had been on the proper mushroom wave length earlier you would have started finding them earlier. Were they just not there or did you just have a failure to see?

OK, where am I going with this? Five more minutes. I just finished a book about gratitude where the author was challenged by a friend to keep a log and find one thousand things that she was thankful for. At first it seemed like a huge challenge and maybe an impossibility really but she persisted. And what happened? She did surpass the one thousand mark and once she got the hang of seeing all the good around her, everywhere all the time, she went on and on and wrote a book about it and most importantly it changed her life!

OK, so that is where I am going. Is it us or what? Are our glasses dirty? Are we too busy, too distracted? Are we looking in the wrong places or just not looking? Are we on the wrong "mushroom wavelength"? Hmmm.

June 7, 2014 / Two Hundred Miles

Peter, Paul and Mary song? I don't know but that is how many miles Esther wanted us to have on our new hiking boots before going to Spain. That's how these Caminoheads think! Wow, I was thinking twenty minutes. But I am happy to report that we are on track to do that 200 miles before flying out of SeaTac, Esther. She will be here in a few days.

Then there is Melania who walked in I forget what year. She came to my talk at the Episcopal Church and then came to walk with me. She came home from her trip and built a labyrinth on her property which she invited us to. In medieval times I have heard they were built to give people who couldn't go on a crusade a chance to have a sort of virtual experience. There is one at Chartres Cathedral that Sister Joyce and Maryka told me about.

Then there is Susan who I haven't met yet but talked to on the phone. She did her Camino in 28 days. Blistering pace, excuse the pun. Then she went on to do treks all over. I asked her if she wanted to do the Camino de Santiago again and she said that she wanted to remember it just as she remembers it which was a wonderful experience. Yup.

Then there is Henry who is twenty-three years old and the son of a dear pastor of Rebecca's and my church in Burton, WA. He walked last summer and came and walked with me recently. He had all his trail clothes and gear and pack on just like the "real" thing. Great young man who I am sure will be up, up and away doing amazing things in the future. His priority on the Camino de Santiago was the camaraderie that he found there. And, of course, some of these same pilgrims are traveling though the NW and he will meet them and care for them here. Go Henry!

Then there is Annie O'Neil. I will use her last name as she is everywhere all the time promoting the Camino documentary and therefore the Camino. Go Annie! Well, she doesn't really need that from me maybe because she runs on some sort of hyper energy that only exists rarely on this planet. She came back from her Camino in '09 and has since has been on fire about her experience and what it has taught her. See her blog: www.everydaycaminowithannie.com

Well, that's all the steam and time I have for today. I'm off to my Bible class, if I can figure out where it is meeting, and then back here to walk on this beautiful day. Buen Camino, Phil.

JUNE 9, 2014 / SCAN

I have a big scan today. I need a scan similar to the last four, God willing. They were all good in the sense that nothing was growing or changing. That's what I need tomorrow. Because I have my plane tickets, my passport, my pilgrim passport and my travel insurance and a bad scan would be a serious complication to untangle before the trip. Prayers please.

JUNE 10, 2014 / IN THE COMFY CHAIR

Well, I have my lucky shirt on and I am off to the big city in a few minutes. I had the big scan yesterday to see what's happening on my inside. Today, I talk to my beloved Doc to get his take on the results. I am seeing this as the last big hurdle to the big trip.

So, my plan is to finish this post at the hospital later today from my comfy chair at the Treatment Center. I will have time to practice on my Kindle and send you the results and thoughts on the results.

OK, see you later alligator, Phil.

JUNE 10, 2014 / . . . LATER THAT DAY

Such fantastic news! I just saw my oncology doc and nurse for the results of the big scan and it looks GOOD! I got the go-ahead for the month on the Camino. All good! Everyone at Swedish giddy.

Doc said that I didn't need my lucky shirt. What did he mean by that? I'll have to get clarification. What kind of world would it be if we all had our lucky shirts on?

OK, have to go and celebrate! Later, SJA, Phil.

JUNE 11, 2014 / BRINGING THE CAMINO

Yesterday's stats –Was in all day treatment and did 1/2 mile in the evening with Esther. 5912 steps for all day.

Didn't sleep much last night but tried. Yesterday was slightly more fun than I usually have. My CT scan that I got on Monday turned out better than expected and on Tuesday I got the "good to go" for a month in Spain. Everyone at Swedish giddy. And yesterday Esther Jantzen showed up to bring us all sorts of Caminoness.

Tomorrow, the 12th, is our open house from 1000 to 2200 (10 PM). Esther will be here to talk with you about the Camino de Santiago and other interesting stuff. Please feel free to come and go. We will do some walking on the Camino de Vashon and show some DVD's and drink some wine. Yup.

Thank you to everyone for their thoughts and prayers for me and my health. You don't know how important this is. I pray for you also. My prayers are usually about giving you strength to face life's challenges. The challenges are here for a reason we know. SJA, Phil.

June 13, 2014 / Learning From Esther

Esther took off a few minutes ago headed for Ashland, OR. What a wonderful visit and what a wonderful person. Great get together yesterday. I missed some of it because of a run to Swedish but it was a beautiful event. Fortunately it was nice, for today is rainy, although we need it.

But back to Esther. When I pulled in the yard a few days ago and saw her car for the first time I did a double take. The same exact car and color as Sister Joyce's. The major difference is that Esther has all the gear for her current nomadic life neatly packed inside and still room to see out with the rear-view mirror.

Rick, Kelly and I did a good job of asking questions about Esther's Camino experiences. She has done it three times now in various fashions. The various fashions due to the need to do research for a book that she is writing. We got a list of "can't miss sites" along the Way. A few of which were not in the guide books.

Well, I could go on about Esther's style but basically it just celebrates the whole notion of the pilgrim moving through the world wherever that might be at the moment. Traveling light and being thoughtful of others and the situation is apparent. Really, I am going to stop there because she is going to get back to tell me that this is ridiculous and unnecessary. But I do feel like Grasshopper picking up tips from the Master.

So, tomorrow we have guests from the big city that are coming to walk here and that will be fun. That's Michele and Tucker. Maybe the weather will be a little more summery for the occasion.

OK, have to go. SJA, Phil.

June 15, 2014 / Father's Day

I have 45 minutes and an urge to talk about my Dad's WWII experience. Maybe it will be too heavy duty for normal ears but remember we are beyond normal these days, at least on this blog.

Fred was a pretty private guy and he is scratching his head at why I would be sharing this with the whole world but. . . . Both of his parent's families came from Prussia in the 1840s due to religious persecution. Their whole town came on a chartered ship to NYC and then up the Erie Canal to Buffalo. There they purchased a large tract of land near Niagara Falls and started a community. They wore wooden shoes and the Native Americans called them "clop clops" because of the sound of their walking (I knew that this was Camino related somehow).

Fred grew up in Buffalo and my image of his childhood is something akin to Our Gang comedy. He joined the NYS National Guard's horse cavalry unit and became a good rider. Later he was employed as a horsemanship instructor during the Depression. He learned to be a watchmaker and was employed at his uncle's jewelry store where he met Mom.

But then WWII steps into the situation and he was drafted into the 77th Division at the age of 35. Figuring that he was able to care for delicate small mechanical devices they trained him to be a medic. This becoming a medic was the turning point in his life and the following war stories will illustrate this journey.

Fred participated in four major battles in the Pacific theater and has a gaggle of bronze stars on his dress uniform. Ernie Pyle, the famous journalist, was killed while traveling with his unit. Finally Fred's luck ran out on Okinawa, the mother lode of all land battles of the Pacific and last engagement before the bomb. These three stories were part of my childhood memories and their harshness or heroism never occurred to me. They were just some of my Dad's stories.

One, we will start out easy, had to do with the idea that the medic is always on call and is always serving. The whole division spent six months in Death Valley preparing to go to North Africa. Then that battle was won by the Allies and the 77th went to the Pacific. Dad's recollection of that era was of a lot of long-distance marches and of him never getting any rest on them. Whenever the troops were allowed a break they would be stripping off their boots and socks and yelling for the medic to help with their blisters. I am reminded of Christ calling us to be servants as he washed feet.

Two was his recollection of numerous times of crawling around out in front of the nighttime defensive perimeter, after the sun went down, trying to locate wounded. Totally hairy activity with the enemy crawling around also. Then finding someone and giving care by feel only and then getting help to drag them back to safety. Very intimate way to fight a war. He always said that you have to steel yourself because you are of no use if you fall apart. Remember that.

Three, was this instance of him having a rush of first aid activity at the front and being soaked with blood. He really didn't know if it was his or the wounded at the moment. After passing the broken soldiers on to be taken back to the aid station he had a break. He was hungry and the only food that he had or was going to have, in his world then, was a chunk of bread in his breast pocket. So, he pulls this out and it is soaked with blood. Whose? His? Does it matter? He gobbles it down, a sort of battlefield communion.

Thank you Dad.

JUNE 16, 2014 / CELEBRATION

Here we are with a brand-new day. A handy bite sized piece of life here for us. Father's Day yesterday and our family was out to brunch to celebrate. Ramon our son-in-law, being a new father, was pretty giddy about his first celebration!

A bunch of us remain giddy over my CT scan that I received at Swedish last Monday, a week ago. To me it is a miracle that this cancer in my liver shrank and shrank and finally got too small to detect. How is that for a reason to be giddy!

I am giddy about things that I hear are happening in my and the larger Camino world. I will have to treat it as scuttlebutt at the moment but know that St. James is afoot doing what he does. It's all good.

Here is a giddy for the future. Esther left us with the name of a French comedy film about the Camino de Santiago. How fun! We have yet to find it but it is out there somewhere. It is *Saint-Jacques La Mecque* and it is with Coline Serreau. So check that out.

I am working on one computer now and right next to me is another with its own monitor as we are in the excruciating process of switching to Windows 8.1. Anyway, Rebecca had set up the way to show our pix on the screen whenever it is not being used. And I am working here on this incredibly important document and next to me images are flashing by of all sorts, all good. And one was of our ten-foot picnic table set for dinner during harvest season last year. This peaks in late August and early September with the corn ripening. This is one of the high points of the whole year. And my giddy thought is that I will be jetting back from Spain on August 25 to be here just then. Not in Spain, not anywhere but right here! Nice. Good on good.

Have a brand-new day, Phil.

JUNE 17, 2014 / CURING VS. HEALING

Part of what I am doing here is supposed to be talking about my cancer hobby. So, today I thought that I would get started on that.

This could all be very lengthy but I really would like to keep it light and moving. What I say is not intended to be glib so don't take it that way. Cancer is a serious disease but having cancer doesn't necessarily have to be all that serious. I have found two things that I stick to and that serve me well: One, do not deny that I have a serious disease and two, do not let that knowledge identify me.

So, they say that I have stage four cancer. There is no stage five. I say that I have an A in cancer. I am excelling in this category!

In a very timely manner I was introduced to Dr. Robert Barnes' book by Michele, my physical therapist at the hospital. The title is *The Good Doctor is Naked*. Dr. Barnes passed away a few years ago unfortunately but the book lives on.

Toward the end he goes into the difference between curing and healing. And I really can't do the topic justice here but just to take part of it and put it to work for me. What I see in this is that curing is working on the body to rid it of the disease, a noble goal. But healing is something that could include curing but doesn't necessarily have to.

Healing, as I see it now, is getting out to the bigger picture. About getting outside myself. About knowing that my physical body is just part of the bigger picture. It is about knowing that I am loved by God and that the cancer is a challenge like other challenges that I have faced, no more and no less. So, whether I am ultimately cured or not appears to me as less important than whether I am ultimately healed.

Saint James is Afoot, Phil.

JUNE 18, 2014 / DID I SAY THAT?

OK, so yesterday Kelly and I had a great walk mostly in what is known as the Island Center Forest. We were exploring various trails and byways. Very few folks actually take the time to be there so we saw very occasional runners, walkers and horse people. Actually, we didn't see any horses but it was obvious that they are present other times.

It is designed to handle horses so the trails are big and wide and two Caminoheads can walk side by side and converse. Perfect! As Annie would say, "Oh, how Camino!"

Annie just got back from NYC and Boston where she was accompanying the Camino Documentary (www.caminodocumentary.org) to do Q and A sessions for the audiences. I didn't hear much about the particulars but she did say things like Hartford was sold out and we had to turn folks away. It seems to be well attended everywhere.

Kelly and I are going to the big city on the 26th to go to the hospital for my three appointments. But before, we are going to REI flagship store to buy a few more items. The big thing is for me a pack but first I have to get fitted for the pack. I thought that my pack problems were solved when I made the outrageous request of Annie to carry her pack across Spain and she said yes of course, the dear. But what did I learn shortly after but in this over-engineered world there are male and female packs. I mean, did pilgrims of the past have to put up with these kinds of complications?

Just one more thought on this post of dibs and daubs. Every time I get involved in the minutiae of the pros and cons of different pieces of hiking gear, which is easy to do at a place like REI, I have to remember the "old" pilgrims. What was their experience, hey? Dodge a few bandits here, swim a few rivers there, starve a little here, flog yourself a little there. Right? And I have to dink around with male and female packs. Doesn't seem quite as heroic. Oh well, such is our modern life.

JUNE 24, 2014 / EUROS

Tuesday again and I am off to Swedish Hospital for treatment. Well, I go every other Tuesday to get it right. This a chemotherapy treatment that pretty much takes up my whole day. And it is the kind of deal that any normal person wants to run away from. Going through the door at the hospital takes a lot of courage. It is not because the experience is so bad, really the contrary. It is just the volume of chemicals that will enter my body this afternoon that I don't want to think about too much.

But beside that it will be fun to see my doctor and nurses. It is a great crew of folks that are fun to be with. I have people that I don't see for two months and we will pick up on the conversation where we had left it. Maybe it's books, movies, sports, movies or wine. All good. I always try and remember to bring some sort of healthy snack for them.

Anyway, I will take the Kindle along and do more blogging from there. I have about three hours of being confined to the comfy chair and if I don't nap off I can get something done. I will think of something fun to do. OK, 'til later, Phil.

JUNE 27, 2014 / THE SHORTEST OF SHORT

I have 15 minutes to do this so a little short story is in order. Rebecca, my dear wife, and another lady had the job once of doing an estate sale. The people whose property was to be sold were some of those amazing folks that lived through the Great Depression. They were very frugal and watchful and never threw anything away it seems. So, Rebecca and Susan are sorting and pricing and displaying in preparation for the big weekend sale. And they come across this cigar box with the writing on the lid, "Pieces of String Too Short to Save." That's it!

June 28, 2014 / Pacific Crest Trail Camino

Our son Wiley is currently on the PCT with a group of buddies from Vashon Island. Three of them started at the Mexican border this Spring and have been hiking north. Wiley flew to Bakersfield and joined them after a tough catchup march. The PCT is its own brand of Camino for sure. There is personal challenge. There is camaraderie, there is adventure, there is a rolling party, there is a chance to get away. There is danger of physical and psychological meltdown. There is physical beauty in spades. Yea. So, we are thinking of these guys and praying for them as they journey onward. They will come back to us inspired, healthier, wiser and new and improved.

To borrow Dr. Seuss' quote from Annie O'Neil's book, "Your mountain is waiting so. . . . get on your way!"

June 29, 2014 / The Three Amigos

The three amigos had their weekly meeting and wine tasting this evening. We had Portuguese wine so I hope that is OK. We checked out my new boy pack. We talked about communications. We talked about how to get pix from a camera to my Kindle and then onto the blog, this blog. We talked about training for the coming week. We talked about how we have only one month to go!

I have talked about Kelly some in the past. He is in his sixties like me. He is a retired school teacher. Now he keeps himself busy helping his daughter remodel her house and he helps with their two children. I started calling him Padre because he has an eerie resemblance to Padre Pio the Italian saint. Kelly lost his wife to cancer a year ago. That is not the reason I chose him to go with me but I used to see him out in the rain and the dark of winter walking alone and I said there is the guy. He is also slower than I am so that is helpful!

Then there is Rick who we both invited along because once he heard about our idea just couldn't control himself. He is like a piece of spring steel physically, seventy years old and walks circles around us two. So, we nicknamed him Mario like the race car driver. I worked with Rick in the past and we always had a good time together. Rick and his wife, Carole Lynn, run a nursery where they grow beautiful landscaping plants. This keeps them busy and in shape. Padre and I figure that with Mario's speed he will be able to sprint ahead late in the day and line up the hostels and dining when we are on the trail!

So, we have a plan. Yea, for once. Kelly and I are flying to Madrid where we land on St. James Day, July 25th. We are busing to St. Jean in France to the start. We will walk to the 17th of August, somewhere around Léon, where Kelly will put me on a bus to run me up the road to the west. Later that day I will get to the monastery at Samos and meet Rick. Kelly will be on his own for some personal inner Camino 'til his son Michael will join him to do the last 100 kilometers. And Rick and I will walk from Samos to Sarria and do the last 100 kilometers. God willing, Rick and I will be at the

Pilgrim's Mass at the cathedral in Santiago at the end of the Camino on Sunday August 24th. Then the next day Rick throws me on the plane for Madrid and then I am off to Seattle. Will be traveling with the time zones this direction and will arrive the same day. Then next day I will be on my way back to Swedish Hospital for an appointment with my psychologist and have a scan later that day. Rebecca will probably have to strap me to a hand truck and deliver me there.

All three of us amigos are practicing Catholics and all along this Camino there will be religious activities and events to participate in. We are planning on the moderate pace of 12 miles a day to allow us time to do this. "It is not a race!" as Kelly, or should I say, Padre reminds us. And our parish, St. John Vianney, here on Vashon has written letters in Spanish for us to announce that we are on official pilgrimage. And at Mass toward the end of July we will be blessed for our journey by Father Marc. All official, right? Let's get started!

July 1, 2014 / We're Running on Miracles

That's what Ivette says about things. And what things are those? Well, it is time to let this cat out of the bag. There is a movement afoot to create a documentary film of my journey to Spain and the walking the Camino there. This all started with the idea that the success of my rehab after cancer treatment is noteworthy and would be helpful to inspire the countless cancer patients out in the world who could use some better training along with their treatment.

The ability for me to even think about this journey is wholly a gift to me. A big part of that gift is the training and counseling that I have received at Swedish Hospital. Another big part is all the support that I have gotten from family, friends, church including the Archdiocese of Seattle. And finally the opportunity that the Camino de Santiago has given me to participate in something that is meaningful, significant and doable for me.

We are terribly last minute with this film idea and we are looking for a miracle to have this happen. And as Annie has told me more than once, we have already had miracles and we need to continue to expect the good. I have a team of people on the East Coast and West that are using all their creativity to bring this together. This is totally shoestring but not outside the box. Possibly we will be able to just capture the raw footage initially. There is much more to the process but maybe it is one thing at a time. People in general are inspired by my story and this will carry the film forward to its conclusion even if it is just one step at a time (sounds like a Camino to me).

Today, after training, I am opening an account at US Bank that will be able to accept donations to help fund this process. I will give you more information on that soon as I know it. This kind of thing doesn't happen without a certain amount of money. Enthusiasm, smarts and creativity will only carry us so far. If you have any ideas about finances let me know, sooner rather than later. And pray for us. St. James is Afoot, Phil.

JULY 2, 2014 / A FLY IN MY COFFEE

I was emailing with Annie yesterday and we were writing about inspirations for blogging. And I was saying that I thought that I did my best work when something was bugging me. That thing could be a bad thing or a good thing in normal thought. But it is something that sort of clings to you and hangs around. It is good ammo for blogging and good probably to get rid of it, which of course, makes room for the next one.

So, very ironic that this a.m. with my well-deserved first cup of joe, what is floating in there but a big juicy fly. I would put that in the category of bugging, wouldn't you? That was minutes ago and right in the middle of my half-baked thoughts about what to blog about this a.m.

Back to that in a minute. What really needs to be done is to write a brief statement for a newspaper ad that will appear in the Beachcomber about a donation drive. Yesterday I blogged about the documentary film idea that is struggling along. A lot of creative work is being done but until we get some financial help behind that we are not going anywhere. Big money from big sources is proving hard to come by. So, we are looking to get local and focused on raising funds from "just folks." Our daughter, Tesia, is going to do the graphics for the add and she asked me to provide some text for the appeal. So, I thought that I would combine that with doing this blog and then there is the fly also. Hmm.

"This morning there was a fly in my coffee. This life there was cancer in my body. What I have learned I would like to share with others who are suffering. How can we rise above our circumstances and do more than we thought was possible? How can we stay inspired and possibly inspire others? We are looking for a way to fund a documentary film about my journey through the medical world, spiritual world and the world of the Camino de Santiago. Please help us fund this small project about the search for healing in. . . . "

There, how is that so far? Not quite there but pretty darn good. Have to get the last sentence hammered out. How about, "Please help us in our search for funds to tell this story about one man's search for healing in a complicated world." Sort of, but too complicated. "Help us to tell this story about one man's search for healing." OK. "Vashon, help me to tell one man's story about a three-year search for inspiration, connection and healing." Not bad. I like saying that to Vashon. "Vashon, please help me to fund this small project about one man's search for inspiration, connection and healing in a complex world." All right, let's see what that looks like all together.

"This morning there was a fly in my coffee. This life there was cancer in my body. What I have learned I would like to share with others who are suffering. How can we rise above our circumstances and do more than we thought was possible? How can we connect to something larger than ourselves? How can we stay inspired and possibly inspire others? I am looking for help to fund a documentary film about my journey through the medical world, spiritual world and the world of the ancient mystical Camino de Santiago. Vashon, please help bring to light this small project about one man's search for inspiration, connection and healing in a complex world."

Well, I think that is good. Need it pruf readed. OK, so I am off to walk with Kelly and Signe in the cool of the morning. Walking seems a soothing rest from the details of life. Saint James is Afoot, Phil.

July 4, 2014 / Roadhead Finds Iron Artifacts

Early morning Fourth of July and just got done helping my American Legion Post put up flags. We put up a hundred flags on eleven flag days each year. And this morning was super glorious weather-wise and it was like walking around in a Norman Rockwell painting! Kind of like Annie talking about in Spain walking around in a postcard. Another part of our Rockwellism is our amateur hydroplane race which starts at 5 a.m. every Fourth and the guys circumnavigate the Island with a racket that can be heard five miles away easy. I hear through the grapevine that Carl Olson won and Paul Hoffman flipped over at the north end but is OK. This is supremely cool totally local stuff.

So Peggy, one of my buddies that works at the hospital told me that Caminohead means Roadhead. She grew up in Panama so she knows her Spanish. I tried to explain that it was a little different but actually maybe not so much. I got into Roadheadism yesterday during my training.

Yea, was doing a six miler on Old Mill Rd. But really on one stretch of the road and it is 3/4 of a mile. So, I go back and forth four times and that gives me the six miles. This stretch has a big open field on one side and is forested on the other. No houses to be seen and no dogs to come out and bark. There are little blue flowers and songs of Redwing Blackbirds that one cannot enjoy from a moving vehicle. Anyway, back to Roadhead stuff. I got into studying the walking surface, the road, well the road and the shoulder. Got it in my head that the they are built with a camber or in other words it is a slightly convex surface made that way to shed rain. So, if I always walk on one side facing traffic or in this case occasional traffic I am always walking across a slight slope. So, it occurred to me to lengthen that outboard walking stick 5 cm to compensate and it made a difference! A little minor tweak that made a long stretch easier.

Also, picked up a couple of "flat tires", as my old boss Robert called them, a 16-penny nail and a drill bit on the road. Yea, a good deed. A few weeks ago I spied an earthworm out in the middle of the pavement and I got out there and tried to pick him up but he was too small and slimy and I wound up flicking the little guy ten feet to the grassy shoulder. This kind of stuff happens when you get older, risking your life for an unendangered species!

OK, have a great Fourth, wherever you find yourself.

July 6, 2014 / Scrambling

Kelly says that we have 19 more days but I'm trying not to count. Rick got a new pack. It is a smaller version than boy pack. We just got done with our weekly meeting/wine tasting. Getting acclimated to the Spanish wine scene is proving harder than expected.

JULY 7, 2014 / ULTIMATE ROADHEAD

OK, so here it is, the ultimate roadhead: Santo Domingo de la Calzada or St. Dominic of the Pavement (road surface). Yea, there's my man! I learned about him from Esther and he is her favorite saint. Esther emailed a bunch of info on him and let me sift through that and come up with a bio. Now, I can see that this will take more than one day so here is the first installment:

The town of Santo Domingo de la Calzada is just west of Logrono. It is considered by some to be the spiritual heart of the Camino. So, Dominic Garcia was born in 1019 AD nearby. He was a shy devout shepherd boy who at some point left to become a monk. He was humiliated later because he was expelled for not being a good student. He decided to become a hermit and lived in the forest there. This forest was infested with bandits who made a living attacking the pilgrims who were slowly making their way on the fledgling Camino. At this time they basically had to follow the setting sun to move westward. There was no clear path and they had to swim the many rivers and were easy prey.

Dominic had a dream telling him to serve God by doing something for the pilgrims and this unschooled simple man became the first engineer of the Camino. He cut down trees to make a trail and built a bridge across the Oja River. His projects were so big for one man that legend says that angels helped! More tomorrow, SJA, Phil.

JULY 8, 2014 / ULTIMATE ROADHEAD PART TWO

So, yesterday we were talking about our favorite guy, Santo Domingo de la Calzada or Saint Dominic Ultimate Roadhead. And we talked about how he did improvements on the physical Camino. But he also helped out the pilgrims personally as in the Miracle of the Cock and the Hen and others.

There was a young German man doing the pilgrimage with his parents. Somehow he became involved with a young local gal that he ultimately turned down. She was not happy about his decision and framed him with a serious crime. Poor Hugonell was sentenced to death. Our dear Roadhead went to his rescue by going to plead before the magistrate who was unfortunately in the middle of his chicken dinner. Not happy with the interruption he roared at Dominic, "If that young man is innocent, these roast birds will rise from the platter and crow!" The rooster on one platter jumped up and crowed and a hen on another rose and clucked! So, young Hugonell was released and sent on his way. Even today descendants of the original birds live in a coop in the church in Santo Domingo.

There is an artistic image that appears at the church of a dog carrying a human hand in its mouth reminding us of another miracle done by our guy. Two men were dueling and in the fight one lost his hand and the dog brought it to Dominic and he reattached it. Pretty cool.

Quite the story about a guy that started out from humble beginnings with no education. What does it take to be helpful in this world of ours? For sure we can't say that there is nothing for us to do because we don't have the fancy training.

Yup, Saint James Afoot, Phil

JULY 10, 2014 / ALL ABOUT ME

Today we start filming for the new documentary. I am off to Swedish to get my portable pump taken off which I have been living with for two days since the big infusion on Tuesday. This is all standard procedure. What is not standard today are several meetings with my docs and physical therapist to have the camera be a "fly on the wall" and try and catch the content and flavor of that. So, I will there most of the day which will be an enjoyable thing really.

Yes, and what could be a more enjoyable day than an "it's all about me" day! This is tricky and needs to be sorted out and thought about. One, it is just a little bit flattering that my personal journey is of so much interest. I have to ask, "Really?" But two, I realize that there is something going on these days that is way bigger than myself. And it is all pointing toward the Camino de Santiago and telling that story. I am blessed by the presence of so many positive influences these days that are buoying me up and sustaining me to be able to do this mission. I really don't know the complete story but I know enough to always keep moving one foot in front of the other. What more can I ask? And this will be, in short, what the documentary will try and capture.

When I came to the Roman Catholic Church I asked them for the "Full Meal Deal" and I got that far and beyond my imagination. Of course this is built on all the other influences that have come before: my family, my medical family, my beloved Bible class, my Protestant friends, my fellow vets, old friends and all the great people of Vashon Island. I feel at home here and now and this is the stable platform from which I am launching.

Sister Joyce says that I am a magnet picking up good things in my environment and weaving them together to build my view. Prayers for Sister Joyce by the way, as she travels to Iowa and for healing for her ankle that she turned. She was supposed to come and walk on my Camino here at the ranch but was prevented by her injury. Anyway, we are thinking of you now Sister Joyce.

I think that at this point it is fair to say that the real emotion and thrust of this effort is going out toward fellow cancer patients, cancer survivors, cancer hobbyists and cancer wrestlers. I have been all four of those. What I am trying to say to them is that get good treatment, get good rehab and hang out with people that inspire you. And then you will inspire others which should be our main goal. Saint James is Afoot, Phil.

JULY 11, 2014 / AH . . . .

Good morning. Just trying to get myself back together after yesterday. We started filming the "Phil Volker Documentary" (working title) yesterday. It revolved around my appointments there at Swedish Hospital. But there was time for coffee break conversations, and joking with the nurses. Big fun. This is for the beginning of the project which will mostly be filmed in Spain which is less than two weeks away. Big, big fun!

So, we are hopeful and prayerful and looking forward to capturing the basic raw material on film.

July 20, 2014 / El Camino Grande

We are off to do our second day of the big training weekend. We did twelve miles yesterday and had a nice dinner and crashed. Just checking out our gear and ourselves. Another twelve today. Up, up and away, Phil.

July 21, 2014 / El Camino Grande Completed

We're back, no blisters, no bedbugs, all good! Yesterday we did twelve miles and went to Mass and came back and slept out in a tent by the corn patch. There were owls hooting and ravens trying to imitate them making weird noises keeping us awake. After our walk we made Vigil Mass and we were given a Pilgrim's Blessing by Father Marc. I wept, which I have been doing a lot lately. Today another twelve miles and it seemed easier today than yesterday. Lots of people stopped for hugs and encouragement.

I am just overwhelmed by the amount of love and support by so many people here and elsewhere. This is the most amazing ad hoc gathering of good energy that I have ever had anything to do with. I just want to thank friends and neighbors, the Swedish Hospital folks, my family and St. John Vianney Parish. Annie tells me that there are people I am not even aware of that are making things happen. Annie also tells me that we will have to list St. James in the credits of the new documentary. Yup, it's an awesome phenomenon.

OK, have to check out for now. Keep in touch as I will be blogging as often as possible for the near future. After a few days in Spain a new routine will develop. Way too many details are swirling around now but focusing on getting on the plane on Thursday evening. Love you guys, Phil.

July 22, 2014 / Last Minute Root Canal, No Joke

I never ran the high hurdles in high school but it seems I am getting my chance now. OK, root canal, no problem. That's tomorrow though. Today it is off to Swedish to see my beloved oncologist and his team and then off to the last treatment. Can't do without my gallon of chemicals, well it seems like a gallon.

July 23, 2014 / At Swedish

Treatment today and I am what is called a frequent flyer here. Don't know exactly what the benefits are but it is generally a good deal. Ivette is here with me. We met a great woman in the waiting room who had a beautiful spirit.

July 24, 2014 / Back On the Fun Train

Passport? Check. Boy Pack packed? Check. Got root canal? Got it! Off to get some sleep and put the finishing touches on it mañana. All good, Saint James is Afoot, Phil.

JULY 24, 2014 / THE COUNTDOWN IN HOURS

God willing Kelly and I will be jetting off at 6:11 Seattle time for the big adventure. Follow us, be with us as the Camino unfolds. It has already been an amazing journey and we haven't left yet. How does that work? Thanks for all your prayers and support. St. James is Afoot, Phil.

JULY 25, 2014 / AMSTERDAM

A little cross eyed at the moment but sitting at Gate C10 where a flight to Madrid will be leaving at 16:50 local time. I don't think we can screw this up.

JULY 25, 2014 / MADRID ON ST. JAMES DAY

Kelly and I checking out the ninety-degree weather. Buying bus tickets for tomorrow . Off to get a taxi to the hotel. So far so good. Phil.

JULY 26, 2014 / SAINT-JEAN-PIED-DE-PORT

Ok gang we are here! Eating dinner with Jessica and Todd. Much to do this evening so need to keep this short. Todd and I met because we were photographing each other, him on the ground and me shooting out the bus window. A good start I would say! Saint James is definitely afoot. Phil.

JULY 27, 2014 / EVERY MUSCLE IN MY BODY IS TWITCHING

We made it over the mountains to Roncesvalles. Unbelievably beautiful and unbelievably grueling. Will try and write more after shower and dinner.

JULY 27, 2014 / RONCESVALLES PLUS

Kelly and I are sitting in the Casa Cabina celebrating our victory. It wasn't pretty but we got it done! And what a beautiful area. I am celebrating also because today's walk is supposed to be the hardest of the Camino and today is my worst day in the chemo cycle. So, what could be better than to get to our destination before dark on a long walk, yes?

This is such a wonderful experience. I wish you all a chance to be here sometime in the future. It makes me want to learn Spanish and move in! Thank you St. James for helping today, Phil.

PS—Today at lunch in Orisson there were fifty eagles swirling around overhead. An omen?

JULY 28, 2014 / ZUBIRI

We made it to the hostel before the rain came. Walked about twenty kilometers to this town of Zubiri. This morning was very private for us but we fell into a great group for the afternoon. Two Dutch sisters, a gal from Sweden and a fellow from Egypt. We talked our heads off and the kilometers went by quickly.

July 29, 2014 / Cizur Menor

We walked over every possible type of surface today but ice and snow and maybe wall to wall carpet. Walked through the beautiful city of Pamplona this afternoon. Also, need some help on the "Br'er Rabbit" song. What is after Mr. Bluebird is on my shoulder?

Hi. Jessica here. Phil handed me his iPad and told me to write. Firstly, Phil and Kelly are cheeky, funny, deep, and absolutely easy to film. Everyone around them is drawn to them. And the ladies we are eating dinner with were naming all the things they loved about Phil and Kelly before they arrived for dinner.

Secondly, I must mention pace. Todd and I are participating as much as we can in walking and are learning just as much as the next pilgrim about pace. Today my pace was jumping off a bridge into water, eating ice cream in the street where the bulls run and walking just a little less than was expected to rest my knee a bit. Pace is everything. Find your pace!

July 29, 2014 / Cizur Menor Again

Todd: hard to put into words the uniqueness and power of this experience. The simplicity and rhythm of the trail has already become addicting. This morning I awoke to Phil shaking me awake, for which I was grateful since supposedly I had slept through my alarm. I was surprised to look around and find that we were beating all the other pilgrims to the trail since they were sound asleep around me. Glancing over at Phil's bed I realized he was already halfway packed for the day. I had the choice to either meet him in his urgency or take a look at my phone to see if I had time to catch another 5 minutes of sleep. I choose the latter. When I read my phone it said 2:05. Check my camera to confirm. Yep, 2:05. Apparently Phil's phone was stuck on the time that he had intentionally set his alarm for. One could be upset at the disruption of sleep, but I was just grateful that I had 4 more hours of shut eye.

July 30, 2014 / Half Day

Taking a short day today since are all in various shades of battered. We went off on a side trip to see a "spectacular" church in Eunate, just west of Pamplona. All good, Phil.

July 30, 2014 / Right Now

Right now Kelly and I are sitting out in front of the hostel under a porch roof. Actually he just ran off with Todd and Jess to film around town. It is 1800 and the sun is still pretty intense. There is an ever-changing scene of pilgrims talking, drying their clothing or drying their hair. The wind is gusty. An occasional car goes by.

Somehow, we wound up with two bottles of wine to drink up tonight as no one wants to carry another extra thing tomorrow. Met a most interesting lady from Ireland today, Máiréad. We were going to meet her to check out the "spectacular" church but we can't find a ride. We will catch up with her tomorrow or the next day is the way to think about it. Discovered gazpacho today. Every day I tell someone about Sister Joyce. Another day on the Camino. Time to say my rosary.

AUGUST 1, 2014 / FIFTH DAY

I had 35132 steps today. Half day yesterday had 17970. Tuesday had 39348. Hot here and we may do half day tomorrow and get done by 1300. Kelly had heat exhaustion here after we got to the hostel but he is sleeping now. Everyone's is looking after him. We left Uterga this morning and are in Lorca now. I think that it was about 22 k with a detour that we took.

The detour was to the Knights Templar church constructed in the 12th century. It was supposed to be open but was locked up. We investigated the exterior. I placed my hand on a small carved cross that is on the right side of the entrance gate. I am finding touching history to be very powerful.

I want to get back to the idea that the pain gets silly that I was working on earlier. Taking this out of context sort of makes for some strange reading but it is what it is. Two nights ago some our party was staying with Maribel in Cizur Menor. She is a Camino Angel who has been working here for close to thirty years. She works on foot problems and can tell the problem before you take your boots off. One of her secrets is to put Maxi Pads as insoles to collect sweat and blister gunk. Yea, works.

Yesterday at lunch Jess and Todd set up this game of rock toss trying to get gravel into my empty boots. They had all of us playing. Then this morning I had both my boots laced up and tied and ready to go and something just didn't feel quite right but since my feet feel so bad on the bottoms I am not quite sure. Sure as heck had an almond sized one in there. But the key idea is that I wasn't sure.

And this after the really hilarious move of putting my glasses in one of my Crocs before bed and then getting up at 0600 and walking to the communal toilet and back with them in there. Again something didn't quite feel right. Hmm. I have managed to fix them sort of.

We caught up to Máiréad. Tomorrow we may lose her again as we will go light with Kelly. But people walk in fits and starts so that finding them again is easier than one would think. I had a great conversation with Todd this afternoon and of course mentioned Sister Joyce, Rebecca, Danger Zone: Dr. David Zucker, Nugget: Dr. Philip Gold, and Dr. Robert Barnes. Todd is getting the Camino experience even though he has all this work to do. Jess is still nursing knee and has been taxiing ahead.

Well, I have to go and find some sleep. Day six tomorrow. Have to say one more rosary for a Camino Angel that brought us out cold cans of Coke as we stumbled by her home. She had beautiful roses and I stopped to smell them I might report. We had nothing to give her so I gestured that I would pray for her and she seemed happy. Buen Camino.

August 1, 2014 / Got My Red Scarf

Big celebration here in Estella, feast day for St. Fermin, I think. Lots of food and singing and music. Running of the bulls tonight at 2030 and I got the red scarf so I am ready. Going for the gusto, right?

Kelly feeling better today. He walked with me after sending his pack forward for a few euros. We had agreed that we could do this occasionally if needed. So he is back with a vengeance.

Tomorrow it looks like we will wind up in Los Arcos which is 21 km down the road. We are on the verge switching over to kilometers from miles. Along the way is a winery that has a free wine fountain. We will have to try and pace ourselves once again.

Well, maybe I will go for a nap while I can. Need to maintain my strength to keep one step ahead of the bulls tonight. Buen Camino, Phil.

August 2, 2014 / Day Six

I must apologize to you because I just lost some valuable entries that people put on last evening. My fat fingers are to blame. But ever onward and we are at the town of Los Arcos after a good walk of 21 k. The morning was overcast and delicious and then the sun broke through and we did our best. We had a pretty good gang of walkers but we got strung out and some of us had to drink a lot of beer in the shade waiting for everyone to catch up.

August 2, 2014 / Double Rainbow

Yes it's true, Todd and I ran with bulls last evening. He was in there with his video camera so there will be some footage of that. It was mostly chaos with hundreds of well-lubed Spaniards. And the bulls turned out to be pretty puny but we didn't really know that 'til the dust cleared. Anyway, if I had a bucket list it would for sure be on it.

Today the walk was really the best yet. We have a group that is coalescing. We are working on getting all the continents represented. We might be short a few penguins but it is fun trying.

Todd is taking some great shots. Captured a double rainbow over the church here in Los Arcos. He is having ball.

OK! I am going to post this before the hostel turns off the Wi-Fi, if they do. They try their best to get everyone in bed at a decent hour. Buen Camino, Phil.

August 3, 2014 / No word For Giddy

One of the little-known facts that I have discovered is that in Spanish or Italian there is no equivalent to our word giddy. Have discovered that in our walking days there are three stages: first few hours of pain as we warm up, then a giddy time when it all seems so wonderful and then finally when we get really tired and there is a sort of automatic pilot situation. But it is all really wonderful.

The idea that we are sharing the experience is very important. It leads to a certain understanding between people that we are in this together no matter where we start from. We are learning how to put up with each other in all things. We are learning to help each other through our hard spots which we have every day.

There has developed a small group of wonderful ladies who are going by "Phil's Angels." Laura, Anna Maria and Alida are going to leave me instructions on how to operate after they leave. It's going to be tough carrying on as they only have a few more days.

August 3, 2014 / Frickin' Heavenly

Well, I don't really know how to describe my evening. Our group, now called the Hotel California, had a picnic on the grounds of a church in beautiful disrepair. Yes, the church was the one in beautiful disrepair. It was for sure a vision of heaven. In the Spanish sunset with a spread of Spanish food with Camino friends. Ah, I'm going to cry just thinking about it. Then we got lost in the rain trying to get back to the hostel before they locked us out at 10:00. We made it and here I sit blogging with a damp shirt and fighting off sleep for a few more minutes.

Tomorrow will come with a walk of 22.5 k through Logrono to the town of Navarrete. We still have enough food left from the picnic for breakfast and lunch. We will be up at 0600 and on the road by 0700. We are supposed to be ready for surprises so that will be our mission.

August 4, 2014 / Phil From USA

Here I am sitting having a beer in Navarrete. There are seven pilgrims sitting here with me and want to introduce them to you: Grace from Australia, Raymond from Netherlands, Cristina from Barcelona, Abel from Madrid, Kelly from USA, Matthew from Netherlands and Cherry from Australia and me. Yup, pretty much an international forum I'd say.

Today we went through the city of Logrono and Grace and I set off to find a phone charger and a stylus. We had a wild time trying to find those simple items. We gave money to all the beggars. I said my first Spanish complete sentence, "dónde está el Camino." Ok, we have to go find the angels, Phil.

August 5, 2014 / Lounging With The Angels

I'm getting the hang of this heaven thing. Kelly and I were filmed saying our rosary in the shade along the trail today. I'm glad that I remembered the right words under pressure; just act natural.

I'm learning to live with my blister, my first. I've been lucky. Dillon named one of his blisters after Kelly today. Another case of giddy.

We lost Alida today as she had to get back to civilization and eventually Miami. Now I'm down to two Angels. Times are tough.

Have to go, love you all, St. James is Afoot, Phil.

August 6, 2014 / "You Can Check Out But You Can Never Leave"

Day eleven and that is from "Hotel California" by the Eagles, right? It is the name of our group but I am quickly realizing that it is something bigger. The whole Camino conquers your heart and you can never leave really.

One more paragraph now because the Angels have arrived and it is lunch time. Laura just came up with another line for the song, "No matter where it takes me, I won't be afraid of walking anymore." Phil.

August 6, 2014 / Just a Quickie

We just checked in to a beautiful albergue and time to shower before sightseeing. The church has a chicken coop in it that symbolizes one of the miracles of Saint Dominic.

He also was the first engineer on the Camino, building bridges and clearing the trail from the forest. Ok, have to go, sorry. The shower calls, SJA, Phil.

August 6, 2014 / Our Buddy Todd is Off Today

Todd has to get back to civilization but may be back at some point. He has been wonderful keeping the project moving forward. He left me with a thought: don't be afraid to let the good get better! Sometimes we all reach a plateau of what we call good and never let there be more. He said that it was like the hills here that we climb and we get to a place where it looks like the top and a few more steps reveal a new summit and this repeats itself over and over. Nice.

Kelly wanted to say to his family that he is alive and well. He is having the time of his life. He complains about the effort it takes to keep me under control though. He feels a big responsibility for my safety and well-being.

Yup that's the way that it is! Later, St. James is Afoot, Phil.

August 6, 2014 / Here at the Cathedral

We have spent half the afternoon exploring the nooks and crannies of Iglesias Catedral de Santo Domingo de la Calzada. This place is all about St. Dominic.

I must talk of Matthew who is here walking for his brother Jan who died of cancer. He is a super walker who is hanging with us even though we are so glacial. I just stomped on his toes with my chair trying to get out of the way of a truck going down this narrow medieval street. Yikes!

I am going to try and give some of these folks an archery lesson without gear this evening. Kind of a mime thing and major fun on the Camino.

August 7, 2014 / Hey

I feel good

August 9, 2014 / El Alquimista

Breakfast on day 14. Things primitive and Wifi marginal. We are planning on being in Burgos later today. Stay tuned, Phil

August 9, 2014 / Lunch Day 14 Cardeñuela Riopico

Salami and cheese on GOOD bread. Fresh squeezed orange juice and a nectarine also.

We have given Grace from Australia the title of Camino Flight Nurse for her work in watching over me these last few days. Yesterday we went together to Mass in a most beautiful church. At the high point of the service we were kneeling and very casually, it felt like, I passed out right on top of her and she kept my head from hitting the stone floor. I woke with the priest and all these people looking down at me. Luckily the same male nurse from Netherlands was on hand that tended to Kelly a few nights ago. It's all OK and working out, don't worry, another day on the Camino, Phil.

August 9, 2014 / Burgos, the Big City

Just went to the Saturday evening vigil at the Catedral. This was the home of El Cid, who I have to study up on. I just slipped in with the locals and took Communion like normal. City people are so good smelling and pilgrims not so much but they for the most part enjoy and shelter us. At the service there was a prayer for us and I got really brave and walked up and got to shake hands with the Bishop after the service was over. How's that?

Tomorrow is another day and more surprises await. Kelly and I will be up early to walk out to the country where we belong. Grace is staying here to freshen up. We will miss her.

Had dinner with a group of Italians who are traveling together. They always look like they are having too much fun. I finally got a cash machine to work, small miracle. Beautiful foggy morning today which was cool for walking. Ok, enough for now, Phil.

August 10, 2014 / It's Not All Fun and Sun

About ready to go out on the Meseta and having an orange juice in the town of Tardajos. I am mourning losing Gracie, Official Camino Flight Nurse.

Gracie agreed with the vision of heaven being the picnic in the sunset in Viana but wanted Sam Cook to be there so yes of course. So, today is starting to unfold and looking forward to more surprises. Kelly promised me an ice cream bar if I can get myself to the next town.

August 11, 2014 / One Dried Out Hummingbird

Arrived at Castrojeriz. Sun hot and we are sheltered at the albergue. Need to shower and wash my sweaty clothes and then find a beer, long day.

I was thinking about it being Monday and some of my friends and angels are back to work in places like Miami and Barcelona. I was singing the official song of Hotel California for you, Vella Chiruca. You are dear ones.

Just looked at my pedometer and have 45,188 steps today. That's ridiculous! Miller Time for sure.

Just want mention the instructions that Phil's Angels left so that I would not get into trouble after they flew away: 1. Eat more. 2. Hydrate more. 3. No drinking after 2130. 4. Remember to take your meds. 5. There are always angels. This is good advice for us all of course.

AUGUST 11, 2014 / JUST FOR THE HECK OF IT

I have time so I will post again. Just developed a new drink sensation—I haven't named it yet but a glass of Spanish beer with a lavender blossom thrown in is pretty darn good. Multi-tasking these days is blogging and drink development. What a deal.

Today I spent a lovely profitable time walking with a lady named Clara from Assisi, Italy. She teaches high school philosophy and history there. Today is the feast day for St. Clara so she was getting phone call after phone call wishing her well. Nice. She went on to San Nicholas to stay because she served there as a volunteer in the past. They are supposed to have good Italian coffee there so we will stop tomorrow and check it out.

Really, I am capturing ten percent of what there is to capture here but hopefully it will do. Things are so rich after you've walked 'til you're giddy and brain dead that it is hard to describe. Of course, that is my job so I will try harder. Maybe time for a pic or two.

AUGUST 11, 2014 / MORE THOUGHTS

Having dinner at a lovely place with some lovely people and I talked them into saying a few words about their day:

Mary from New Zealand here: We met these two crazy guys Kelly and Phil last night at the pilgrim's meal at the albergue in Rabé de las Calzadas and they have followed us all day today. It's been a good day however; the scenery has been beautiful and the weather much cooler. What more could one ask for. And after a good night's rest we will begin the walking all over again. It's an amazing community of people walking this Camino with us. Go well, all you pilgrims, whatever your reason is for subjecting yourself to this experience. We are like one big happy family.

Clara reminded me of something today and I thought that I would pass it on. They say that your Camino begins when you get to Santiago, meaning the real challenge is returning to your life and applying what you have learned. Ah, what will that look like? OK, have go and prepare for tomorrow, Phil.

August 12, 2014 / The Meseta

The Meseta is the high plain in central northern Spain. It is a place of too much sun, too much wind, too much a lot of stuff. Not like Sleepy Hollow, not like anything but the outback. It ground me down today. We walked twenty km okay which should be an easy day but it beat me up.

This is the first time that I don't recognize anyone around here. You know how much fun your friends can be and when there are none you can get depressed. So, I am fighting to get to a good mood.

Okay, so that is all I have for you today. Just missing my angels and good buddies. Off to Carrión de Los Condes tomorrow. Love, Phil.

August 12, 2014 / Evening Here

We have been getting up earlier and earlier each morning so that we can get more kilometers in before the afternoon sun.

August 13, 2014 / Carrión de los Condes

In town and ready to shower. Back in groove again after two hard days. More good people to inspire me. That's our job to inspire each other, right?

August 13, 2014 / 2129

There was one minute to go before my wine curfew this evening at 2030 and I had to finish, oh, let me stop there. Well, new angels have arrived and we haven't had this much fun since summer camp in seventh grade.

OK, so, we went to Mass this evening in this town and it was most beautiful. They had a wonderful pilgrim blessing afterward. There were probably 75 pilgrims there most of whom were Italian. There are big groups of Italian seminarians that are walking.

Todd is back after a quick trip to the States to film a wedding. Jess and Rebecca are fine. Mary Margret and Angela are on board for the walk tomorrow. It will be a long day tomorrow with few towns and few ice cream sandwiches. Love you all, Phil.

August 14, 2014 / Amazing, Hey?

That's Australian from Angela. Long day today but we are here in Terradillos de Los Templarios. New friends Alvaro from Madrid with the smiling eyes. The Sheriff is here (Sherif from Egypt).

Today was very long in the hot sun but we had amazing conversations and views. We are planning a birthday party for Angela on the 16th. We cobble things together as we go, of course.

I am going to post this quickly before the wifi disappears. Love you all, Phil.

August 15, 2014 / In Sahagún

Alvaro, Kelly and I sitting in the shade having some refreshments. Back on the road in a minute. Thinking of all you nurses, friends and angels, Phil.

August 16, 2014 / A Blistering Pace

We are in Mansilla de las Mulas after a 24k hike. I was with Todd and Kelly. Had a very high-level talk with Todd and then there was Kelly. He feels so responsible for my well-being and is so afraid that I will go astray after I leave him tomorrow that he insisted on giving me the big lecture. Yikes! It was full frontal Kelly. I mean what trouble could I possibly get in?

I know that he is going for a raise so he is trying extra hard. But really, he has been the best buddy for me. Tomorrow we will say goodbye for I will be busing ahead to meet up with my other buddy Rick at the monastery at Samos. Ever onward!

Well, the Sheriff just rode in to help me get this evening's party started. He is turning into my favorite Egyptian! Well right, I don't know that many. And I was hoping that we would catch up with Angela but I hear that she is up ahead. OK, best wishes Angela!

Cherry just showed up and Kelly. We have an international forum cooking. Laurence from England who operated on Kelly yesterday is here. I'm sorry that I miscalled him a German, but oh well. Mary Margret is here so anything could happen!

Todd is going to do some interviews momentarily. We did some amazing filming this morning. The rising sun was beautiful along with the local countryside and architecture.

All good. Ever onward and all that. We miss you Angela. I think that I will publish this before something unexpected happens. Love you all, SJA, Phil.

August 17, 2014 / Samos

This is incredible and totally unexpected. Todd, Rebecca, Jessica and I rolled into town to meet my old friend Rick from home who is going to walk the last 100k. Yes, but who did he bring with him but his beautiful daughter, Maryka! She walked with me back home in Vashon in the snow and rain. We have fun.

Kelly should be in Léon lounging around in a hotel. He pinned a note on my shirt for Rick. In other words, he figured that I would mess that up. Kelly, really?

Galicia, is totally green and lush. A real change from the Meseta, that we had grown to know and almost love. OK, so, that's it for now. Love you all, Phil.

August 18, 2014 / Ora et Labora (Pray and Work)

Rick, Maryka and I are in Barbadelo, just west of Sarria. Very lush here compared to the desert I was in yesterday morning. I am looking at oaks, poplar, birch and a laurel hedge; looks like home.

Kelly is lounging in Léon. Ladies, a tip. In Léon I spent an hour and a half sitting by the Cathedral waiting to say happy birthday to Angela but she was on the road somewhere Caminoheading along. But it gave me time to place all the stones and build the thing. But I came up with more questions than answers. How did they do this and how did they do that? Oh well.

I lost the stylus that cost me 5 euro and an hour of searching around in the big city with Gracie. Oh well. Rick just handed me an extra one that he stole from Kelly. See how it works?

Annie, message for you. Maryka had a dream last night in the albergue that you will have a big lucky windfall. So keep your eyes open!

OK, have to shower and do laundry. Maybe take a nap. Say a rosary for my stone pile and pilgrims struggling along the way. 'Til later, all good, Hotel California.

August 19, 2014 / Two Drops in a River

I was walking with Maryka today and she said that the two of us were like two drops in the river of pilgrims. It is getting very crowded as we get closer to St. James. But I love it as it is all part of the story, right? People are sleeping on the floors of the local school classrooms and gymnasium. I heard that in Santiago they are rearranging the Cathedral to accept a thousand people at the Pilgrim Mass each day. It's massive!

I asked Maryka to help me today. The question is whether I am experiencing an internal hallucination or whether there is really something happening here that is exceptional. Well, she says that even on her first day that she sees that there is truly something happening here. Rebecca from the film crew says that it is a combo of internal and external. Yes.

We are going to finish eating dinner and go for an evening walk (paseo). We are in Portomarín which is on the shore of a reservoir, very beautiful, of course, what else right? Need to sign off for now, love you, Phil and crew.

August 20, 2014 / Another Great Breakfast

San Miguel and Magdalenas, which translates to beer and sweet rolls for breakfast is what started us out this AM. Todd says that it is choose your own adventure day so I'm signing up for the Giddy Dilly Dally Adventure Package. So here we go! Phil.

August 20, 2014 / Gonzar

Stopping for an orange juice and a chocolate croissant in the town of Gonzar. Very crowded and hard to hold a decent conversation. Lots of individuals, families and groups walking the last hundred kilometers. Us guys that have been at this for a while seem pretty gnarly compared to the newcomers.

Sixteen kilometers to go before our rest. Phil.

AUGUST 20, 2014 / 71 KILOMETERS

We just pulled in to Palas de Rei and it is 1711. So many things have happened that I feel like I have captured ten percent of it. Maybe I can glean a few more important items.

I have some cooking/food thoughts that I could throw in here. 1. Gazpacho rules and is really a blend of tomatoes and peppers, onions maybe cucumbers. Then it needs some croutons, oregano and a little olive oil floating on top. 2. Olives, peppers and anchovies on sticks was one of my favorites. 3. Crunchy bread with olive oil and salt. 4. Tortilla Española is good and easy. It's egg and potato pie.

Maryka just got some of her grades: three A's. So we are celebrating, cerveza grandes all around. She is laughing and having a good time after all her hard work.

OK, I have to go do some serious stuff now. Shower, laundry and troll for dinner. Love you all immensely, Phil.

AUGUST 21, 2014 / DAWN POST

It isn't light yet but I thought that I would say hello. I love this place in all its funk and glory. Have an extra ordinary day. Love, Phil and Team Wifi and Hotel California.

AUGUST 21, 2014 / FORDING THE RÍO ISO

We forded the Río Iso at Ribadiso da Baixo where we have a room. This is a working farm a little off the Camino. Things are so crowded that facilities along the trail are full.

Kelly and I always said that we had to ford or swim across at least one river to celebrate how the old guys did it. No bridges back then. We heard that Kelly is doing fine winning friends and influencing people back there somewhere west of Léon.

I am working on some homework that I need to get done before going to the Cathedral in Santiago. Clara explained this to me as we walked a while back. When one goes to St. James to ask something of him because he is such a big powerful saint one is better off having a short list of items to ask of him instead of one thing. That way he gets to choose the one he thinks is the best for that person. So I will work on that and report back.

Love, Phil.

AUGUST 22, 2014 / FARM BREAKFAST

Orange juice, coffee with warm milk and sugar, cookies, toast with jam. What no sardines and chocolate? On the road in a few minutes. Still dark. Love, Phil.

AUGUST 22, 2014 / ANIMO!

It's an encouragement in Spanish written along the Way today. We are sitting at our hotel having a grande after covering 36 k today. My longest day and 58,294 steps! Just a few kilometers to go.

There's a Spanish family here on the steps of the hotel taking family pictures. They're pretty cute. They're breaking up now, kissing each other and lingering slightly before they all jump in their cars. Nice.

Maryka here: the Camino does unexpected things, opens you up, beckons conversation, wears you raw, pains in places you never knew, but all the while there are fragrant roses along the way, surprises around the corner, and best of all: ice cream sandwiches at 3:00. Phil is keeping me in pace and I am so very grateful for that.

A kid on a scooter just went by. It had a very strange design and I am too tired to try and describe it, sorry. Love, Phil.

AUGUST 23, 2014 / EARLY MORNING DILLY DALLY

Maryka and I having fresh squeezed o.j., toast and jam and cafés con leches. Having a dilly dally because there are only a few more kilometers to go to meet the film crew for the final sprint into Santiago.

OK, I am trying to get my thoughts together to meet with St. James. I can feel the energy building as we move along in the flow of pilgrims. See you later today, Phil.

AUGUST 23, 2014 / MONTE DO GOZO

I completed my petitions for St. James for tomorrow. This is a method that Clara described and involves having four candidates and letting St. James pick what he wants to pick. OK, I'm with the program, so: 1. I am asking for a blessing for our world that we may continue to work toward reconciliation and peace. 2. A blessing for the people of Spain for hosting us on our Camino. 3. A blessing for my family, doctors, nurses, angels, friends and advisors that have supported me on my journey. 4. A blessing for my personal Camino wherever it goes from here and for all those who carry a cancer burden. There that looks pretty darn good.

Later, love, Phil.

AUGUST 23, 2014 / ITALIAN MASS

I just went to a little informal Mass. It was just a priest and maybe twelve people gathered outside by the place we were eating. I just walked over and joined them and they welcomed me warmly. It was beautiful and simple.

We are off to do some filming at sunset with the Cathedral in the distance. OK, love you all, Phil.

AUGUST 24, 2014 / SANTIAGO!

The promised land! Earlier we got our Compostela and now we've just gotten out of the Pilgrim's Mass. That was spectacular. There was Romanesque architecture complete with squinches. We had communion which was a general mob scene but good. There must have been a thousand people there. Then they did the big incense burner that swings the length and height of the cathedral.

So we are catching some food and drink before afternoon activities. I have to get back into the Cathedral to talk to St. James which is the important thing. Have to pick up a few gifts here also.

I am crawling at this point, pretty exhausted. Have the feeling that I will collapse when I let myself. Will be on the plane tomorrow and can sleep then.

OK for now, Phil.

August 26, 2014 / Vashon, WA 98070 USA

Home for the night and then off again to Swedish Hospital now. Am getting aboard the ferry and I will have twenty minutes to hammer out a post. Well, just had to talk to two people about the trip.

I spent way too much time on planes yesterday. Did the whole trip from Santiago to Madrid to NYC to Seattle in one long day. At one point was lost in the airport in Madrid and was saved by a Camino Angel that I met earlier.

Had some fresh corn from our crop for lunch today. Harvest time. It's the best time of year, I think, and I am back for it. Everything around the ranch looks pretty good for not being touched for a month.

OK, we are coming into the dock. Keep going, love, Phil.

August 27, 2014 / Uber-Fortitude

That's what we need right now, those of us off the trail. It's a phrase coined by Mary Margret. It's not a happy time. Somehow we have to navigate through these rocks and shoals and make something happen.

I had a post written on this topic but I just threw it out. Maybe I will try a new approach. Maybe I will put my ideas in the form of questions as in what ifs. Maybe we could try things and share. What do you say?

What if we joined a pilgrim organization? US has American Pilgrims chapters that have regular outings in your area to meet other pilgrims and share ideas. Other countries have co-fraternities.

What if we got a lavender plant or a fragrant rose bush for our house? Or what if we got a whole bunch of them and planted them all around? Smells we all know are a pathway.

What if we learned Spanish cooking? This sounds like a winner to me. And it doesn't look all that complicated; it's doable. And combining that with good wine or brewskis (sorry, beers).

What the heck, what if we learned Spanish? Clara (a history teacher) was quoting some king from the past who said that if you want to talk about politics speak in Italian and if you want to talk about love speak in French and if you want to talk to God speak in Spanish. Sounds like a plan. Maybe French too.

OK, enough of that for now. Right now I am sitting in front of a big picture window getting my chemo treatment at Swedish Hospital, Seattle. Not a cloud in the sky. Learned that my scan yesterday showed that the spots that I have are unchanged and there is nothing new so that's a good thing. Today is the first treatment in a new series of twelve treatments, six-months' worth with the same drugs as before, which is keeping the cancer from spreading. What fun. Oh, I forgot but I got an official weigh-in today here at the hospital and I lost eighteen pounds since last month at this time. Man, and I ate like a horse on the Camino!

"It is the time when all the presents that the Camino gave us will become useful." That's Lucia from Sicily. I like it. Let's think about that. Love you guys, Phil.

August 30, 2014 / Laughing and Crying Our Way Across Spain

It's a rainy Saturday morning and am hanging out in the quiet trying to figure out things. I know that it is not going to come all at once and that I should not force things to happen at a faster pace. I know but I just don't want it to be Paradise Lost.

But we are Caminoheads, right? We keep going, that is what we do, one foot in front of the other. Part of going is recording what we do know, like taking photos along the way. What do we know?

I thought of three things that I know. That not only happened but hugely happened, you know what I mean? Over the top happened in unexpected ways and at surprising moments but happened enough times where I said yes, I got the message.

One, my connection to the earth was vastly strengthened. Sometimes this was the most beautiful landscape in a cloudless sky, say. Beauty was over the top for sure to the point where I didn't know what to do with it, no existing category. But yet I am talking about something else. What I am getting at is the link that we have with the earth in the way that it provides us with sustenance. Obviously, the Spanish are no slouches when it comes to agriculture, as we saw every day.

Start with the vast oceans of wheat and sunflowers that we walked through on the Meseta. And the vast fields of corn, sugar beets and potatoes that we saw along the rivers where irrigation was possible. Then there were the ever-present backyard and empty lot family gardens in city and country with beans, lettuce, cucumbers and tomatoes. And the huge piles of straw bales going off to be bedding for cows and pigs. It was all very impressive and Spain must be feeding half of Europe and us as we ate in the cafés along the way. Yea, totally underestimated the power of this.

Two, was the amazing connection and bonding that happened between folks. Folks from Netherlands, Italy, Australia, the States, Spain, you name it. We even had a great fellow, Sherif, from Egypt in our group. People sharing ideas, insights, fears, you name it. People doctoring each other's feet, sharing food, water, funds, carrying someone else's pack when they couldn't anymore, you name it. People watching out for each other (you would never leave anyone alone on the Meseta). Yea, totally underestimated the power of this.

Hey, and not to mention all the situations that we got in in all the albergues with their weird bathroom and sleeping set ups. Endless variety of awkward deals. At night at least eight people snoring, at least eight people rolling over on the squeaky springs, church bells ringing all night long. I remember having one ear plug and trying to figure out which ear to put it in. It forced us to realize that yes we irritate each other at the very same time that we need each other.

Third, my relationship with God was vastly improved. Not a sort of theoretical or far away feel but something close up and in the moment sort of improvement. In Spain along the Camino with all the pilgrims moving there almost always is a reminder of God and his posse to be seen—on a person, or fence or building or shrine or a church or hilltop. Just a sort of constant reminder that God is always present in my/our lives. Once again totally underestimating the power of this.

Wrap that all up and you got a bundle. This is what I feel with the rain still coming down outside and my eyes saying how about nap time? Love you, Phil.

August 31, 2014 / I Want to Dilly Dally With You

Dilly dally—waste time through aimless wandering or indecision. Hmm. I think that definition could be improved, don't you? Let's see, how about: aimless wandering with little indecision as we relate outside of time? Better.

We are back from the trail and we are wondering just what kind of freight train hit us. This is not business as usual but we will figure it out eventually.

Rick, my walking partner, is coming back to Seattle this evening. We are supposed to have dinner tomorrow so I will fill you in on how he's looking. Maryka is either in Seville or is back in NYC. Kelly is with his son Michael somewhere around Sarria and are on their way to do the last 100 k.

OK, the sun is out and I am going to get outside to do some chores. Everything good just slightly confused lately. Yours always, love, Phil.

September 1, 2014 / The Smallest Remembrance

I want to get outside, as it is beautiful. It is Labor Day, a holiday here in the States. It makes for a long weekend and sort of the end of the summer season.

I just wanted to relate a little story about a little piece of soap. Yea. One day at some nameless albergue (hostel) I had used the toilet and was at the sinks to wash my hands and was looking for the soap dispenser on the wall since I hadn't bothered to bring my kit in. No dispenser, no soap, oh darn.

Sometimes along the Camino things happen in such little ways at times that normally would seem little or empty or sparse or just plain ordinary and easy to overlook as anything meaningful. Anyway, there were four sinks in a row and on one I spied something tiny. Look at that, a piece of soap that someone left just for me! It was the size of my littlest finger nail. And I washed my hands carefully with that little piece of soap and look there is still some left for someone else. Just the littlest, tiniest of miracles. Love, Phil.

September 2, 2014 / Big and Breathtaking

Well, yesterday I talked about something tiny and today I thought that I would get to something really big but we will see. Lots of happenings and details to tell you about.

Rick returned and we had dinner with him and his wife Carole Lynn at our friends' lovely home here on the Rock (a nickname that we have for this island that we live on). Rick was full of stories of his adventures since I saw him last. After Santiago he had walked to the ocean to see that area, which he thought was great except for the rain.

I have never sufficiently talked about the fact that Matthew was walking the Camino for his brother Jan who had died of cancer recently. I could tell that he really loved his brother and I volunteered to take his place as we walked. We had much great conversation over three or four days. Thank you, Matthew.

I want to get my walking schedule figured out for the "backyard Camino" here. I had some serious regular walkers before Spain and I need to connect with them. Thinking that should be something like 0900 to 1000 maybe three or four days a week. Give me a few more days on this.

OK, well, we successfully dilly dallied around enough to not have time to work on the "big" topic. Or maybe this is the "big" topic, hard to say at this point. SJA, love you, Phil.

September 5, 2014 / Buen Camino!

I remember the first few days on the way out of St. Jean Pied de Port we said to each other "Buen Camino" and it felt good like yea, we're real pilgrims now. But it didn't take long for the novelty to wear off and the aches, pains, blisters, sunburn to start showing up to the point where we were hurting bad, discouraged and maybe laid up for a few days. Getting broken in I suppose is the term. And somehow some way we kept going and then when we looked each other in the eye and said "Buen Camino" it really meant something. Something more like yea, we are still here still doing it.

Somehow, I am feeling that again this morning. I just want to say "Buen Camino!" to you and to myself. This reentry is tough and yes, I/we were discouraged but heck look at us, we're still doing it, right? Our amazing resilience is something that we know. This realization is one of the gifts of the Camino that Lucia was talking about. A gift that we can employ to move forward. So, "Buen Camino!"—Phil.

September 7, 2014 / Warning

I want to warn you that my inner romantic has escaped and is, well I don't know where he is now really. He may have first left in early August around Estella in Northeastern Spain. The last thing that he said was something about running with the bulls.

Be careful with him if he appears. Not that he is dangerous really but he has a tendency to be beyond normal, to talk poetically, to promise you anything. He is often outside of time and will trap you in endless dilly dally. He thinks that God made heaven just so the three of you could be together—imagine!

I just found a few paragraphs recently that he wrote and they may be helpful:

"I went to Spain to do the Camino with openness, with room for it to join with me. That's all, really. And what I got in return was a hundred-fold.

The Spanish people: I remember an old woman begging outside of the Cathedral at Burgos, dressed all in black, she was so beautiful. I gave her some money and kissed her; I couldn't resist. I remember a woman who brought us cold Cokes as we stumbled past her house in the heat. We didn't have anything to give her but I made a motion with my rosary that we would pray for her and she understood and was happy. I remember a farmer herding his dairy cows down the road and I wanted to shake his hand. He made a motion like his hands were dirty so I kissed him on the whiskery cheek, nothing more, nothing less. I remember walking with a Spanish pilgrim who pulled out a candy bar and broke it in half and was in the process of handing half to me and it fell down into the dust of the Camino. I picked it up and he said that it was OK that he had another but I felt a need to eat that one as a communion with the trail and its millions of pilgrims. His smile signaled to me that he understood.

Then there was the scenery that was knockout beautiful. And the agriculture which was ever present, robust, varied, feed the world awesome. There were the ancient stone bridges, stone buildings, roads and fountains to remind us that plenty of people had worked very hard to make us comfortable.

The Camino attracts a certain set of people that come from all over the world and each has a story. Some are pilgrims to start with, others become pilgrims. You can communicate with them more or less according to your combined language abilities and this is major fun. I don't know about major fun but a lot of communication takes place through the universal language of hunger, thirst and pain. In the end all sorts and flavors of people meet, talk, share, eat and drink with you. They listen and encourage and inspire you. They are your angels getting you from shade to shade or water to water or from town to town. Just as you are their angel.

There are huge cathedrals at one end of the scale and little simple churches in all the small towns. OK, I was ready for that. But what else was every size, color, shape and variety of material reminder that God is present in the form of crucifixes, statues, shrines, collections and you name it all along the way.

And I went into every church that was open, went into monasteries, convents and other meeting places. Prayed with nuns and brothers. Took Mass in a cave, outside, inside in small churches and Cathedrals. Passed out from heat exhaustion at the high point of one Mass and was caught in the arms of a woman named Grace. Falling into the arms of Grace, no joke. Shook hands and talked with the Bishop at Burgos. Was blessed along with my fellow pilgrims by priests in numerous places along the route.

OK, so this is the evidence of how I flirted with, danced with, cavorted with and got drunk on Spain and the Camino. And in the end we made love."

Yea, see what I mean? Look, if you run into my inner romantic would you please tell him to check in. We need to talk; you know what I mean. Thanks, Phil.

September 8, 2014 / I Carried This the Whole Way, Just For You.

I picked this half piece of paper up early on in a quiet church. There was an old nun sweeping and smiling. It was there for the taking and I didn't know it at the time but

I brought it for you. I will try to copy it word for word and not change anything; it is so precious.

The Way: Parable and Reality

The journey makes you a pilgrim. Because the way to Santiago is not only a track to be walked in order to get somewhere, nor it is a test to reach any reward. El Camino de Santiago is a parable and a reality at once because it is done both within and outside in the specific time that it takes to walk each stage, and along the entire life if only you allow the Camino to get into you, to transform you and to make you a pilgrim.

The Camino makes you simpler, because the lighter the backpack the less strain to your back and the more you experience how little you need to be alive.

The Camino makes you brother/sister. Whatever you have you must be ready to share because even if you started on your own, you will meet companions.

The Camino breeds community: community that greets the other, that takes interest in how the walk is going for the other, that talks and shares with the other.

The Camino makes demands on you. You must get up even before the sun in spite of tiredness or blisters; you must walk in the darkness of night while dawn is growing; you must get the rest that will keep you going.

The Camino calls you to contemplate, to be amazed, to welcome, to interiorize, to stop, to be quiet, to listen to, to admire, to bless . . . nature, our companions on the journey, our own selves, God.

September 9, 2014 / The Flipside

This is the other side of the piece of paper. It is not knowledge that is secret but it was gotten at some sacrifice and is a benefit of taking that less used road.

The Beatitudes of the Pilgrim

1. Blessed are you pilgrim, if you discover that the "camino" opens your eyes to what is not seen.

2. Blessed are you pilgrim, if what concerns you most is not to arrive, as to arrive with others.

3. Blessed are you pilgrim, when you contemplate the "camino" and you discover it is full of names and dawns.

4. Blessed are you pilgrim, because you have discovered that the authentic "camino" begins when it is completed.

5. Blessed are you pilgrim, if your knapsack is emptying of things and your heart does not know where to hang up so many feelings and emotions.

6. Blessed are you pilgrim, if you discover that one step back to help another is more valuable than a hundred forward without seeing what is at your side.

7. Blessed are you pilgrim, when you don't have words to give thanks for everything that surprises you at every twist and turn of the way.

8. Blessed are you pilgrim, if you search for the truth and make of the "camino" a life and of your life a "way", in search of the one who is the Way, the Truth and the Life.

9. Blessed are you pilgrim if on the way you meet yourself and gift yourself with time, without rushing, so as not to disregard the image in your heart.

10. Blessed are you pilgrim, if you discover that the "camino" holds a lot of silence; and the silence of prayer; and the prayer of meeting with God who is waiting for you.

OK, there is it. Love, Phil.

Healing holds a lot of silence

SEPTEMBER 10, 2014 / MY FLAN REPORT

Yes, got the flan made this AM. Right, last minute. And Rebecca said to make sure to tell you that it was Jello brand in a box. OK, right, but the directions are in English AND Spanish so that should count. It took me twenty minutes from box to refrigerator, not that it is a race.

I have a quote for you from church on Sunday here on Vashon. There was a response that we repeated I think three times just to make sure . . . "If today you hear his voice, harden not your hearts." You may have heard this but I am passing this on, just in case.

It has come to dawn on me that my Camino is starting to talk to me here just as she did in Spain. She says that I have too much going on and I have to slow my pace to avoid injury. So, I am going to try and do something with the blog to give me a little break for ten days. If I did a post each day coming up on one of the ten Pilgrim Beatitudes it would be less effort and still fun and profitable.

And I did hear God's "voice" last night in between sleeps. I put that in quotations because he just occurred rather than I heard something. The message in paraphrased form: "Your Dilly Dallies on Earth are only tapas. Your complaint that there is not enough time to DD sufficiently with everyone will be solved in heaven because time will be unlimited forever." Yea, that's what I'm talking about!

So, here we go off again. Love to you and yours, Phil.

SEPTEMBER 11, 2014 / THE BEATITUDES OF THE PILGRIM #1

BLESSED ARE YOU PILGRIM, IF YOU DISCOVER THAT THE CAMINO OPENS YOUR EYES TO WHAT IS NOT SEEN. The Camino is a walk designed to give you an experience if you are open to it. It has been going on for 1200 years and all those millions of pilgrims that have walked over that time speak to its power.

Camino Repair and Towing Project #2: starting today and for one week put a Band-Aid (plaster) on one of your feet even if you don't need it just to celebrate healing. And maybe even put it on top of your foot where folks can see it and wear it proudly!

OK, have to get to work and then to the hospital. So, so long for today, Love Phil.

SEPTEMBER 12, 2014 / THE BEATITUDES OF THE PILGRIM #2

BLESSED ARE YOU PILGRIM, IF WHAT CONCERNS YOU MOST IS NOT TO ARRIVE, AS TO ARRIVE WITH OTHERS.

Or as Kelly would say, "it's not a race, people!" Yesterday we talked about the idea that the Camino is not just a walk but it is a walk with a purpose. Today we are adding the idea that that purpose is not one of competing. The idea is not to win over someone by increasing the distance between you but to decrease the distance 'til you are with that someone.

Who might that someone be? Your hiking partner or a pilgrim that you are familiar with or is it someone intriguing that you caught a glimpse of yesterday or a week ago perhaps and lost track of or is it someone that has just shown up "out of the blue" or is it possibly yourself?

Whoever it is, everyone will prosper. Maybe that will be in some small way but maybe in some huge way, you never know. Don't be shy, it's all good in other words. Love, Phil.

SEPTEMBER 13, 2014 / THE BEATITUDES OF THE PILGRIM #3

BLESSED ARE YOU PILGRIM, WHEN YOU CONTEMPLATE THE "CAMINO" AND YOU DISCOVER IT IS FULL OF NAMES AND DAWNS.

In this document, as it is written, every time the word Camino is used it is in lowercase and in quotation marks. Interesting. Have been thinking about this and working on it. To me at this point it is so beautiful and mysterious that I would rather not clutter it up with words. Couldn't we just let it float in the breeze and admire/savor/wonder? OK, I'm glad that you are with me! Love, Phil.

SEPTEMBER 14, 2014 / SATURDAY EVENING

Kelly's back! I just talked to him on the phone. He, Rick and I will have a meeting tomorrow evening, well, meeting and wine tasting. Let's see what else is new? Rebecca and I had a great dilly dally this evening. Just to sit with someone you love and have a glass and tapas and put the day in context is priceless.

I am going to try my second adventure with flan in a few minutes. Yea, I got the Royal brand (directions in Spanish) which makes twice as much as the Jello brand for the same price. Making it for the Camino meeting with Rick and Kelly. Will give you the full report.

Love, Phil.

SEPTEMBER 14, 2014 / THE BEATITUDES OF THE PILGRIM #4

BLESSED ARE YOU PILGRIM, BECAUSE YOU HAVE DISCOVERED THAT THE AUTHENTIC "CAMINO" BEGINS WHEN IT IS COMPLETED.

I think about the Camino in Spain as being an international spiritual boot camp. That is, it is training in things spiritual in which a lot happens to many pilgrims in a

it is not morning yet and I am awake

very short compressed period of time. That is why we all feel like just got run over by a big truck and we have a tough time talking about what happened.

But the important thing is that the Spanish Camino gave us "presents" to use in our walk now and tomorrow wherever that leads. Let's work on discovering those and putting them to use to make things easier and more meaningful. And beyond that I am no longer thinking that I should bring little trinkets from the Camino to plug into my "real" life but just the opposite--the Camino is the new paradigm for me, for us.

Words from Laura, "Above all, we are lucky, aren't we? We've been there . . . we've experienced . . . we've tasted . . . we've enjoyed . . . we've felt it." Yes. Love, Phil.

September 15, 2014 / Sparked and Up Early, Part 1

Couldn't sleep, thinking, moon coming on, remembering, the morning is not here yet. Something has got me moving.

I feed my dog, Sture, and make breakfast for myself. French toast comes together from slices of stale baguette and very fresh eggs from a neighbor. I fry that up with olive oil and put a big spoonful of Rebecca's blackberry jelly on top. And with coffee, nice.

But this isn't about breakfast or cooking. Last evening Rick brought Kelly over for a reunion and that is where this all started. Remember I said that I would give you a report. Yea, the Three Amigos together again after our various Camino experiences. Kelly and Rick looked great.

We talked Camino and Rebecca joined us. News of great people, places and events were shared by Rick. Kelly, the last back, had news about folks that I had met, some who I had heard about and some that were totally new to me. I served the flan that I had made earlier in the day. That was my second flan adventure by the way and it turned out good though slightly different. But this isn't about French toast or flan or cooking.

Rick talked about his walk after leaving Santiago. We all had catching up to do.

After the guys had taken off, Rebecca asked how I thought it went and I told her that something was odd although I couldn't put my finger on it. Something was off. Kelly and Rick had been there in the flesh and blood with us a minute ago but something was different and it was disconcerting. Things were slightly off. And that is what had me not sleeping and up early and writing to you and, well, to myself.

What had happened was that we had changed, slightly. We were there in our physical bodies but it seemed that we weren't the Rick, Kelly nor Phil that we were when we were last together in July. Dawn is here. Sture is wondering why his master is slightly off.

But also something else showed up that has sparked my interest. Both Rick and Kelly touched on topics that got me thinking and moving early. What they said independently was related as they talked about the same thing, I think, although they come at it from different angles. Interesting.

Kelly talked about real people on the trail by name. Names included Sherif, Cherry and Anse. I am going to borrow those names from Kelly to try and describe a

WALKING IN THE MUD

dynamic here so bear with me. I hope that the real people don't mind but this is pretty factual. Ready? Here we go: So, I talked with Sherif on my first or second day but didn't walk with him 'til later. Cherry came in and we met and at some point walked together. Kelly walked with her. Then Sherif and Cherry walked together and had big adventures. I walked with Kelly a lot but not all the time. Kelly and Emily walked a lot together or was that earlier? Then I had to bus ahead to meet Rick. Kelly stayed to keep walking and then Anse, from Netherlands, showed up. OK, are you thoroughly confused? Yes, good, I was successful. Keep reading please.

Then Rick brought up an observation, that we pilgrims never talked about the towns that we had gone through that day. I protested saying that we dilly dallied around for hours in the evenings discussing the day, how was that possible?

Well look, Kelly will be here in half an hour to get me up on my feet and walking again so have to go for now and get ready. Sorry to leave you with this cliffhanger but we will have time to bring it together tomorrow. OK? Thanks, I knew you would understand. Love, Phil.

SEPTEMBER 16, 2014 / SPARKED AND UP EARLY PART 2

One hour is all that I get today to wrap up these thoughts. We can do this. So, one thing was the idea that we were all changed by that experience. And I think that generally it is subtle. Ok, we may come back wearing the Camino T-shirt but what about all that deeper stuff that is going to ooze out in time. You know that it is in there. Yesterday I fried up my French toast with olive oil which I never would have done "before." That flavor is oozing out to compliment the other ingredients and to make the whole subtly different, better.

Back to Rick's observation. It looks like to me that he got really into the land and the way that the trail laid on the topography. And he got into learning how to correctly pronounce the names of the towns, rivers and other features. Awesome. He can now describe a particular climb or descent in these vivid terms. Very cool. And yes, now that I give it the thought that it deserves, he is right. I for one and a lot of those around me tended to not do that. We didn't sit at the end of the day and really talk about it in those terms. That hill that we climbed to me is remembered by who I was with at the time that was talking me up, sometimes almost step by step. I remember my eyes lighting on heart-shaped rocks that would occur at the most amazing times to be a message that we were loved.

It is said that the Camino is a living thing and a complex living thing with many ways of looking at it and all good. Just a testament to its richness. So, yes let's see just how many ways that we can look at it. And back to the paragraph from yesterday where I confused you with all the names and the comings and goings. It is confusing if you try and keep track of it by what individuals did or didn't do, yes? But when you consider that each one of those great unique individuals while bonding with their fellow walkers formed a fabric, a flow, a river. Each held it together for a short period of time with those around it. And they moved across the landscape making that line on the map.

Later, in the flow of pilgrims from Sarria on, when I was with Maryka, she said that she felt like we were two drops in a great river. Exactly. But really drops only exist when they are out of the of the river, right? And the river by that time in August was in flood stage and overflowing its banks and overwhelming the system. And we weren't bonding as easily with those around us because it was such a rush. We were all swept along.

So, I am musing about this and remembering looking at maps of the Camino, before I got there to experience it, when the trail was a thin line of unvarying width as it went across the topography. But now to see it as a living thing it looks and acts more like a river to me. Sometimes it is just a trickle and sometimes it is calm and moves peacefully but at other times and places it gets unruly and overflows its banks and cuts new channels. And the towns are along its banks and you can swim in to visit a café, church or water closet when you want, but it flows on regardless.

OK, I am just about out of time and I have to work on my taxes as they are due in by Friday. Maybe I will find some heart-shaped rocks to cheer me on as I climb this particular hill. thanks for putting up with me. Love, Phil.

September 17, 2014 / The Beatitudes of the Pilgrim # 5

BLESSED ARE YOU PILGRIM, IF YOUR KNAPSACK IS EMPTYING OF THINGS AND YOUR HEART DOES NOT KNOW WHERE TO HANG UP SO MANY FEELINGS AND EMOTIONS.

Yes, yes and yes. Tears of joy are rolling done my cheeks right now. And if I had to pick one of these Beatitudes as the one that spoke to me the most, this would be the one. This right here was the big realization for me.

The things that you carry from the beginning of the trail in France at some point start to became more of a hindrance than a help. I mean the total weight, and you start seriously looking at your gear daily to cull stuff out. You learn that there is a price to pay for your being attached to these things. Your body pays and then that starts working on your mind and it starts paying and then your spirit starts to pay finally if you let it get that far.

Right, you need some of that stuff to maintain yourself. Yea, but which stuff and how much of it? The more I can jettison the more I will be able to do and see and participate in the next day is my evolving thinking. And isn't the doing, seeing and participating in what I am here for anyway and why I paid thousands of dollars, speaking of paying? Are we supposed to be beasts of burden?

And the more you can lighten your load the more that you can participate and therefore take in. Maybe lightening will allow you to take that side trip where you will. Maybe the lightening will let you be awake and aware enough to catch someone's eye. That is the someone who will carry your pack or doctor your feet or have that little bit of information or have that really big bit of information that you have been looking and hoping for quite a while now.

Anything could happen around the next corner and usually does. It is said that the Camino is full of surprises and you start looking for surprises. Yes, people and places that will speak to you. And sunsets and moonrises, little snails and giant fields of sunflowers, thirst and refreshment, pain and smiles, crowds and emptiness, hellos and good byes. You will become open and looking to see what will happen next.

If you are ready like this you will start to collect experiences and memories. Your pack is becoming lighter and your heart is filling with what you had been hoping for long before you had ever heard of this walk. My thoughts today and praise the Lord. Love, Phil.

September 18, 2014 / The Beatitudes of the Pilgrim #6

BLESSED ARE YOU PILGRIM, IF YOU DISCOVER THAT ONE STEP BACK TO HELP ANOTHER IS MORE VALUABLE THAN A HUNDRED FORWARD WITH-OUT SEEING WHAT IS AT YOUR SIDE.

This kind of thing was happening constantly along the Camino. Sometimes you would be going back, or waiting for someone to make sure that they made it to shade and water. Kelly developed one of his famous quotes which goes, "Shade Thyself." Which means protect yourself (and the guy next to you by extension!).

Watching out for each other became an important activity especially out on the Meseta and the mountains and other remote places. Kelly kept me going on to town numerous times when I would be dilly dallying when I should have been walking, distracted by something instead of getting out of the heat. Later, Rick would range ahead to get lodging and then walk back to carry my pack for a few kilometers at the end of some days. Angels they were. And sometimes I would be a help to them.

I remember one Korean woman what was alone and having trouble that Mary and Angela and I kept our eyes on. And people I didn't know kept their eyes on me/us. And maybe we didn't have a common language but we were communicating on the most important things. love, Phil.

September 19, 2014 / The Beatitudes of the Pilgrim #7

BLESSED ARE YOU PILGRIM, WHEN YOU DON'T HAVE WORDS TO GIVE THANKS FOR EVERYTHING THAT SURPRISES YOU AT EVERY TWIST AND TURN OF THE WAY.

It will sort of pick at you. Or nudge you. Or trip you up. Or suggest. Or trick you. Or show you something. Or invite you. Or draw blood. Or give pain. Or take away pain. Or give you something. Or have you meet someone. Or . . .

As I reread this Beatitude now, again and again the phrase "to give thanks" jumps out and is my surprise at this turn. Have I done that? Have I done that sufficiently? It is showing me something.

I hope that there are some clouds to shade you as you walk today! Love to you, Phil.

September 20, 2014 / The Beatitudes of the Pilgrim #8

BLESSED ARE YOU PILGRIM, IF YOU SEARCH FOR THE TRUTH AND MAKE OF THE "CAMINO" A LIFE AND OF YOUR LIFE A "WAY", IN SEARCH OF THE ONE WHO IS THE WAY, THE TRUTH AND THE LIFE.

This to me is the overarching message of our walk. That we will be blessed if we take our experience and make a life of it. And this life will be a journey, a search for the one who said, "I am the Way (Camino in Spanish), the Truth and the Life." This is Jesus talking to us. This is my interpretation of the situation.

Throughout the Pilgrim Beatitudes the word camino is used five times and it is always in lower case and in quotation marks. I think that the author is using this to refer to the physical walk, the el Camino de Santiago. And this thing/experience is a facsimile of the real Camino, or the Way that is following Christ. It is a training ground to get us started in the right way.

OK, that's all for now. Love, Phil.

September 21, 2014 / The Beatitudes of the Pilgrim #9

BLESSED ARE YOU PILGRIM IF ON THE WAY YOU MEET YOURSELF AND GIFT YOURSELF WITH TIME, WITHOUT RUSHING, SO AS NOT TO DISREGARD THE IMAGE IN YOUR HEART.

If I am not mistaken this sounds suspiciously like Dilly Dally here or Smelling the Roses. Or maybe more random acts like jumping off a medieval bridge into the river on a hot afternoon or howling into the emptiness of the Meseta. Strange but true.

The Camino is not supposed to be all work. Make room for FUN. Make room for the JOY. Make room for ICE CREAM. Make room for SURPRISES. Make room for the UNPLANNED AND THE YET UNDISCOVERED. Love you guys, Phil.

September 22, 2014 / The Beatitudes of the Pilgrim #10

BLESSED ARE YOU PILGRIM, IF YOU DISCOVER THAT THE "CAMINO" HOLDS A LOT OF SILENCE; AND THE SILENCE OF PRAYER; AND THE PRAYER OF MEETING WITH GOD WHO IS WAITING FOR YOU.

This best describes the time alone that you spend walking. There is time to contemplate and commune even in August which is the busiest month there. Toward the end, after Sarria, finding the time and space for this was harder in the dense flow of pilgrims. But as we know, God is always present and it is just us that gets distracted with the busyness around us.

But there is plenty of silence and time in most of the earlier parts of the trail. The Meseta is the best. A lot of people tend to by-pass this part but it is the best for being out in the middle of nowhere. Kelly said that this was his favorite part and I would have to agree. Of course, the whole Camino is good in its own way but for silence the Meseta is priceless.

Well, we are at the end of our Beatitudes with this being number ten and it is getting time to move on down the trail to other things. Just a few last-minute items for you. I hope that this has been helpful and thought provoking. It has for me. There are a lot of riddles in there to chew on. There are little puzzles to contemplate. I am currently working on this phrase, "the silence of prayer." And we must say thank you to the author whomever that may be. It is an unsigned gift to us and we are grateful. Ever onward, love, Phil.

SEPTEMBER 25, 2014 / PHIL'S CAMINO

I really need to get my walking trail open again on a regular basis. I miss my local folks and the fun that we had before that darn trip to Spain. Anyway, so here is the schedule to start with and we will tweak it as we go along:

> Monday 0900-1000
> Friday 0900-1000
> Sunday 1000-1100

I am not going to have sign ups. Just come and walk.

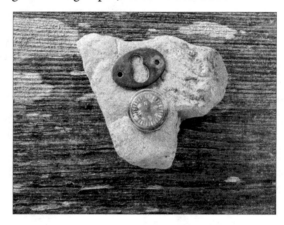

This is a photo of three artifacts that I found within a half-hour as I was working our corn field getting ready to plant this Spring here at the ranch on Vashon: an excellent palm sized HEART ROCK accompanied by a working COMPASS (as in finding north) and a brass KEYHOLE plate. A message do you think?

So yea, let's get walking again wherever we are. Love, Phil.

SEPTEMBER 26, 2014 / HI

I just wrote an email to my old Caminohead friend Annie and I said something to her that I had to look at again. Maybe marks a new level in finding my way back home after Spain. I wrote, "My reentry is sorting itself out."

Liking that so much. This is one of the new gifts of the Camino for me and for you maybe. We can't effect reentry all by ourselves, we have to give it a life of its own so it can do what it needs to do.

I got to see Sister Joyce yesterday. What a joy she is. She always leaves with the feeling that we are all in this together. And that is very comforting. Love to all, Phil.

Camino as the el Camino de Santiago

SEPTEMBER 27, 2014 / THE GRAINFIELDS

We are on an agricultural theme today because I ran across this passage in the Bible from Matthew 6:1, "One Sabbath Jesus was going through the grainfields, and his disciples began to pick some heads of grain, rub them in their hands and eat the kernels." We would grab a snack in the same way. Sometimes it's a long way in between towns. You could eat the wheat like that or eat the bread when you got to the next town which is made from the same stuff.

So, thanks for joining me in this little remembrance. Have to get out to the outdoors. Love, Phil.

SEPTEMBER 28, 2014 / CAMINO GIFTS

Little gifts are coming at me. I am doing my best to catch them and to examine them and be thankful for each. These are realizations resulting from seeing my surroundings, physical and otherwise, from new viewpoints, new perspectives, I think.

Remember when we were walking and we were in the middle of nowhere, and we were in that stage between pain earlier and tiredness later. That's right, the giddy stage. We had mastered pain for the time being and we still had plenty of energy left to walk and learn about each other. We talked and we had time and we explored each other. Is that sounding too weird to say? Somehow in that process I was not only hearing your story but magically I became your story. And maybe you became my story, I don't know for sure. I was seeing things through your eyes is maybe a more conventional way to say it but it was stronger than that. It was more than an intellectual understanding. And maybe when one does this with enough people you just get the ability to lose yourself which I think is what I am experiencing now.

And this is part of being a Caminohead, don't you think? And maybe part of the reason I think so much of you. SJA, Phil.

SEPTEMBER 29, 2014 / IT'S FALL IN THE NORTHERN HEMISPHERE

I know, the Fall Equinox was a few days ago but it started feeling like Fall for real for me this AM. Had the first real fire of the season in the wood stove. Time to take the screen doors off so it will be easier to get the firewood in and anyway the bugs are gone mostly.

That all sounds very local which is good for me to express as it is a reflection of my progress to get back home after Spain. But at the same time my walking buddies from Australia and South America are in my thoughts and who are maybe home by now and welcoming Spring there. Love you guys and you are always welcome. All good, Phil.

SEPTEMBER 30, 2014 / VERY VERY LOCAL

I was just in the kitchen trying to make breakfast for myself and I clumsily broke a wine glass that was on the drainer next to the sink. It fell into the sink with a crash!

And that's pretty loud in a pretty quiet house, just me and the dog up and he is quiet and content after being fed.

Yea, so? Well, the other part of the story is that this is the time and place where most of the blog writing gets done and this morning, like very recent mornings, I was having trouble. Topics have been hard to find. They weren't just lying around on the surface to be casually picked up the way that they were earlier. So, I was thinking about that actually when crash the wine glass went falling into the sink and woke me up.

Let me try again to describe it with what I felt. Ok, so crash, the beautiful and delicate glass that was happily sitting on the drainboard, meets the not so beautiful and not at all delicate sink.

Yea, so? But what's important really is my first thought. What about people coming to Dilly Dally? What about those great people that have been coming to share afternoon tapas with us? What, now we are down to three wine glasses. This will never do!

Love, (do I need to say that? Yes.) Love, Phil.

> PS—the walking schedule for the near future:
> Friday the 3rd 0900-1000.
> Sunday the 5th 1000-1100.
> Monday the 6th 0900-1000.

(This is here at the ranch. Just show up with your boots on. Would be great to see you!)

October 1, 2014 / Yesterday, A Boaty Day.

Boaty is sort of a word that I used in Scrabble one time and Rebecca rejected it but she has since seen my side of it, I think. Anyway yesterday I walked on the ferry boat with a few tools and my friend picked me up and we went to a marina in Seattle to work on his friend's sailboat. That's two boats. We worked as long as we could and took off to get me on the ferry again to get back to the Island on boat three. Then I met a dear friend that I haven't seen for a while and we caught up and while that ferry was close to the Seattle shore we watched a man fly fishing from a red canoe, boat four. I could see fish rising in the water around him. Finally we got too far out to see him and at that point he hadn't caught anything yet but he remained hopeful. Of course, I am speaking for him there and I don't know him but I know fishermen, and that is what fishing is all about, yes?

Please remain hopeful, love, Phil.

October 3, 2014 / Found Them

Zowie! I found another half dozen wine glasses that are the same as our set that was down to three since I so handily broke that last one. And I forget the description on the box that they came in but it was something like oversized or wide or grande or over the top. I like the idea of that. If we are going to dilly dally let's be generous about it all, don't you think? Love, Phil.

October 5, 2014 / Kelly To The Rescue

I don't know how many times Kelly saved my sorry butt on the Camino in Spain. I owe him so much and he was the perfect partner on our journey. Just one example: he always said that we were Slow and Steady. Here on Vashon in training I was faster than he was so I got the nick name Steady. Then somewhere in Spain we switched and he took over being Steady. Let's say that we complemented each other beautifully.

Thank you Kelly for the help that you gave. Thank you for your friendship. Thank you for your smiles. Thank you for your "Kelly's Quotes of the Day." And maybe most important, helping me deepen my faith. You're the best buddy, thanks for putting up with me. Love, Phil.

October 7, 2014 / Rick To The Rescue

Somewhere along the trail Rick picked up the nickname Quick. And he was and is quick for sure.

Rick is from here on Vashon Island. Kelly trained with him a lot and I trained with him some before Spain. I say some because it was harder for me to join Rick because of scheduling. And one time the three of us did get to walk together which was hilarious to the max.

But in Spain we were never together like that either. Kelly was with me for the mountains and the Meseta and then Rick was with me from Samos Monastery westward to Santiago. I was blessed to have them both, for they kept me organized and moving in their own ways.

Rick's way was to help me by figuring out the lodging for us, which was problematic in the last 100 km due to the robust flow of pilgrims. He enlisted his daughter Maryka, who speaks Spanish, to help with cell calls out to potential places. We even stayed at a dairy farm one night that he engineered. Quick Rick to the rescue!

One day we walked a long way to a town that we thought had bunks but was full up and we walked on another ten km to the next town. It turned out to be our longest day, 35 km, I think. But anyway Quick hiked ahead to that town, left his pack and came back to help me. And he carried my pack the last 1 1/2 kilometers. What a guy. Rick to the rescue once again! You're the best, Phil.

October 8, 2014 / I Try To Stay Sober . . .

"I try to stay sober and then I see a beautiful flower." This is one of my thoughts that I wrote down on July 8th and just found. This was before Spain. I was already getting in the zone here on Vashon.

A good robust response to beauty is a beautiful thing, yes? And I know that we all felt that because we all laughed AND cried all the way across that beautiful country where we were in and out of beautiful churches, and met beautiful people and had beautiful surprises. That looks all good to me. Love, Felipé.

OCTOBER 9, 2014 / SOMETHING SHORT AND SWEET

I'm off to a busy day in the big city so I need to talk with you now.

You know along the trail when one of us or anyone was having a bad time, a bad stretch of personal road we would be there for them, no question. Well our beloved Anamaria is having such a time right now. Her personal road is hard because she, the wonderful girl, is heart-broken over the death of her beloved friend.

We are all connected by bonds that we don't always understand but regardless we feel them. I am reminded of that old Sam & Dave song "When Something is Wrong With my Baby, Something is Wrong With Me." Please be there for Anamaria now in your own way.

Yes, what could be more important than that? What are we here for if not to support each other on the Camino. It still goes on, yes? You're the best, Felipé.

OCTOBER 10, 2014 / WHAT IS LIFE WITHOUT TAPAS?

Now there is a Kelly-quality quote. I came up with that. Yea. Maybe we will explore its meaning soon. But for now I have to be brief. I am walking in a few minutes and if I am lucky I will have some company.

Rebecca purchased a leather couch yesterday. It is not new but it is beautifully broken in, burgundy color and very Spanish looking I think. She is redoing the living room. Thanks Rebecca.

I got a message from Anamaria and she is feeling better. So, whatever you are doing, keep doing it for a while yet, please. You guys are the best, love, Felipé.

OCTOBER 12, 2014 / CAMINOHEADS?

What the heck is a Caminohead anyway? Good question, let's work on that. Maybe I need to back up and give you a little history of my thinking. Within the last year I heard a quote in Spanish that went, "The Camino is a drug, it will hook you." And that entered my thinking and started roaming around.

Then one day about six months ago, back before Spain, I needed a name for this blog and a few things came together to gel and form Caminoheads. One obviously is the druggy sort of connection. There are potheads and all sorts of heads, so why not? The other component, you are going to laugh at this one, is cheese. There is a brand of string cheese (mozzarella) that we started buying to put in the kids' lunches when they were in school. There is a little Cheesehead guy on the wrapper that looks like he is the more energetic brother of the GoDaddy guy. He's got a crazy smile and crazy string cheese hair. So the addictive notion of the Camino combined in my right brain with this guy and the result was, well, you guessed it.

I think that we could continue this thread tomorrow. I want to try and hammer out a definition of Caminohead but for now the sun is out and maybe I could get some tractoring in. Thanks for being here. You guys are the bestest, love, Phil.

October 13, 2014 / Caminoheads??

Hi. What if we continue on with what we were talking about yesterday. As Kelly would say, "Let's review." I don't know how many times he used this on me, as I am a slow learner apparently. So, I was telling you the genesis of the name Caminoheads and how that got started.

I am going to jump ahead and go for the jugular on this and say, at the farthest reaches of my thinking, that a Caminohead is someone that has a longing for God and has been attracted to the Camino because of it.

And look, in between those two ends we can conveniently fit all sorts of folks with all sorts of ideas, thoughts and motivations. The last thing that we need is an exclusive club, right? This has to be a club where the readers come together and learn from each other, support each other and celebrate each other.

Well, we made vast progress. Maybe we can gather a few more ideas and then tomorrow boil this down to something workable. I have a walking date in a few minutes and need to go for now. How about tomorrow? Love, Phil.

October 14, 2014 / Caminoheads???

Good morning or whatever time it is there where your body happens to be at the moment.

Back to our pursuit of a definition of Caminohead. Let's review: a Caminohead is an individual that is a hiker at one end of the spectrum and a pilgrim on the other. And additionally he/she is someone who is interested in what the Camino de Santiago means, offers, facilitates. And further, this is not an exclusive group. everyone is welcome that comes with a willingness to open themselves up to possibilities. Yes?

You know what, my Camino calls and have to close for now but we are making good progress and things are becoming more clear. And more clear is good. Love! Phil.

October 15, 2014 / Caminoheads????

The Caminohead is not necessarily a veteran of walking part or all of the Camino. The Caminohead is someone that, as the Pilgrim Beatitudes talked about, learns about how to make their life a walk, metaphysically speaking. So, being a Caminohead really is a state of mind, a path, a way to think about and navigate through this world, this life wherever he is physically.

And there is no denying that the ultimate way or The Way is following the path that Jesus has taught us. That is the twelve-hundred-year-old draw to that trail. That is the reason why the whole thing is so saturated with the Holy Spirit's magic dust. You can't go ten feet on the Camino without some getting on you. And the pilgrim walking next to you is dusted with it. And then a whole group of you walking together gets covered with it and it starts working on you and them. And the whole trail is covered with it. If you could see it, it probably is drifted up like snow in places as the wind blows it.

Wow, that was fun. And I promised you that we would finish this up today Oh, well. OK, tomorrow then. Love you dusty characters, Phil.

OCTOBER 16, 2014 / CAMINOHEADS ?????

This is turning into my favorite time of day. It is barely light out and I am on my second cup of coffee, the dog is fed and flames are dancing in the wood stove.

According to my good friend Ivette, when you are looking at an artist's painting and you see an area of the canvas that the artist has reworked and has obviously struggled with--that is the point of growth, I think she called it. It is the place where growth is happening and has the most potential for breakthrough. It is the spot where a lot of energy is being focused and it has high potential. And we all have spots, moments or areas where we struggle, rework or fret about, yes?

This definition seems like that for me. There is something important about it that will clarify things or focus things. It is something similar to creating a mission statement, perhaps.

How's this: Caminohead--a person with the state of mind that makes a walk of their life following the possibilities that the Camino de Santiago teaches.

Wow, I've just spent a lot of time working and reworking that here but that looks pretty darn good for now. Let's let it rest for a while.

OCTOBER 21, 2014 / FALL COLORS

Fall is such a great season. I know that some folks are lamenting the end of the Summer. It is special for sure but I've always enjoyed Fall the best. Something about the clarity of the air and nature's fireworks show of the hardwood leaves. Of course there is the adventure of hunting season.

I'm at the hospital now for my treatment. But on the way I have a Fall thing to report. The filberts, also known as hazelnuts are ripe now and the crows are having a field day. They fly the nuts to the roads and put them down so that the cars and trucks crack them. Works slick. And they don't just put them anywhere on the road but just in the track where the tires roll. Amazing example of animals using tools.

OK, time to go for today. It's been great being with you. Love, Phil.

OCTOBER 23, 2014 / A REMEMBRANCE CONCERNING MARYKA.

I had the great pleasure to be with my Vashon buddy Rick (Quick) and his lovely daughter Maryka for the last part of my Camino de Santiago pilgrimage. I got to spend a lot of time with her just doing what we seem to do best, walking and talking. And it was just a continuation of our walking and talking that we did in the rain and the snow during the winter here on Vashon.

And this is my remembrance: We were up early, from I think the monastery at Samos, and it was dark and foggy. We were walking mostly along the shoulder of a paved road with some occasional traffic. It was a little hairy since the footing was questionable and with the real possibility that we would miss a sign and be headed off in the wrong direction. Rick was ahead or behind on some scouting mission. Anyway, Maryka and I got on the topic of Patience. Don't remember how it started but we were throwing our best most inspired thoughts into the mix of our conversation as we felt our way along in the fog.

I remember talking about us Americans being so impatient, being a spray-can society. If we can't do it quickly and easily and just by pushing a button we are not interested. The conversation went on and I was talking about how we would put our money in the Coke machine and if things were too slow or non-functional we would start kicking it, like that was going to do some good. And no sooner did that come out of my mouth than in the distance we spied this weird red glow. And as we got closer It grew in size until we recognized it as a, guess what, a Coke machine. No joke just there with nothing else around it and with an extension cord running off into the fog. It was the first one that I saw that had the Cathedral at Santiago image on the front. We just stood and stared at it. Message, you think?!? Love, Phil.

October 25, 2014 / It's 0700 and . . . .

It's 0700 and I have a roaring fire in the wood stove to warm our hearts. It's been a rough few days for us here. I had a health scare which fortunately has been figured to be the lesser of the evils. Good but exhausting. Then last night our son had news that one of his high school classmates had taken his own life. Someone we knew. We have had a rash of young people taking their lives in the past few years. Hard to handle for me and for us.

You will remember that when I was in Spain I had three of those wrist bands on to remind me of things. One was for a wonderful young US Army Officer that was killed in the recent fight against terrorism. I knew him. Second was a wonderful young man that took his own life here in the neighborhood and I knew him. And the third bracelet was from the hospital to remind me to talk to people about colon cancer. Somewhere on my way back from Spain I cut these all off because they . . . .Well, they were too heavy for me, if that makes sense. I had bought the pilgrim bracelet and I had to go with that for a while.

Please say a prayer for our neighborhood. Ah, I look up and the fire has died down and we need some more wood. Let's keep it all burning. Love, Phil.

October 26, 2014 / Come In . . . .

Come in, I have a big fire going. We will warm up, yes? Glad that you could make it.

How are your feet and legs? Could be better, yea right. It's amazing what kind of situation that we can still walk on. Well, just kick your boots off while we have a bite to eat. Yea, change your socks, that's always good.

You got some sunburn too I see. Right, the tops of your ears get it the worst. No hat? It blew off? Well, just hunt around in that big box over there and maybe you'll get lucky. What's that? Not your favorite team? Well it is now. Ha-ha.

You want a big glass of agua? Then you have some soup and a glass of wine, how's that. I made chicken stock and I had some garbanzo beans in the pantry that I threw in, you'll like it. There is carrots and parsley. Everything tastes good to a hungry pilgrim. Well, yea, some of that ham is pretty bad. You mean that stuff that you can repair your sandals with? Ha-ha. Yea.

OK, here's your soup and some toast. We take care of you good. There's plenty of salt in there, you taste it first. Good, good. You want red or white? Red, OK.

So, dessert? We have some flan, homemade. Yes, good, here. More water?

Feel better? Right, not too many pilgrims in October. We are about ready to close for the year. We had a record year and August, you should have seen August. That's the worst or the best, depending on how you look at it. Yea, Saint James is happy.

So, you were crying before you came in? Tears of sorrow or tears of joy? Oh, it's an anniversary of something. A death, I see. Well, I will pray for your loved one and pray for strength for you precious pilgrim. OK, lace them up well, you have some ups and downs ahead before you get to the albergue.

There, you look better. A smile and a hug, what a lucky man am I. OK, see you next time.

November 2, 2014 / All Souls Day

> No man is an Iland, intire of it selfe; every man
> is a peece of the Continent, a part of the maine:
> if a Clod bee washed away by the Sea, Europe is the lesse,
> as well as if a Promontorie were, as well as if a Mannor
> of thy friends or of thine owne were;
> any man's death diminishes me, because I am involved in
> Mankinde; And therefore never send to know for
> whom the bell tolls; It tolls for thee.
> JOHN DONNE

Somewhere east of Burgos is a monument at the top of a mountain marked 1937 or 1939 for men killed in the fighting there during the Spanish Civil War. Maybe more of a hill than a mountain but the important thing is the monument and what it stands for. I was waiting to run across some such remembrance along the trail. I had read Hemingway's "For Whom The Bell Tolls" twice by then and roughly I knew the story of the war.

And near the monument are three or four picnic tables where Kelly and I had some food and rest. While sitting there I noticed a wooden fence with a gate close by so I walked over to investigate. Inside the fenced area is an area about fifty meters by four meters that is bordered by rocks and beyond an interpretive display. So I continued in to see the display.

What was going on was that it was a gravesite or actually a former site. The information described the project done in the early 1980's of digging up the 104 bodies that were there and running DNA tests on them to identify the remains. So the bodies were ID'd and returned to the families in their home towns. All the little and big towns that you had just walked through or were going to shortly had someone or more. The project took place shortly after the death of Franco, the Fascist leader of Spain that died in 1979 when finally the country returned to normalcy.

So last week I started to read the Hemingway book to get me in the mood for this topic. Just wanted to include it somewhere as it was a part of our walk and this is the appropriate day. Not exactly cheery but a story of reconciliation which is a good thing. Love, Felipé.

November 4, 2014 / Do You Think That We Had Too Much Fun?

There are points where a casual observer would think that we were having too much fun on Camino. How about a few things that I could come up in a minute: the sunflowers, the swallows, the eagles, the roses. The picnics. The free wine fountain, the tapas, the wine with every meal. (The waiter would bring you wine almost automatically but you had to ask for water).

We did laugh a lot when we weren't crying. Sunrises, sunsets, clouds to shade us.

OK, I am having way too much fun writing this.

November 5, 2014 / Great Day, Strange Vegetable

Yea, I have to admit that my personal Camino has been a little rough lately. And I know that is the way it is and I need to be present, keep walking and it will flatten out again. Right, that is the way it is set up, that nothing lasts forever. Laura says that we need Patience (always capitalized now). I have to quit kicking the Coke machine looking for faster results.

So, yesterday, my stars were really lined up I guess, and a great day appeared out of nowhere. The trail flattened out for the time being and I had a great time with great people. Yea, the old great people thing again. We need to hold each other close as it is amazing how much good influence we can exert on each other.

It started out with a Skype with Gracie in London. It was a short one because I needed to run off to Seattle for my big chemo treatment day. She is such a sweetheart and never fails to get me going. Then at the hospital my doctor, the receptionists, the schedulers and the bevy of great nurses never fail to give me the chuckles. So, I got about five hours in a comfy chair while the strange chemicals go coursing into my 175 pounds. But I always bring stuff to do and drink coffee and take advantage of the time to work on the blog or work on a book or try to flag down a nurse that has computer savvy to get some free advice. Then I get done at 4:30 and jet out of there to beat the worst of the afternoon rush.

So far so good, right? So I get to the ferry and I get to cut into the line because I have a pass from the hospital (special dispensation). And who do I run into but my old hunting buddy John, who is incredibly talented as a writer, song writer, musician and other stuff. He is our resident fisherman poet who I never get to spend enough time with.

I make it home and Rebecca has whittled out some great looking tapas which I characterized as rugged and she laughed. She laughs a lot. And she brought this strange new veggie. I'm calling it Intergalactic Broccoli. It has the most amazing geometry based on the spiral. And some try to tell us that there is no God.

For dinner we have venison in mushroom sauce by Rebecca and a glass of red and the phone rings and it's another of my favorite people who, like John the fisherman poet, is Stephen the cowboy chef. So, he says, "Lucky, I just made this deer liver pâté and I'm bringing it over so you can check it out. Are you going to be there?" Man, my stars are members of the Indiana University Marching Band.

No coincidences right? It's all in the plan, right? Just have to be Patient and let things unfold, right? Something that we learned on the Way of St. James, right? Hold me close, love, Felipé (aka Lucky).

November 6, 2014 / Tapas (Short But Tasty Topics)

The intergalactic broccoli has been sitting in water on our table for a few days now and I am totally fascinated by it. Notice how the big cone shapes are laid out in spirals and lines of the cones are orientated in two different patterns, both spirals. And then on those cones the smaller cones that cover those are laid out in this interlocking pattern of intersecting spirals. So cool. And then on these little cones the same thing occurs in miniature. And maybe on and on.

This is the same interlocking pattern that is in the layout of the seeds on the sunflowers in Spain that we walked endless kilometers through. Look at the pics. And this is the pattern that is used on some of the great old cobble stone streets in the cities there. Remember? I'll have to look through my photo album for that. Kelly was always taking pics of the walking surfaces. Last Sunday we had Will and Jasper from Green Man Farm over for dilly dally and din-din and Will put a name on that phenomenon, calling it an interference pattern.

So, in a recent post I was describing Rebecca's tapas as rugged. That was just a word that shot out of my brain on first glimpse. It was because she had some delectable goodies on the plate but some were standing up giving it this great 3-D look. My tapas are always very lounge-y. Like the little slices of cheese and the olives are having a little dilly dally of their own after a long day in the frig. Very relaxed but maybe slightly giddy just because they enjoy each other's company.

OK, you lounge-y tapa characters, I love you immensely! You're the best, Felipé.

November 9, 2014 / Alida's Flan Recipe

Flan! A great day for making flan!

> 1 14oz can of sweetened condensed milk
> same measurement (measure in the empty condensed milk can) of milk (I use 2 percent but you can use anything)

3 eggs
1 tsp vanilla

On the metal pan, melt about 2 tablespoons of sugar, stirring constantly so it doesn't burn, until it's golden caramel. Set aside

Blend mix in blender for about 1 min, until it gets a little foamy. Pour over caramel.

350-degree oven for 1 hr. Let it cool and put in refrigerator. I like flan a little cold.

Yup, got it in the oven with 25 minutes to go. I have been making this recipe in eight little ramekins so I had to experiment with the time. I am down to forty or forty-five minutes, still playing with it.

The beauty of the sunset is an indication of how beautiful the day was. See, it doesn't always rain here, just most of the time. I find myself staring at beautiful things lately. Staring maybe isn't the right word. But just trying to soak in as much as possible. More has got to be better, right?

OK, I am going to save this for Sunday morning. Awesomely awesome guys! Love, Felipé.

November 10, 2014 / El Cid

Kelly came over for dilly dally and dinner. Then we watched the 1961 El Cid with Charlton Heston and Sophia Loren. One big Spanish history lesson. I saw a Sophia quote the other day where she said that, "Everything she had she owed to spaghetti." I'm thinking on that one.

So, Kelly says to me that it's all my fault. Well, that the walk was my idea and I invited him to go along. And now he thinks about it every day and can't get rid of it.

We are walking in a few minutes so I am going to give you the lean and mean version this AM as time is short. Wiley is coming as well as Ross, a young man who has been afflicted/ blessed with blindness. He is a rare fellow. I enjoy his company.

OK, big and empty is a good place to leave you. Perhaps we can fill it with our positive energy, good spirits, prayers, thoughts, wishes, hopes, hoops, yells, hollers, memories. Excellent. Love to you, Felipé.

November 12, 2014 / Nine Months Later

Last evening Quick, his wife Carole Lynn and I went into the big city to see *Walking the Camino, Six Ways to Santiago*. Lydia B. Smith is the wonderful person who is the filmmaker and driving force behind this amazing work. Thank you Lydia for your many-year effort. I wonder what the "B" stands, for blistered, beautiful, bountiful, beneficial, best documentary ever, yea, that's it.

We had to fight our way through downed power lines and tree limbs to get there and back, almost like last February 7th when we saw the film the first time and it was the middle of a snow storm. Anything for Lydia I guess. Another thing that was the same was the fact that I wept all the way through the darn thing twice now. It so captures the pain/ joy/wonder/ camaraderie/ blessing/ work / play aspects of the trail. Absolutely, a must see!

And! And we walked out with our own DVD's of it. Ha! The much-awaited day. We so want to share it with friends. Almost better than Christmas.

Lydia did a great job of introducing the film last night and then after took some questions. The crowd seemed to enjoy hearing about what the six walkers were up to five years later. They seemed all to have pitched in to help with some aspect of promotions or translating for their home audience. The film has been subtitled in ten languages.

Then at some point in this she said, "Is Phil here?" And I groaned and stood and thanked her and gave a short talk on the "Phil's Camino" project. What a deal, the limelight. So, it is all moving ahead in strange and mysterious ways.

OK, second cup of strong coffee. So, Gracie has the flu and is feeling all alone in her room in London. What can you do about that? I told her that she was definitely not alone. Please send her what you have.

Obviously I am in love with you all, Felipé. XOXOXOXO

November 15, 2014 / It's Friday

The big news is that our beautiful dog , Sture (pronounced Stura) has come down with something that looks like some form of liver failure. I spent a large part of the day at the Vet's office working on that. Bummer.

I did get my walk in this morning and I want to remind you that I am still doing it three days a week now. That's Monday from 0900 to 1000, Friday from 0900 to 1000 and Sunday an hour later. Just come and walk and talk.

Falling asleep. Love Phil

November 15, 2014 / Smiling Sisters and Gnarly Dudes.

Late Saturday morning here on Vashon. The sky is blue as a result of the high-pressure system and should remain so for more days ahead. Things colder than we are normally used to. I'm here babysitting my sick doggy. The Vet did some stuff to make him relatively comfortable. So he is hanging out.

The really good news is that I was over at my friends Dick's yesterday and he kind of lost it and made five apple pies. Nobody does that. So I got a piece to bring home which I shared with Rebecca. She immediately calls Dick up to say that it is the best pie she has ever had. So today, Dick gives me a WHOLE pie with the message that flattery works. Yea, see.

Anyway back to the other Camino. Kelly came up with a pic of the Sister who was at the gnarly old church on the hill where we got the Pilgrim's Beatitudes. The church itself was in a grove of trees and you walked to it. No road or driveway or parking, old school.

And the Sisters were always smiling, well not always-always, but you know most always. Whatever they would be up to no matter how mundane or ordinary they were smiling away like they know something we don't. Hmm.

Then the topic of really gnarly dudes that you would see occasionally walking like they just live on the trail. Sometimes they would be walking the other way, the wrong way which always attracts attention. Yea, these guys were the cool grad students on campus and we were the dorky freshman, like you can't even approach them. I bet they had some stories. Needless to say that I don't have any pics of them although they closely approximated the archetypal St. James Pilgrim look, if you can picture that.

OK, Thanksgiving holiday is coming up here in America when we are thankful to God for the rich bounty that we enjoy. You guys are peachy, Love, Felipé.

November 17, 2014 / Sunday, Sunday

Today was memorable. Kelly, Rick, and I put on our long-awaited Camino slide show at our church. We had about fifty folks come to hear us and watch the slides. Even Sister Joyce was there. It's always fun to try and put the Camino into words. Although impossible, we are somehow getting closer with each try.

Hope that your day is going smoothly. It's cold here and I find myself longing for the heat of Spain in August. A hot cup of tea will have to suffice for now. Love, Felipé.

November 18, 2014 / Olive Oil and Salt

I think it was Mary Margaret that said when she travels she carries a little bottle of olive oil and a little bottle of salt. So she can always buy bread, a tomato and some cheese or whatever and be set for a meal. Nice. Almost seems too simple.

The other day I went exploring in the oil department at the local super market and came away with the really expensive stuff. Well not the most expensive but the second most. The most expensive brand bottles were dusty and they were over their expiration date. I just want to taste some really good stuff. And it was really, really good needless to say. Too expensive to use for general cooking purposes but great for on bread or salad.

And in the process of reading the labels I got the idea of the different characteristics of the different oils from different locales. So I have a lot to learn and a lot more fun to look forward to. This particular brand that I bought has a resin pine taste that I like. It is from Tuscany.

Well, have to go for now. Saint James is Afoot, Love, Felipé.

PS—I didn't say anything about salt but what can be said?

November 18, 2014 / Stretch of Bad Road

My trail is rough right now. I'm sitting in the comfy chair at Swedish Hospital getting my big two-week chemo treatment. It's not what you would call fun but that is not what is bothering me at the moment. I think I mentioned that our beloved dog Sture was sick, and that was bad enough, but now we know that it is a terminal situation. He is suffering from liver failure and we need to put him down. So, we are having a family meeting tonight when I get back to make a plan.

So, if you will forgive me, I think that I will sign off for today. I am totally distracted and need to attend to the situation. Tomorrow, being another day I will try again. There is a reason for this to occur right now so maybe that will become apparent. Thanks, Love, Felipé.

November 19, 2014 / Wednesday Morning

Everything in the Universe is going according to plan. Wow, how is that for starters? Sometimes this stuff just jumps out, thank you Holy Spirit.

This weekend Rebecca, Jessica and Todd of the infamous film crew will be here. And Annie and Maggie, who have been tirelessly working on the *Walking the Camino* documentary film, will be here. Annie has been producing *Phil's Camino* which is in the construction stages, all good, with St. James helping Annie at the helm.

Sunday afternoon and evening we are having a Camino party and film shoot. 1400-1600 walking, 1600-1800 potluck and 1800 on a bonfire gathering. We have shelters, tables and Coleman lanterns.

Yea, and our crisis with our beloved dog Sture has been eased through meds and procedures. But his basic bad problems remain. We are happy that perhaps we will have a few more weeks with him. Having a problem come up like this just before the film crew arrives is reminiscent of me having to have a root canal two days before we flew out to Spain in July. But all part of the big plan I know.

Have to go, love you all, Felipé.

November 23, 2014 / Reunion!!!!!

The film crew has landed here on Vashon Island. They are at Kelly's albergue for the night. They had dinner there last night and a big old dilly dally happened afterward. Rick and Carole Lynn and Rebecca and myself were there. What a great bunch of people. We were a few short of a cosmic quorum but we had a great time anyway.

Annie O' Neil will be joining our merry band and we will descend on Sister Joyce's office in Seattle for a film shoot later this morning. All good. Spent two hours with Sister Joyce and then back to Vashon to film outside along the Camino in an unexpected sunbreak.

We had a big dinner with all of us at our place and talked and laughed 'til we couldn't anymore. Then off to bed and another day awaiting. Really hard to write this post when there is so much going on but of course that is the way it was in Spain. Love, Felipé.

November 24, 2014 / He Partied with Us and at a Certain Point Got Up and Left

We got to the Island on Saturday after being with Sister Joyce and we spent the rest of the afternoon capturing a couple of hours on the Camino here at the ranch. And the weather, although stormy and rainy in the morning gave us those hours with beautiful sunshine.

Then yesterday after church we were busy again with sometimes two cameras going at once to get everything in the remaining hours. A little crazy at times but it was a great opportunity as the weather cooperated again, which around here at this time of year is a miracle. So the afternoon progressed to the evening and people arrived to be at the potluck. And we were still filming into that and doing a last-minute interview with Dr. Zucker and me and Annie and me. And it seemed like the super heavy topics were there at the end. And finally it appeared like we were talked out and we could go eat and relax.

Dinner was great as we had provided chicken and Italian sausages cooked by our dear chef friend Stephen. And Rick and Carole Lynn had made paella and Kelly a chocolate cake and there were salads galore. So it is dark by now and our son Wiley has the bonfire going full bore and finally everyone is having a drink and getting in the mood.

So this whole time Sture our beloved dog who has had end-of-life type issues with his health was cruising through the crowd looking for leftovers just like normal. He was next to Rebecca and myself and he just keeled over and was gone in a minute, like dead in a very short minute. Yea, right there so quick and easy right with us and right in the midst of the whole gathering. Amazing.

We carried him out on a quilt made by my grandmother and put him in the back of my truck where he loved to ride. We laughed and we cried.

Love you all, Felipé.

November 25, 2014 / Found My Santa Hat

I know that it is a little early but I just donned my really cool camo Santa hat that one of my archery students gave me. Need something to cheer me up at the moment. Sture being gone is leaving a pretty big hole in our winter evening. Well, it feels like winter.

So, we are all cleaned up after the big reunion weekend. The pilgrims have come and gone. They travel so lightly and well that they don't really leave much of a footprint.

Watching the flames dance in the wood stove and thinking about your warm hearts scattered around the world. Join me, won't you. I am going to propose a toast to the prince of dogs: Thank you Sture for your tremendous heart, love you, may we all be as robust as you.

Love, Felipé.

November 26, 2014 / A Highly Successful Dilly Dally

Before I get started on that I want to put my walking schedule in here:

> Mondays 0900-1000
> Fridays 0900-1000
> Sundays 1000-1100

This is here at the ranch. Wear your boots. Come walk and talk with me and whoever shows up.

My Rebecca belongs to a group called the Vashon Free Range Folk Choir. And last evening they were singing as part of a multi faith gratitude service. I got roped into going to the service, but it was lively and just what I needed to start getting out of my doldrums with the death of Sture. Somehow Rebecca and I wound up going along with a small group afterward to one of the local restaurants for a drink. Besides the two of us there was a dad of one of my archery students, the local head guy with the Sufis, the abbot of the Zen Center and the abbot of the Russian Orthodox Monastery. Also included were two folks that I really wanted to touch base with who are the parents of a young man that recently took his own life. What a crew! What a dilly dally! It was extremely jovial and informative. I am so glad that I was there. It was really high and the parents said that it was the first time that they had smiled since the death of their son. It is hard to see how that all worked but it did beautifully.

So yea, the trail goes on, the surprises continue and the dilly dallies are there for the taking. Amazing. Dilly Dally love to you, Felipé.

November 27, 2014 / Turkey Day 2014

It's Thanksgiving today, a truly American holiday.

> "To speak gratitude is courteous and pleasant, to enact gratitude is generous and noble, but to live gratitude is to touch Heaven." —Johannes A. Gaertner.

November 29, 2014 / Thanksgiving Weekend

Well, we all survived the holiday. It is fun to gather and toast. Hopefully your group keeps politics and old worn-out history under control. At its best it is a giant dilly dally with the emphasis on gratitude, which should sound familiar to pilgrims of all flavors.

December 1, 2014 / Two Courageous Camino Characters Checking In.

Just chatting with Mary Margaret and this new word popped up. Yea, alperfect. Spell-check likes it with one "l." OK. Man and machine work out compromise.

I am looking out the big windows here at the hospital and it is a beautiful day. The view is to the west and a quarter of the sky is covered by mare's tail clouds that predict a change in the weather. Yup.

Alperfect loves, Felipé.

December 3, 2014 / Alvaro Where are You?

The Camino becomes a traveling, "all the world's a stage" situation. I don't mean that people are playing anything other than their selves but as we all got ground down, our inner selves began to show. And these characters began to interact with each other. This was after the beginning when we were settling into the rhythm of the daily routine and developing a passable pilgrim's walk (limp). And shedding makeup, deodorant, more than one kind of soap and other niceties which gave us that really cool pilgrim patina on our skin, wind-blown hair, and that natural aroma. Which didn't seem to matter much with all that fresh air.

This is when we were really doing it, and when we greeted each other with the "Buen Camino" it wasn't a cliché but had a meaning that, "yes we have sunk our teeth into it and we are still here." "Still here" should probably be written with caps to express the idea that we understand and are committed.

In the late afternoon after getting a bunk, showering, laundry, we would be ready for tapas and liquids at the daily dilly dally. A chance to say to each other the same thing, that we understand and are committed. All with a splash of fun and banter. We rehashed the day's journey and put it into context.

Thank you all for your impact on me, love, Felipé.

in a state of alert relaxation

DECEMBER 4, 2014 / ALERT RELAXATION

This season is Advent where we are to prepare for the coming of Jesus. I heard it expressed recently that we are on a pilgrimage to Bethlehem. Can we relate to that?

Or my Rebecca who most times seems to have a different take on things than I do says that she is in a state of alert relaxation. As in Jesus will come to her is what I see there. And why not? Be open, be faithful and he knocks on your door. I guess I am always doomed to do things the hard way. God bless my Rebecca.

So, in a little while I am off to the big city to the hospital and to meet with Sister Joyce for an hour. The snow and ice have mostly melted and the roads are clear. I will say hello to Sister Joyce for you. She loves you all.

A funny thing happened the other day. I was emailing to Annie about the upcoming visit of her and the film crew to Seattle and Vashon Island. And I had written something about getting into SJ's office. I was taking a short cut and meaning getting into Sister Joyce's office. I forgot that over the last year we were using those initials for Saint James, who is the patron saint of not only Spain but Western Washington State. Sister Joyce's office is at the headquarters, the Archdiocese. So Annie was impressed, to say the least, that I was checking in at the Big Guy's office. That was Big fun.

OK, enough of this, I have to get ready to go. So remember about the pilgrimage or the alert relaxation, whichever suits your fancy. Love you, Felipé.

DECEMBER 5, 2014 / WITH SISTER JOYCE

I got to spend an hour with our Sister Joyce yesterday. I don't know how I get to hang out with such quality folks as SJ. AND she has a bobble head rendition of our beloved leader, Pope Francis, on her desk! A bobble head pope is a concept that could stop you in your tracks and there he is to greet you as you walk into SJ's.

SJ is my spiritual advisor. As a new Catholic I have questions. And then I have other questions about this and that. And then I have things that I bring to her that are truly knotty. You know, those "who you gonna call?" questions. And I feel like there isn't anything that I could say that would shake her. She's been around the block eight times before me. Is that reassuring?

I'm back, was out walking the Camino. The bird feeders needed attention, so I did that. Everyone is hungry this time of year. And it's pretty outside in a rainy sort of way.

So, the important thing to know about SJ is how truly joyful she is. She will be talking heavy stuff and her brow takes a particular topography but always the sea calms afterward. And my hour is up and I am on my way recharged. I hope that is not too wearing on her.

Yup, so remember that at this moment somewhere there is a Pope Francis bobble head in action. I think that Bobbling along must be similar to Caminoing along. Pope Francis is saying yes continually with each bobble, yes? That just occurred to me.

Yes love, Felipé.

December 6, 2014 / Christmas Cards, 'Tis The Season.

Right now at the moment I feel 180 degrees out from Spain, from Caminoing along in the heat. Somehow at the moment I am caught half way between these two worlds, Spain and here. Yea, linking them up would be the trick. "Heat Wave", the great oldie, just came on and is playing right now for me on a CD. That sounds like my Spain experience to me!

In shortly over an hour I will be at my Bible class studying the parable of the feeding of the five thousand in Mark 6. This is where Jesus and his disciples fed the huge crowd with five loaves and two fish and had more in leftovers than when they started. Yea.

And here we are in this time of year waiting for the yearly coming of Jesus who came two thousand years ago to show us the Way. We are waiting for the winter solstice to mark the beginning of the season of light and warmth. The season, the Heat Wave is coming! Hang on, love, Felipé.

December 9, 2014 / A Rescue Mission Has Been Undertaken.

Well yesterday, with all my worries, turned out pretty well except for one detail. I wound up taking the ferry and driving into the University District of Seattle because it was the only church that I could find that had a mid-day Mass yesterday so I could fulfill my obligation. It is a beautiful church and it was a beautiful service and I as usual got all wrapped up in it (wrapped up in it, nice) and as a result left my faithful lucky hat in the pew. You know--the red one!

So, this morning I called my faithful friend who lives a few blocks from there and he found it and just called back a minute ago that it was in his possession. Not that a night in church was a bad thing and not that losing my old hat would have changed our walk. But it is good to be reunited. Anyway, thanks to my friend, Captain Phil for the successful mission.

OK, off to hit today's trail. May you find something lost, love, Felipé.

December 10, 2014 / Two Potatoes, A Remembrance.

Somewhere east of Burgos and west of the Pyrenees I was walking with Gracie and we found two potatoes in the road. They had fallen off a wagon recently. They weren't beautiful really, just two potatoes. I put them in my pants pocket and I carried them there for four or five days. I would bring them out when we would dilly dally and we would all laugh about it.

Everyone at that point in the journey was intent on shedding weight to make things easier or maybe we should say possible. I remember seeing a beautiful feather drift down in front of me and refused to pick it up. I don't need to carry another thing but yet I still had the spuds. There always was this thought that we were going to sleep out some night when the albergues were full. And the potatoes would come in handy, maybe.

Then finally somewhere near Burgos we decided that we could plant them next to the trail and that would be the fitting conclusion for my little pommes de terre. So that is what we did.

A nice little story, don't you think? It's all in how you look at it, love, Felipé.

December 11, 2014 / American Pilgrims

My Rebecca says that I should go. It is a coffee chat meeting of this association, American Pilgrims, that is happening relatively close by. I just have to take the ferry off the south end of the island to Tacoma and it is right there. I really don't need something extra to do these days but this is a good exception.

I continue to be blessed with many things. For instance there is a priest from along the Camino that is trying to get a hold of me to talk on Skype. I look forward to an awkward conversation with this dear man. I think that our Skype skills are probably matched by our foreign language abilities. Things like this are fun and the more effort the more rewarding usually. Also, my birthday party is coming up Sunday and am planning on trying to get a few friends over and maybe showing *Walking the Camino* and have pizza. It will be the anniversary of the opening of Phil's Camino, the trail here and we are still walking.

Thanks so much for reading along as we walk our lives wherever you are at this moment. It is a small world when we can get together so easily, yes? You're these best.

So I will leave you now to get ready to go and have café con leche with some other scruffy pilgrims. Keep walking, love, Felipé.

December 15, 2014 / Getting In The Mood

Yesterday I went to two Christmas events, a pageant and a concert and in between saw Sister Joyce. Actually, Rebecca, went with me to see SJ. I picked up some new insights on the pilgrimage toward Christmas.

First, we were singing carols at the pageant and I had to write down the second line of "We Three Kings" which was very Camino-y: fields and fountain, moor and mountain. Nice.

Then at the concert last night we listened to some great music. And one of our new friends, Jasper, sang in the performance and not only sang but SANG! Wow. Sometimes people can just blow you away unexpectedly. Nice.

Then I wanted to report on what Sister Joyce said in answer to my question about how do we prepare for Christmas. She laughed when I had my little notebook out to try and capture her thoughts but I was on the job for you. Here is what she said in paraphrased form: "If we can find the HUMILITY we will enjoy the SIMPLICITY that will put us closer to the MYSTERY." Nice.

OK, it all continues. Take time for the important things, love, Felipé.

December 17, 2014 / Does It Make You Shiver . . .

It's the start of a line from a blues song by Nina Simone which I have been playing lately. The whole line goes "do you shiver from your head down to your liver?" Funky little line but it points to something that we should get. We can get brain shivers pretty easy with all the information that we can access these days. But what about those rare really important things that speak to our inner being? Let's be on the lookout.

Last night due to Rebecca's and mine individual schedules conflicting we didn't get to have our normal dilly dally at 1700 and then dinner. So I got back here at 2100 and built some tapas and broke open some red wine thinking that she would be back soon. So I got that set up and I lit a small candle for Alida, our friend on the Camino. And I got a larger candle recently for the Lady of Guadalupe with the image of Mother Mary on it and I got it lit up. That all looked so bright that I turned off the electric lights.

I said my rosary and started to contemplate on Mother Mary. She is one reason that I was drawn to converting to the Roman Church two years ago. I was looking to find comfort. It seemed like my whole life comfort was in short supply. So last night I had this session with Mother Mary with tapas at Dilly Dally that shook me to my liver. It didn't take long, it didn't cost much, all I had to do was figure how to invite her in. Yea, that's my report.

Love as always, Felipé.

December 25, 2014 / All Day Long

Merry Christmas to you and yours! With you, Love, Felipé.

December 30, 2014 / A Fat Little Hummingbird!

It's a she and she is in a little patch of bamboo in a planter outside the window here at the hospital. Hummingbirds shouldn't be here this time of year but people feed them and they figure out how to get through the cold weather somehow. It's a gorgeous day today which means that it is cold. Cold and dry or warm and wet is the drill for Seattle. She is nervously fliting from one perch to another. Hummingbirds are pretty nervous and this may be just her version of rest or my theory is that she sees her reflection in the window and it is making her agitated. She sees a rival.

She sat on the same branch for three minutes, an eternity, but is off again. Even while she is sitting in the same place she is constantly dinking with the leaves around her. What a nervous creature.

The sun is starting to go down and it is 3 o'clock in the afternoon. The days are getting longer supposedly but hard to see yet. It Is pretty right now out the window to the west and will take a pic unless I can get a shot of Queenie. I named her.

New Year's coming and it is hard to imagine a better year than 2014 but heck lets go for even better. What do you say? Alperfect, Felipé.

December 31, 2014 / More About A Fat Little Hummingbird

First of all I have to apologize to Queenie because she is not fat but has her feathers all puffed up because of the cold conditions. Sorry Queenie it was just my first impression. And then Rebecca said those are the Anna's Hummingbirds that do winter over. OK.

I broke out my two trusty bird books and checked on what was written about the Anna. The Peterson said it was basically an Oregon, California, Mexico bird and casual (means marginal) up to southern Vancouver Island, Canada. And the *Audubon Guide* said it stays year around near Victoria which is at the south end of Vancouver Island which is a little north of us here in Seattle. OK, so it seems given the right micro environment and some food source which I suspect has to be human provided would suffice to hold them over this far north. So, Queenie's color, size and markings lined up with the Anna also, not that she knows that word. For habitat the Peterson said chaparral, broken woodlands, gardens. Maybe add hospitals, don't you think?

Why is this even remotely important I had to ask myself? Did I just need something to blog about? Am I boring my readers with random baloney? I really had to think about this last evening. And what I came up with was that one of the lessons of the Camino was that everything and everyone that we come into contact with on our daily walk has a message for us. First, we have to recognize that fact and then second, we have to learn how to decode it and then to interpret it. Some things are as easy as getting handed an orange by a smiling pilgrim that you don't know. Or have the tip of the perfect pyramidal rock come up though your boot sole and line up perfectly with your perfectly painful blister. Yikes isn't really the word that you scream. Or maybe it's something more subtle, like coming across a perfect little patch of shade or the perfect or imperfect wildflower.

Maryka, the dear, reminded me of the heart rocks that would appear as you walked and especially on tough uphill stretches would they be welcomed. They were saying that you have the heart to do this, keep going. Thanks Maryka.

So, what does Queenie say? Here I am stuck at the hospital on a beautiful day getting a gallon of chemo cocktail pumped into me and feeling pretty marginal. And just out the window is this little fat hummingbird living her life on her species margins and doing her very best. Aren't we kind of "birds of a feather" as they say? I like it, can you tell?

Hey, it's New Year's Eve here but Brisbane and Sydney are about three and a half hours into New Year's Day. Yea! Looks like Sherif is next in Cairo. OK, it looks like we should just give a big global Happy New Year at this point. Love you all wherever you find yourself now, Felipé.

PART II

What Can Come Out of One's Backyard?

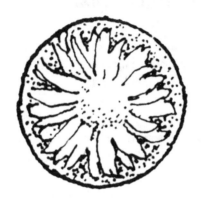

JANUARY 12, 2015 / EXTRAORDINARILY ORDINARY

Monday morning here which is looking pretty ordinary. Outside the kitchen window the climbing rose's branches are all dripping from the last shower. Close to the ground fog is thick. But when I look up at a higher angle there is some blue sky in place of the usual ordinary winter overcast. Is that sunshine hitting the top of the fir trees? Maybe not so ordinary after all. Nice.

When Henry was here the other day he was telling me how extraordinarily ordinary I was and my scene was. It took it as a compliment. I could be ordinarily extraordinary just as easy. This all reflects our "walk and talk" conversation which was inspired by a quote in the kitchen from Albert Einstein, "There are only two ways to live your life: one is as though nothing is a miracle; the other is as though everything is a miracle."

Isn't this one of the things that we learned as we walked through Spain's ordinariness? You would look and see ordinary people, places and things all along. And then the next minute you were struck by the extraordinary beauty of it all. So beautiful you didn't know what to do with it, no existing categories. Overwhelmed with the ordinary extraordinary beauty, truth or holiness of things that you cried your eyes out.

Well, I just walked three laps around the backyard Camino, sort of an ordinary place. I filled three of the bird feeders along the way and then said the rosary for the last lap. Praying for my friend David who is having surgery today and for all the other stones on the pile. And the sun disappeared at some point just as mysteriously as it appeared earlier.

But that's the way it is. As long as you know that the sun could come out, we will be OK. It doesn't even have to be out on us in this particular spot. It always helps to see a sunbreak in the clouds and the rays are pouring down on a hillside five miles from here. Yea, that's good, it's their turn and we may be next or maybe tomorrow.

But things are possible in our world is the important thing to remember even in the seemingly most ordinary of times. You could remind me and I could remind you. OK, off to my day. Reminding you loves, Felipé.

JANUARY 13, 2015 / I THOUGHT THAT I WOULD WRITE ABOUT CANCER

It's my every-other-Tuesday and I'm at Swedish Hospital Cancer Institute again. It occurred to me recently that I don't talk enough about my cancer. It is an important part of who I am these days and maybe today is the day to work on that since I am here at the epicenter.

But first, my whole morning has been lovely. Like the weather is beautiful, the traffic was reasonable, I got all my errands done and things just generally ran smoothly like maybe this is my kind of day. Which is great really because I have been a little burned out by the hospital routine as of late and sort of forcing myself to smile about it. And today the universe is conspiring to treat me well even with my grumpy attitude, how nice.

This is delightful actually, as I am in a good mood to tackle this hard topic. Well, let's forge ahead then with such an auspicious beginning how can I go wrong? Cancer, yes.

Well, it's not cancer in general but just my version, which I can talk about. I can talk about my experience mixing with other patients who have a variety of situations that I know little about medically. And really I know little about my cancer either. I mean by that that I could be way more studious and read up about studies and research. But I have a life to live and trust my doctors and nurses to cover my backside.

The basic idea, my modus operandi, is that I have to know that yes I do have cancer, yes, but at the same time with that in place, I can't let cancer define me. I think that I have to accept it totally to be able to be free of it this way. It is a workable situation for me.

So, the cancer was the catalyst for ninety five percent of what is going on in my life now but remarkable it only takes up five percent of my consciousness. I have to say that another way. Cancer knocked me off my horse, so to speak, but I got right back on another, a superior one. Life goes on for me in a better way really.

How that happened and what that is is a long story that hopefully the documentary will get into. Maybe that will explain it to me too, haha. Well, I still haven't talked about my cancer but I have talked about it as an instrument of change and the ultimate challenge is how to make that good change.

Change for the better loves, Felipé.

JANUARY 17, 2015 / YESTERDAY WAS A HAPPENING

In the morning Kelly, Mary Margaret and I were here walking Phil's Camino. MM got a taste of the locale through that. Then in the afternoon Kelly and Rick showed up to walk and be a part of the photo shoot for the *NW Catholic* Magazine article coming up in March. Stephen and Ellen were here from the Archdiocese for a number of hours taking shots and trying to capture the flavor of our effort here. Then at 1700 tapas began and dinner somewhere around 1800.

The meal was delicious and the wine drinking was also. The table was strewn with all the evidence of that and also the Bible, other books, an icon, a map and other reference materials. Conversation was spectacular. We approached the realm of being louder than the Italians. What pushed us over the top was the opening of a champagne bottle with just one slash of a big kitchen knife by MM. We were swashbuckling our way through the universe at that point! So yea, the Camino continues.

Then we had a few hours' sleep and Kelly and MM are off to Seattle this AM to tour the Pike Street Market and then head to the airport. I am just positive that MM's trip was a total success and that makes me feel good. We all connected beautifully and this is a gift of the Camino to be able to do that so easily. Yup, reporting from the epicenter, connected love, Felipé.

MARCH 1, 2015 / NOT JUST ABOUT GETTING SOMEWHERE

Just back at the beginning of the trail. A jay is scolding. Can you hear him? I'll put a rock on the pile with a prayer for you. Well, that lap took 45 minutes when it usually takes 15 minutes when I am just walking and not blogging along the way. But it just goes to prove that it isn't just about getting somewhere. Buen Camino, love, Felipé.

MARCH 6, 2015 / WALKING FRIDAY MORNING

It's going to be a bright morning here at the ranch. Cold though, approached freezing overnight. I have a little time before 0900 when I need to be out ready to walk. Sometimes people show up to "walk and talk" and sometimes it's "just me." I've gotten in the habit of writing that in the logbook when no one shows up but it is hardly just me.

I should find a better way of communicating that because it is not accurate really. What about the six bird feeders along the trail and all the songbirds and squirrels that attracts. Then there are Scout and Tia, the neighbor's dogs that check in. Then bumping into members of the local deer herd happens. We have coyotes here and very occasionally black bears but I haven't seen them, although that is a possibility.

And what about my inner Camino? What about the ever-increasing population of saints that I learn about and get to know? I read a blog post last night by Reverend Bonnie Barnard about the Communion of Saints and maybe that is what is flavoring my mind. I just feel like my inner life is being populated by more and more very interesting and inspiring characters who have gone on before. My big brothers and sisters that I am getting to know and appreciate their stories. Ones that I have focused on recently are Francis and Clare of Assisi and Patrick and Brigid of Ireland. And good to know that Francis and Patrick have equally as interesting female counterparts. I'm learning.

Are we ever really alone? Thinking of you and how you are not alone, love, Felipé.

MARCH 29, 2015 / CALLIGRAPHY

I was off walking on the backyard Camino with Dana today. We are just getting to know each other although we are close geographically, as in she is just around the corner. But we discovered that we have this mutual interest in calligraphy which I'm not sure that I have a handle on what it all means.

It is basically the art of handwriting but handwriting sounds so simple and art seems complicated. See? I don't think that I could have said that better if I had tried. That just sort of typed itself. And then on to typing and keyboards and talking to each other as we are communicating right now.

I remember my dad teaching me lettering and a love for communicating in that fashion. I don't think that we knew the word calligraphy but we had the spirit. Then the excitement in fourth grade to learn cursive (longhand) with the Palmer method. This all sounds like ancient history. But it gets even better!

The elementary school that I went to in Buffalo, NY was in two old buildings. The steps were cupped, Camino-like, from billions of little feet. You have seen pics with the desks that were wrought iron and wood and screwed to the wooden floor in rows, each had a hole in the top for an ink well. The ink well was a little glass container that once had held the liquid ink and was used with a straight pen to write. The student would dip the nib of the pen in the ink and write a few words and dip again and continue. This is one step more modern then writing with a quill, a feather, gang.

And our teacher somehow got into an old storage area and found enough of the pen nibs and holders and blotters and wells to outfit they whole class and we used that stuff the whole year. Timewise people were just in the transition between fountain pens and on to ball point pens then in the 1950s. And here we were with this ancient stuff to learn to write cursive with. I was in heaven.

So now when I notice a person with a "nice hand" or in other words who takes joy in writing and communicating in that fashion I make sure to compliment them. I think that is what Dana and I clicked on as we walked the Camino this AM, it was the joy we shared for that particular form of communication.

What does this have to do with the Camino anyway? Well, maybe we are talking about taking the time, when we can afford it, to communicate in an artful manner. To say to our audience that besides wanting you to get what I am saying, I value you. I am taking my time to be with you. I am "spending" my time with you. Isn't that what we did on the Camino where we walked on our blistered feet ever so slowly across Spain.

I'm weeping, sorry, love you, Felipé.

PS — thank you Dana.

April 13, 2015 / The Best Idea Of 2015

It's true, yes, I am announcing this with the year barely started. Every once in a while something extraordinary happens and you have to go with it; you have to say yes this is obviously the big one. And although we have a slight bit of confusion as to whose fault, ah, idea it was, the event of a POTLUCK TAPAS PARTY occurred and it was a thing of beauty.

I think we had fourteen participants and some folks made more than one thing. And most of the offerings were recipes that we all enjoyed for the first time. Exceptional event and my words are not doing it justice. But a highly recommended activity for Caminoheads everywhere, none the less.

And early on Sunday, with less fanfare, a man named John came to walk with me and who is going to Spain in August. We fired each other up as we Caminoheads tend to do. Lovely man. He gave me a rosary that he made. It is one made with all knots, no beads, I call them fisherman's rosaries. Very beautiful but too new and clean. It will reach its true beauty with use and the patina that brings. Thanks John. I gave him the shell that both Annie and I carried across. Alperfect.

"Heat Wave" playing! Yea, that's it gang! Love you, Felipé!

May 5, 2015 / An Hour Early

What could be better. Just time to write to you. I'm in the waiting room with other cancer patients, some might be cancer campers, I'm not sure. I came up with this term a few days ago. A patient is someone who is just that, defined and situated. A stump could do that. A rock could do that. Campers are those who achieve some sort of peace and are active with coping with the situation. As a camper maybe sunburned and bug-bit but happy and mostly on top of it. That's a good place.

Lately I have been chafing at the boundary of this category. What's next? How can I make a difference or how can I cause some trouble or how can I help others? (Somebody just said something funny and made me laugh, that's good.) I came up with the term commando to describe this next level. I'm liking it, Cancer Commando. Here is a definition of commando: a small group of soldiers trained to make quick and often dangerous attacks inside enemy areas, or a member of such a group. Yea, we could do that.

love, Felipé.

May 6, 2015 / The Really, Really Good News!

Yes siree Bob, had my good news yesterday. This was the report on my scan of cancer sites in my body. Everything there remains stable so there is no change in treatment. We seem to be doing all the right things, nothing is growing or moving around. Yea, now I can relax for another three months.

This is in regard to what we were talking about yesterday in the hospital waiting room. Was searching for a commando pic on the web but didn't come up with anything appropriate. Too much weaponry, or too sexy, or just too. A commando is "too" by definition but it is different and more than all that garbage. More than half of it lies between the ears in terms of honesty, smarts, bravery, creativity and endurance. It used to be known as woodcraft. That's what we are looking for, the rest can be learned. You got what it takes camper?

What is the enemy? It is anything that robs us, you and me, of the joy that we were meant to receive today. We are looking for the full meal deal around here.

Nine o'clock and I need to go. It's all going on out there: the good, the bad and the old ugly. Navigate through it 'til we meet again. Commando loves, Felipé.

May 18, 2015 / Soaking It In

We just had tapas and dinner outside on the deck and I am enjoying the evening here with the twilight and the noise of various songbirds. Of course wine is a factor. The air is full of sweetness as all the plants are celebrating. I find myself lately asking myself in any given situation what is the most beautiful thing around and let me stare at it as long as possible to soak it in completely. It could be the color of the wine. It could be a particular row of trees. It could be the pretty lady. Right now as I sit here, I spy a patch of blue iris flowers that are particularly attractive. Ah, Chris took a pic of them on Friday and I could get that for you. Japanese iris, I think.

And the air is cooling down and I feel it on my cheek. I just finished off the wine, a rosé from Portugal.

Thinking of you there where you are. Wondering what the most beautiful thing in your view is? Don't forget to soak some in, love, Felipé.

May 26, 2015 / Report On A Special Day

Sunday we finally got Sister Joyce, my spiritual advisor, to come and see Phil's Camino. Jennifer was here to help me host her. Basically we enjoyed each other talking away. Then I thought that we should show Sister Joyce the trail and she said that she couldn't walk that far. So, Jennifer got this great idea to have her ride the mower around for a half mile, which she did. She is such a good sport!

May 28, 2015 / The Buddy System

Well, we tried it out yesterday for our chemo treatment day at Swedish Cancer Institute. We as in Jennifer and myself. We are both here on Vashon Island and it was just a matter of time before the island grapevine got us together. And we do what Islanders do when faced with the big city, we carpool. And actually it is beyond that to a budding buddy system relationship. We found that we had the same docs and treatment pathway but she was being treated one week and I was on the next week. Anyway with a little help from folks at the hospital I changed my schedule to hers and now we can team up on it.

Also, what is important about this is that I have been doing this for going on four years and have grappled with many things that I can hopefully coach her on. And vice versa--she is seeing the situation with new eyes and coming up with some new angles. (listening to my Soul music and Laura Lee just had a line that might be apropos, "I'm going to slap him in the face with the unexpected!" Putting cancer in its place!). Jennifer is just starting with chemo and this is a totally freaky prospect. It's all so foreign and difficult. I am happy that I have some extra energy at this point to help out in some small or large way, who knows.

And with me at this point the endeavor of keeping the cancer to a dull roar is an endurance race at best. Being able to keep my health in other areas to give me a strong base to work from is important. And then to be able to keep one step ahead of the chemo side effects and carry on is important. Then to keep the whole person, me, intact with the help of prayer and advisors and strong family. This blog is part of it also. I have a mission with the Camino and you the Caminoheads to help keep things burning that gives me a focus and helps keep me alive. Thanks for reading and being here for me and Jennifer.

Yes, but the world is chock full of different realities. This was just a little glimpse into this little backwater. Good luck with your struggle where you are. Buddy system loves, Felipé.

June 3, 2015 / "We Must Never Forget . . . "

My good friend Father Tom emailed some material that I just got to this morning with first coffee. I've been calling his forwards "Tom bombs", as they are heavy, on target and ultimately chock full of good stuff. Yea, this one I was working on this morning was partially about what should be Catholicism's view of the other religions that surround us. Pope Francis had a great quote, "We must never forget we are pilgrims journeying alongside one another."

We can relate to that, right? And the Camino works like that. We all not only journeyed alongside but we actively helped each other along in all sorts of ways. We popped blisters, bandaged blisters, soothed, encouraged, intoxicated, inspired, bothered, irritated, underwrote, watched out for, made time for, pushed, pulled and moved each other along down the dusty trail. We kept each other going so that we could reveal our personal witness to each other, partially. Right?

I can tell that I am in good territory when I blog with my vision blurred with tears. Yes, here we are. So my take on the Pope's quote is to encourage, to befriend, to keep judgements to a dull roar and to keep moving. Thanks, love, Felipé.

June 11, 2015 / Cancer Camino Not A Cupcake

The Cancer Camino that I have been walking for almost four years is no cupcake but that is not to say that it doesn't have miracles happen and precious high points happen. And these stand out maybe more brilliantly because they appear on the contrasting dark background. So, to begin my story I have been joined on my Cancer Camino by another. And this has been very special and a big breakthrough for me.

And along comes Jennifer. She lives on the Island, has the same doc and we figured how we could get our hospital visit in sync. So now we commute together. And just as being joined by someone, a complete stranger, on the dusty or muddy trail in Spain after maybe too much time alone, you marvel, how much fun is this? Where have you been?

So, yesterday a miracle occurred or maybe we just heard of it as it happened earlier. But I have to back up a few notches to fill you in. On Tuesday Jennifer went in for a scan to look into her insides. This is a valuable tool that our oncologist uses to check what going on. Sort of as close to boots on the ground as he gets. So she gets one every two months and this marks a place, once the scan is looked at and interpreted where strategy and/or dosage is likely to change. The doc can tweak things depending on what he sees on the report on Wednesday and talks it over with you.

From the Cancer Camper's (patient's) point of view this is a totally nerve-wracking, sleep-losing, nail-biting process. Life or death seems to hang in balance in the mind. This is the second scan that she has had and the second time through the wringer. But in spite of all the mental gymnastics that she went through this one turned out to be very, very good. And combined with excellent numbers from her blood work it looks very positive for her. So we are losing no time toasting to her health and the miracle revealed.

So, we walk on through the ins-and-outs and over-and-unders of the Cancer Camino, never a dull moment. Cupcake loves, Felipé.

June 17, 2015 / Playing Around With Death Some More

I am not trying to bring you something morbid but something truly joyful. Organically joyful, bubbling up from the depths joyful, it was always there but you just realized it joyful, all that. Oops, have to go photograph roses, perfect light, see what I mean?

So, where were we? All of a sudden I am deep in thinking about the Cancer Camino and maybe trying to separate things from the Camino Camino or from the Catholic Camino. It reminds me of being questioned by my oncologist and trying to separate chemo related side effects from the bumps and scraps of everyday life, hard to do sometimes. Things get entwined (beautiful word) or maybe they were born together long ago, all in the same litter.

But even though I think that my cancer was an amazing catalyst for change, dealing with it has been dealing with death. Not death as an impersonal creature but the personal variety. I am thankful for that. I have made peace with it and I feel secure.

I hope that I am making slight sense. So, encountering the dragon Cancer (and surviving so far) has been a vital learning experience. And I don't feel like it is my duty, my place to kill it or conquer it or anything it. I have sat at its feet and learned.

Time to go, love, Felipé.

June 21, 2015 / The Tapas Of My Life

I was thinking of a person's life as one day. You know you are born at dawn and you grow up in the morning and the whole thing proceeds to death/darkness. Yea, we have heard it before except this time I realized that personally I am in tapas right now. Huh, now I know why I have been having such a great time and feel in the groove lately. Cool or what?

You have a glass and do you want red, white, or rosé? Love, Felipé.

June 24, 2015 / Cancer Commando's First Mission

It's my chemo treatment day and I am early to the hospital. The traffic was really light for some reason and I just zoomed in. Jennifer is showing up soon. We didn't come in together as usual. But we will cause trouble here shortly.

I did my turn at the jigsaw puzzle here in the waiting room. I try to do at least one piece. Did three today, hurrah. It's where it is happening here. It is the best way to strike up a conversation and get intelligence. Other than that, people are moping around and it is hard to approach them.

Last time I was here I did my first mission as a cancer commando and it had to do with the puzzle. I'll have to tell you about it. I came over to do my usual piece and noticed that the puzzle was the same one that was there two weeks before which is odd since there is usually a faster turnover. Not only that but it seemed still to be two thirds done like somehow nothing had progressed in two weeks. And it didn't take too long of staring at it to discover that it had numerous pieces missing. People realized that and lost interest quickly but the big thing is nobody did anything about it. It just remained.

So, I got it in my head to deep six it with permission of course. It felt so great to slide the pieces off the table and into the wastebasket. I was striking a blow for the other patients coming after. It sounds a little silly but it was a case of realizing the value of a positive action no matter how small. And the value of getting out of my personal "rut" and participating in the bigger picture.

Well, it seems like a dinky little thing but it is part of something bigger, something that could grow. Just getting organized and getting the hang of this cancer commando calling. It feels a little like *One Flew Over the Cuckoo's Nest* if you can remember that. That was from the seventies; I don't know if we can remember that. Later, love, Felipé.

July 9, 2015 / Cancer Commando Caper Confidential

Jennifer and I were at the hospital today, long day. One thing is that we have been working on our lingo. We have swapped out the word mission for the word caper. So, Cancer Commandos will perform Capers instead of missions starting today

St. James is Afoot. Love you, Felipé.

July 9, 2015 / Caper After Action Report

This is highlights only. This was yesterday, our every-other Wednesday great big infusion of medicine/chemicals/poison. So there is that side of it and the other side is to work hard to make that fun. I think that we got slightly (?) carried away but what is life for anyway?

I brought a little cooler with tapas for lunch. I'm thinking about adding wine to that in the future. We had dropped off Jennifer's friend Ellen downtown so she could shop so J and I had a couple of hours to play music too loud, look at pictures of gardens in magazines, think that playing charades would be a good idea and have time left over to eat tapas. Drinks as coffee, tea, nutritional shakes and soft drinks are available at the little cantina. We had time to schmooze with our nurses and Doc Gold (call sign Nugget) kept circling through checking on our behavior but trying to look like he wasn't.

JULY 16, 2015 / TWO CENTS

Just got back from my Thursday morning walk. No one came to be with me so I said my rosary for a few individuals and the rock pile. I love saying the rosary on Thursdays because that is the day of the week to ponder the Illuminating Mysteries. These are a set of teachings/gifts that as it says "light the way" for us.

JULY 23, 2015 / WEDNESDAY AT THE HOSPITAL

This entry may come slowly, paragraph by paragraph, as our treatment goes on. Jennifer is here to participate. She is looking especially spiffy with a special headpiece of daisies that My Rebecca wove for her. She is celebrating completion of her set of twelve treatments. Good job!

The day is moving on. Things come and go and those things have more or less weight to them. Some things are totally subjective, totally as seen from this very chair and some stuff is more universal. But we navigate and make our way onward. I realize that is very vague but some things are more confidential than others. But the mission of the Cancer Commandos is to push the fun lever as far forward as possible at any given point and we do a mighty fine job of that.

AUGUST 11, 2015 / WHY ARE WE HERE?

Or why do we stay here? Why do we hang around when things get bad? How would we as Caminoheads answer that?

If we start with the idea that we are not in charge of things that would be good. If we see ourselves as totally unique individuals that would be good. If we see ourselves living the manifestation of this unique personality that would be good. Then all we have to do is to do our best to be ourselves, right?

Are we not living (walking) for each other? Are we not here because we need each other? Who can do this walk alone? Who wants to do this walk alone?

The sun is going to set and our day is mostly over. Some days are harder than others but we persist. Some days I carry your pack and some days you carry mine. We persist. I love you immensely, Felipé.

August 15, 2015 / Itsy Bitsy Spider

I'm sitting at breakfast and the house is quiet. I'm up early as usual. My Rebecca and all our company are still in bed as they got in here at something like three in the morning, just a few hours ago. I'm working on finishing up my first cup after bacon and eggs.

And there is this little itsy-bitsy dot in my vision. OK, what the heck is that? Is that in my eye, in my brain, one foot away, twenty feet away? It's appearing and disappearing, oh man, not another new chemo side effect. Then there are more of them, and I realize they are tiny, tiny newborn spiders repelling down off the lamp hanging over the table. Here we go with Life in the Country or Wild Kingdom, whichever is most.

What if we as newborns dropped down ropes into the Grand Canyon just for something to do on our first morning. Yea, I have to shake my head and admire God's handiwork and admire the bravery of those itsy-bitsy creatures. Let's see, which part of Mother Teresa's message would those guys fit into best? How about, "Life is an adventure, dare it."

Just a little itsy-bitsy message from little old me, love, Felipé.

August 16, 2015 / Camino News Near And Far

On Camino news near, we are opening up another walk "in Spain" right here at Phil's Camino today. We have been walking regularly here but it has been just walking without keeping track and linking it to where we would be in Spain if we were there.

So today at 1600 we will hike out from "St. Jean Pied de Port" on the first day of our pilgrimage. I don't think that we will get terribly far but it is a start. So we will keep you posted.

August 19, 2015 / On Assignment

It's 1:39 in the afternoon. We're all snuggled down in our cocoon of chemotherapy. Jennifer had fixed a great picnic lunch for us, it was her turn. We are hanging out as the sunshine pours in the big windows. Sort of savoring things at the moment, happy to be alive and alive in a happy way.

We will be back on Vashon in a few hours to our regular existence. On second thought that could be debatable, the part about Vashon being regular. Mainland people have their thoughts about island people. There is a popular bumper sticker around, "Keep Vashon Weird." Then there was, "Keep Vashon Wired." And then, "Keep Vashon Normal." And as Our Anamaria said last year after her first visit to the Camino, "What is normal anyway?" Yes.

Corn is normal. Let's remember that. Love you, Felipé.

August 25, 2015 / Another Day In Paradise. What To Do?

It's a common greeting between Vashonites, well, in the good weather of summer. "Another day in paradise" sort of the Buen Camino of our local walk. It becomes more rich as the days of summer become more rare. It's the end of August now and September can be very beautiful here also but we begin to savor the situation.

Savoring the situation, that's nice. Why don't we run with that for a while. I find myself more in this sort of zone as my own personal walk progresses. Glimpses of truth, goodness and beauty become important, vital. Relationships become important. My fellow walkers progress becomes important. Many things have lost their value, their attraction. I find the timeless values of the Camino to be fertile ground for me and others. How fortunate am I, are we, to have stumbled across this jewel after all this time of wandering. Thank you to you St. James, compañero of the Christ.

Oh me oh my, I'm a fool for you baby. Love, Felipé.

AUGUST 31, 2015 / MORE ON THE POSSIBILITY OF GOULASH

I tend to gather broad landscapes and try to boil them down to their essence.

All mechanisms have a central underlying idea. Getting to that and understanding it and ultimately putting the concept to use seems a way, a method, a guiding principle. Sometimes I find a part of something that seems to explain the whole. Maybe like finding a table of contents to a book will give you a pretty good idea what is going on. Yea, so?

Well we were talking about the phenomenon of cancer and our ability to deal with it on a personal level. Personal is the keyword here. That is how I am viewing my Cancer lately. It is very, very personal to me now. It does not have to do with anything external to me. It's all mine, every single cell. It's my own body run amuck, a loose cannon, an onboard fire. Somehow I created it, caused it, encouraged it, kept it going. I did? I did.

That's mysterious. Just why would I do that? I don't know the answer to that but realizing that I did so much to put me in this particular situation may mean that I also have some room and ability to start to heal from the inside out so to speak. In other words if I have the ability to move in one direction maybe I should stop and see if I can move it the opposite direction. What would that look like or mean? Does that make any sort of sense?

When I look at the goulash of possibilities in the area of cancer cures presented to me I glaze over. There are so many and they mostly seem plausible and on top of that they seem to have a certain amount of success individually. How can one choose in this goulash of treatment ideas? And how come they all seem to have a certain amount of success that keeps the idea alive? Is just sitting still and smiling also in the goulash?

Somehow I am guessing that the individual, the cancer hobbyist, is a big factor in all these equations. His or her very personal makeup, energy, thinking, being, fear, is the center of gravity around which the other factors revolve and are influenced by. I'm on thin ice here but there is something going on and I am hot on the trail of it.

Oops, time to go walk and get to Roncesvalles on Phil's Camino. Thanks for putting up with me and my half-baked goulash, love, Felipé.

Everything is a miracle

SEPTEMBER 8, 2015 / BLOGGING FROM THE HAMMOCK

This morning as I stumbled around the kitchen I came across this quote attributed to Uncle Al that I have taped up to a cupboard: "There are only two ways to live your life: one is though nothing is a miracle; the other is as though everything is a miracle." —Albert Einstein.

Well, doesn't that seem to snuggle into the conversation so well. And somehow from a heavy hitter like Uncle Al I can lean on it more than the usual quote. Somewhere out there in the universe there is a place where the hard, cold facts of science kiss the warm spirit of God and all is well. Uncle Al has been to that place I think or close enough to it to live and come back.

I'm weeping, I know that this is a good blog, love you, Don Felipé.

SEPTEMBER 24, 2015 / SLOW THOUGHTS

Before I start on my thoughts, just want to report that we had a wonderful time last evening. We wound up at the Phoenician Restaurant at Alki Point in West Seattle. Had a wonderful meal and wine outside overlooking the water. Then we walked a few blocks for a gelato and ate that on the beach. But here is a great funny thing that happened on the way. I wanted to stop at a pharmacy to get some of my meds and while we were there both Rebecca and I snuck off to the greeting card aisle to get an Anniversary card for the other. We met on the way to the checkout discovering that we had picked out the same card. Nice. We had a good laugh. As Annie says, after a while we can't help it.

So I was off walking this AM trying to get to Pamplona. I was alone although I know that is not true really. It was beautiful with sun and blue sky. So, I took some pix. I said a rosary on one lap. But what was coming at me this morning was the notion that this pace of walking is the speed we are supposed to be moving at. This is the pace we were made for biologically speaking. And spiritually this is the pace of the Old Testament and the New. This is the speed at which things start to make sense. If we spend enough time there maybe we can start figuring things out. Just a thought.

OK, off to tractor around the ranch. That is moving pretty slow also so I think I am good. Later, enjoy yourself, love, Felipé.

SEPTEMBER 29, 2015 / THINKING OF THESE PEOPLE

I received an email from Moira a friend of Our Jennifer's, actually it was addressed to both of us. And she was telling us about this friend of hers that lives up in Victoria, BC, Canada and who for the last ten years has spent three months each year working in an orphanage in India. But this year she is doing something different, walking the Camino de Santiago. She started on September 25th in France and plans on being in Santiago on November 1st, her 80th birthday!

We will think of her and pray for her as she makes her way across the autumn landscape of Northern Spain. We think of her and pray that her near eighty-year-old body moves lightly over the paths, roads and trails. We think of her and pray she has companions both young and ancient that buoy her up in the hard spots. Bless you dear as you walk towards your birthday celebration, awesome!

And Our Jennifer is off to the hospital today walking her Cancer Camino to get a scan of her insides. We are back there tomorrow for our chemo treatment and she will also get her interpretation of the scan from Dr. Gold. Leading up to this meeting is the peak time of anxiety.

We will think of Our Jennifer and pray for strength for her to face the facts as they come in to her. We will think and pray that she will keep the big picture in mind as much as possible as she moves across this strange landscape. We think and pray that the realization that Saints and Angels are walking with her always is always fresh in her mind. Bless you dear one.

Ah, it's a weeping blog post today, the best kind really. Deep feelings come to the surface at these times and we let them massage our being. Always good, love, Felipé.

September 30, 2015 / The Interpretation

Sunshine out the window here at the hospital. Alperfect.

Jennifer's scan went well is the great big happy news today. The first thing she said to me was, "I guess I'll have to start making plans for my life." She is kind of getting the idea that she will be around for a while longer. Nice. We are happy for her. Your prayers were awesome, thank you.

October 2, 2015 / Got All My Life To Live, Have All My Love To Give.

That's from the Gloria Gaynor disco song, "I Will Survive," remember? Ancient history now but the line is sticking in my brain this AM. This could be my theme song lately.

Speaking of lately when our son Wiley was young, he's twenty-seven now, I asked him, "Have you washed your hands lately?" And he shot back, "Don't call me Lately!" Hehe. Good man.

One thing that I wanted to tell you about was this story about this guy in prison that created his Camino around the prison yard and is walking it. I need to talk with him!

October 11, 2015 / Brierley And The Pilgrim Guide

Yesterday I went into the local second-hand store and I found two Camino books there waiting for me. One was a copy of Brierley's *New Lightweight Edition Pilgrim's Guide* (2007). And we all know Brierley, the most ubiquitous darn thing on the Camino Frances next to blisters.

And this book is hardly lightweight. I mean for a library reference book it is lightweight but that's all I can say for it. So, I have heard that there are 200,000 pilgrims walking each year. What if 100,000 carried this guide all the way across. Just a very rough guess since lots don't make it all the way across in a single year and not everyone carries it. So, it is just a wild guess. So now we have 100,000 times 2,193,840 ft/lbs. equaling 219,384,000,000 foot pounds of energy.

So what does this mean? Well, I don't know but it's a lot of energy. Perhaps that's enough to move the Santiago Cathedral one hundred meters. Or perhaps it is enough to move the Vatican one meter. I don't know why we need to do either of those but if we did . . . Or perhaps it's enough to launch an albergue and put it in orbit around the moon, a place to stay. That makes more sense.

October 13, 2015 / A Mix Of Confidence And Desperation

I have spent a lot of my free time lately trying to visualize the tumors within me and asking God to provide for them to start shrinking in size. Medicine has kept them confined in number and slowed in growth. I am thankful but realizing that as time marches on they will catch up to my well-being.

Dr. Zucker told me at our last meeting that in non-medical terms God is keeping me alive to fulfill my mission. And when I think about that it is a miracle already in itself that has already happened. Althankful, love you, Felipé.

October 15, 2015 / A Pickled Prawn Picnic

A wow that needs reporting on is lunchtime at the hospital yesterday. This is the respite in the big day of the Cancer Camino for Our Jennifer and myself. In the spirit of having as much fun as possible and keeping our weight up we decided that having a picnic lunch along would be an excellent idea. I think that this is our fourth try at it as we take turns surprising the other with yummy content and grandeur.

On Jennifer's menu was deviled eggs, Buffalo wings with blue cheese sauce, pickled prawns, assorted olives. There was a drink but I'm not sure what it was although sometimes it's white and sometimes red and sometimes sort of an in between rose color. Anyway dessert was homemade delicious cheesecake. Then coffee and gummy bears (health food for the nails). I probably left something out, oh yes ambience, of course. Have table cloth and battery tea light along.

That was all Our Jennifer's doing although the tablecloth and candle were my responsibility. So, yea, but how am I going to top that two weeks from now? Better start early hey? OK, I am going to try and do another post (didn't get one in yesterday) and breakfast in the next hour. Walking at 0900. Miss you, love you, Felipé.

October 18, 2015 / Off To Mass

Off to be at the early Mass at St. John Vianney's at 0800. We'll get our spiritual batteries recharged.

I hope my day is reasonable. Yesterday I was really fatigued from the chemo. Could barely work the TV remote, that's bad. Feeling half way decent at the moment.

Maggie showed up big time on our radar screen several days ago thanks to a friend of Our Jennifer's. Thinking of Maggie, 79 years old, on the Camino west of

Léon. What an inspiration for us, yes? I wish I were there to roll Compeed out ahead of her like a red carpet.

Go get 'em Maggie! Can't wait for her musings on her pilgrimage.

One of the readings today was from the New Testament book of Hebrews. It just jumped out at me concerning having confidence to pray for oneself and one's own needs. This is from a very modern version called the Message. Hebrews 4:16 says: "So, let's walk right up to him and get what he is so ready to give. Take the mercy, accept the help."

This has to do with my struggles described in the October 13th post: A Mix Of Confidence And Desperation. Well, that's all I have for today. Still feeling tired. The best to you, love, Felipé.

OCTOBER 19, 2015 / MONDAY EARLY

Remember in Spain the metering of water and electricity? Here at home I turn on the tap water or the light switch and it just goes whether I really need it or not. There along the Camino at least the water taps ran for a certain time and then shut down. Ah, including showers! Including the public fountains for valuable drinking water out in the middle of nowhere, which made a lot of sense. Water conservation all around. And similarly the electric lights mostly ran on motion sensors which lead to some interesting moments in water closets and stairways. Electric power conservation all around.

All that took some getting used to but I sort of got in their groove after a time. The intermittent shower was my least favorite though. Here at the ranch we are used to watching our water use during the dry summer season anyway. So back home here I have made some difference in our electrical use by seeing light in a different way. Instead of lighting a whole big space evenly better to light the points where people gather. If there is just one group then bringing the light in just to them makes them special, an ambience thing.

Bringing this all back to "Monday Early", the title of this post, I was up early, 0630, and had made myself breakfast. I was just sitting down at the kitchen table after having just turned off all the extraneous lights. Just the one over the table was burning and I was grooving on the ambience thing while getting ready to enjoy my breakfast when . . .

My Rebecca is a substitute teacher in the local school district. She has an old-time certification that says she can teach in K through 12 which is the whole thing from youngest to oldest. So, she is the perfect substitute. She is perfect in another way which I will attempt to describe.

So, yea, the phone rings at 0700 and it is Barb the secretary at the Middle School. She is trying to find a substitute to fill in last minute for a sick teacher. I wake My Rebecca and she can make it from a dead sleep, to cold pizza breakfast to the middle school classroom in less than an hour on a Monday morning. Now that's perfect! I guess I have given her good training putting up with me. Amazing.

Just a description of our morning. Me trying to snuggle into cozy Spanish ambience and My Rebecca zooming by me in a cloud of dust to ride herd down the road.

OK, then, I can finish up this post and do a walk at 0900. The rain has stopped but I will need boots in the wet grass. Good luck getting your week started, love you, Felipé.

October 24, 2015 / Step Out Of Ourselves

I randomly picked up the local *Northwest Catholic* magazine that had run the article back in March about me and my pilgrimage and read a little article about local pilgrimage. About places to go without going half way around the world. Are there opportunities all over?

As Pope Emeritus Benedict XVI said in 2010, "To go on pilgrimage really means to step out of ourselves in order to encounter God where he has revealed himself, where his grace has shone with particular splendor and produced rich fruits of conversion and holiness among those who believe." (October 2015 edition)

Yup, just thinkin, love you, Felipé.

October 27, 2015 / My Purpose

At some point during the night's waking moments I had one of those crystalline thoughts that I immediately realized I needed to write down. But no, fell asleep again, as I was exhausted. Remarkably the thought persisted though and I could examine it twice more as I had my random awakenings and here it is morning and I still have it!

Fodder for these thoughts come from my own questioning and from conversing with cancer campers and commandos who I am in constant contact with. Seems we are preoccupied with the "big" questions. Why this or why that, right?

But OK, my thought was, "My purpose (earthly purpose) is not to try and live forever (earthly life) but to try and complete my journey (my purpose)." Am I fulfilling my mission as opposed to just trying to lengthen my life for its own sake? The stress, the emphasis should be on the journey that gives my life meaning and not on keeping this old body going at all cost.

If I surrender to God's will I can move beyond this trap of worry about the importance of my own days. What are my days anyway if I give up on my journey, my mission? They are only important in terms of what I am doing with them!

Thank you for being with me here, wrestling in the goulash I call it lately. And this opens the way to being able to pray for myself better now. "Give me the days to fulfill my mission!" seems like a prayer that makes sense to me here and now.

Off to breakfast and work. Thanks for being here for me, love, Felipé.

October 28, 2015 / Will Work For Tapas

Well, that's what it's come to, I guess. One day you watch the *The Way* then soon you are on to *Walking the Camino*, the documentary. Before you know it you are buying hiking boots and a pack and ordering plane tickets and using one of those goofy camping toothbrushes. And the end of all that is that now my big daily thought is how do I just make it to tapas.

Hehe, this has been my downward or upward spiral of the last three years. I know I have talked about this before but tapas still remain the high point of my day. And we had a great tapas yesterday. We have a new friend walking with us and enjoying tapas. He made a comment on how our group looked like something right out of *The Way*. Yea, we both have a common ancestor. Anyway I just threw my hat in the air to celebrate that news.

This "will work for tapas" occurred to me during the night. Maybe our thoughts and talks have gotten too deep and heavy and we needed some comic relief? That's what I am thinking.

And tonight we have a Belly Laugh Theater session scheduled. I'm still laughing over the last one where we watched *Naked Gun 2 1/2*. Yea, laughing is good. Off to lunch. I made mac and cheese for our hospital picnic lunch. Yummy loves, Felipé.

October 29, 2015 / High Pressure—Alarm, Alarm, Alarm!

That's how my day started out, no joke. You know, everything has alarms or rings, or ringtones, seems like EVERYTHING. I'm reaching a critical point where I am starting to block stuff out and not pay attention. Is it all really that critical?

But OK that was a rant. But this morning my portable chemo pump started alarming all over the place: High Pressure, High Pressure, High Pressure!

Yea, and all before coffee. Gee, I don't know, can I ignore it? Well, I guess not. So I call the magic 800 number and after answering a bunch of questions finally get the go-to-gal in North Carolina. And she starts asking me questions like what is the name of your pump and I say "Pancho." And she says huh. She doesn't know who she is talking to, obviously. What she really wanted to know, which is of lesser importance, is that it is a CADD-Legacy Plus. So, it didn't take her long to pinpoint the old problemo. In tracing the plastic line that connects Pancho to my port I came across the point where I had pinched it off with my suspenders clip where the tube ran out of my clothing and across the top of my jeans. Yea, right there where a fella clips things together.

This is all before coffee, mind you.

Well, that's how it all started out but things improved. Love you, Felipé.

November 1, 2015 / In Between Mass and Football

We are in between storms here too. It's been raining and blowing like heck for a couple days and more to come. Have a walk this afternoon and we are starting earlier because of the darkness. The afternoon walks we are moving from a 1600 to 1530 start for three months. I don't know maybe we will have to back it up another half hour in December. All my walks the first time we hiked "across Spain" were in the morning and we never had this problem.

Probably have to walk the alternative trail today. The regular trail I call the "Mary" trail and it goes through the woods. But when it is stormy we stay out of there. Falling limbs are called widow-makers around here. So we have the "Joseph" trail that is safely all out in the open.

OK, we will be safely out of the storm and Maggie will safely be in Santiago. Sounds good to me. Later, love, Felipé.

November 4, 2015 / War Weary

Woke up in the early morning dark feeling exactly that, war weary. The chemo forces and the cancer forces duke it out constantly, all day, all night. There is some ebb and flow to it but it goes on and on and on. They are at each other's throats right now as I try to maintain equilibrium in the bigger picture.

Keeping the battlefield cordoned off to just the body seems a full-time project. They keep tumbling into the mind but I always manage to push them out with some considerable effort. My major fortune is that they will never reach my soul. They may occasionally cause disruption in my mind but that's as far as they can get. Ooh, I like it. Never verbalized that before.

Take care for now y'all, love every inch of you, Felipé.

November 5, 2015 / One Little Bean

Last evening we had a private showing of *Phil's Camino* here in the living room of Raven Ranch house. Our Wiley worked miracles to get us linked up to it out there somewhere wherever it resides. We Skyped with Annie, producer and director, while we watched. It is 27 minutes long and the twelve of us watched it twice clutching Kleenexes and champagne flutes. Wow!

It is beautiful, soulful, poignant and funny here and there. To me as having been involved with much of the component parts it is amazing to see the whole (95 percent there). And the whole is a beautiful story and much larger than the pieces. I am so, so lucky to have somehow been a part.

This early morning I was up at 0530 and scurrying around the kitchen making a fire and coffee and cleaning up the leftover party mess. I got to sweeping the floor of debris and had a little pile to scoop up when I spied one little dried bean there amongst the crumbs, toothpicks and leaves. I knew exactly what it was by its distinctive shape, size and color as one of My Rebecca's precious "Yu Hoh Wong" bean seeds that she faithfully collects and dries and saves for her next year's garden. How easy it would have been to sweep that pile into the dustpan and on into the fire. But that one seed was crying out to get my attention. It started by telling me of its winter sleep that it was just embarking on with its deep subtle mysteries. It told me of the miracle of spring coming and a wonderful growing season full of such joy and promise. It told me of a bountiful harvest and how one seed would multiply to be a hundred provided with a little food, water, sun and protection. It said that its nourishment would help my family and friends prosper and that would ripple outward into the Universe. It said that after a beautiful summer it too would experience a meaningful autumn of life just as I was now. Its beautiful framework would dry and get ready to go back to the earth but first it would give forth one precious pod that would contain the future provided that someone would pick it and dry it and save it.

OK, OK I picked the little guy up and put him with his buddies in the little brown envelope there on the kitchen counter. A lesson from one little desperate Yu Hoh Wong bean seed, right? One seed is much, much more than one seed I learned.

But it is so much like our desperate little 27-minute film. Somehow, someway it has gotten this far through thick and thin. It has survived on meager rations and a little moisture where it could find it. It begged, borrowed and stole. Saint James noticed it struggling and appreciated its intention and shortly afterward the Universe began to conspire in its strange convoluted way to push it forward to this point. We are so lucky to be here to ride along with it. But most importantly it is a little seed that promises much.

Happy to be a small part of the whole, love, Felipé.

NOVEMBER 7, 2015 / THE DOC, THE DOCUMENTARY

Way back in the early summer of 2014 we were so focused on getting to Spain and the filming there. That was where everything was headed and where the story was we thought. We had done a little filming at the hospital before going but not much was happening outside of that. And that was my idea of how the movie would read, all about Spain. But as it turns out the evolved story is more about my inner pilgrimage and all that went into that and all that resulted from that. And that is as it should be perhaps because so much has been published on the trail in Spain and its trials, camaraderie, beauty and so forth.

So, as I think about the movie now that I have seen it and digested it somewhat the story of the Outer pilgrimage has been eclipsed by the story of the Inner pilgrimage that resulted from it. And as the maybe hundred hours of raw footage was winnowed down to the half hour of the movie so many things had to be jettisoned to effectively tell the evolved story. Am I making sense? This is the major challenge of editing, to get down to the essence with the pile of raw material. What are the rock-bottom things that tell the story most effectively?

Realizing that constraint I still long for all memories of Spain and the wonderful folks that really made it all happen for me that would be too numerous to mention. And folks here, too numerous to mention and at the same time so important to me. But you guys know that you dwell in my heart as always. So, onward we go to tell folks that weren't there or maybe never will get close, the story, the story of how a dreaded disease as cancer can be a catalyst for positive change for this guy, the average guy.

Time to bake some cornbread for breakfast. Wiley and I off after that on our third day to finish the old two-day job. Thinking of you, trying to pray for you as often as I can think about it. Alperfect it is, althankful we are, love, Felipé.

NOVEMBER 8, 2015 / ONE LITTLE MOSQUITO

So, I'm making a fresh pot of coffee this early AM before picking up Catherine for Mass. I had just been sitting at the kitchen table wondering about what to write on today's post. In that zone of uncertainty when this little mosquito flies by me. Sort of odd really and caught my attention. Wrong season, right? It's November and well into it. He is flying zigzag as in looking for something or uncertain about where to land, kind of tentative. And then I think OK does this little guy have a big lesson for me, like things have been occurring lately? We've had little spiders and a little bean with big lessons.

He really didn't talk to me but the lesson started when I tried to capture him with a word and came up with "stranger." He was showing uncertainty, was out of place or better out of time. This stranger thing snapped me back to a walking conversation I had with Dana recently about the origins for the word pilgrim being that very idea of a stranger or a foreigner as my dictionary has. Either way same thing. It says from the Latin "peregrinus" meaning foreign.

Dana was talking about the idea that being a pilgrim is supposed to be or puts one in the position of stranger. Aside from the striving for the goal stuff the basic experience is one of experiencing stranger-ness and that is the space intended for you. In other words it is supposed to be a facsimile of life in a Christian sense where one belongs in heaven but we are temporarily wandering on this earth. A stranger as viewed from worldly perspective. Being in and not of, I have heard it expressed.

The short book *Pilgrim's Progress* written in the 1500s I think, talks of this. It was a book that was required reading until maybe mid twentieth century when we became too cool for such stuff. But my little mosquito is still onto it.

Hey have to go. Off to a luncheon potluck. So stranger loves to you today, Felipé.

November 10, 2015/ I Called A Meeting

Seems like since Daylight Savings moved my sense of time around, I have an hour each morning to pray, meditate, wonder, get inside. My brain is waking up at. 0530 because the light is the same as 0630 a few days ago. Don't have me explain that but let's say sleeplessness has its benefits. Now I have to back up to the Camino last year to tell you of the benefits that I came back with. It was a huge sack of plunder but the biggest prize is maybe the subtlest. The biggest prize is the knowledge that God is always next to me, so very, very close. I didn't need a lot of words to pray anymore as in the past. Before Camino God seemed to be always a distance away and a lot of words were needed to lure him in but not anymore. As I think of it, we were so breathless and desperate at times that we didn't have the luxury of all of those words, did we?

Another very important part of my situation was a workshop that I had the very good fortune to participate in recently. And this was a course taught by three lovely and capable women on what I would call Natural Horsemanship. It was all about communicating with their highly trained horses with one's intentions. Yea. If we are without inner conflict and clear we can "talk" to a horse and get him to "dance" with us with our intentions. It was a very transformative experience is how I would put it but hard to put into words.

Well, what does that have to do with anything? It has to do with the idea that if God is close by and I just need a word or two to communicate what does it mean to communicate with God with no words, just my intentions. And if there are no words involved it must mean that God is very, very close, yes? And this is where I have been lately working with this.

But let's pull all this together if we can. This is all going to sound very "out there" and yes, it is but follow along. So, also recently I have been trying to visualize and talk with my eleven tumors in my lungs. Can I convince them to start growing smaller, relinquishing their power? In that process I am trying to meet with the Soul of Cancer, that essence, that force that we dread. So, this morning with confidence and desperation I called a meeting with my Cancer, my God and Myself inside me. Yes, it happened!

Something has to give. We have to work things out. Cancer and I both have missions to complete. How is that going to work? Does one of us win and the other lose? Do we both become meaningful because we are locked in opposition? Do we both win? Do we continue to try and live together beating each other up? Hmm. And that is why God was there to start to sort this thing out. I don't know anything beyond this at the moment but we got started and that is the news!

I am off to see Dr. Zucker this a.m. We will have some good stuff to talk about. So, keep tuned, more to come. Thanks, love you, Felipé the Pilgrim.

November 16, 2015 / Yea, So?

Off for a morning walk. It frosted last night for the first time this fall. The water in Raven Creek is starting to run across the Camino. Changes happening, love unchanging, Felipé.

November 26, 2015 / Giving Thanks For All The Good Souls

That was Our Jennifer's Thanksgiving prayer in an email that I just opened. We both had a hard day at the hospital yesterday. But like her prayer says we had lots of good souls hovering around us to make things easier. Besides treatment we had our interpretation of our scans. Things could have been better with both of them. Doc Gold put us on heavier chemo drugs, Jennifer starting yesterday and I will start in the Spring. I wanted to wait for her to recover from her series before I started. Anyway, that's what it looks like in a very general way.

It's all dicey, yes? But Cancer Commandos hang tough. Stuff happens and pretty soon we're making lemonade, one way or another. I was up in the early hours with the nervous energy from the steroids in my cocktail. Did an hour and a half of writing. Started to develop a list of "Findings", important things that I found in 2015. I can't take credit for thinking up anything much originally but can pick up things off the "spiritual ground" and fit them into the Cancer Commando Code. I'm good at that.

Well, have a great Thanksgiving, and live that gratitude tomorrow and the next day. Love you all immensely, Felipé.

November 27, 2015 / My Rebecca's Thanksgiving Meal

To start with it was a thing of beauty, so I don't forget. Earlier in the week she was whining about it just being the two of us present but then we were present to each other and that's the magic.

Katy, the nurse who I was with the most, was amazed that Rebecca was making the cornbread to make the cornbread stuffing. Then I said that we had grown the corn and ground the meal and that is when Rebecca received the *Little House on the Prairie* chef award, right? She also cooked the real pumpkins, that Catherine and Dana had grown (neighborhood farming), to make the pie. She did buy the real whip cream in a spray can but we let her go on that one as we don't have a cow to milk. The turkey was a gift from Colin, a friend of Our Wiley's.

So yea, kudos to Rebecca on this one. Just like we learned on The Camino, be present, work hard, improvise, pay attention and smile. Oh, and give thanks!

Bless you dear friends, Felipé.

December 1, 2015 / I Just Saw It

The ending to Monday Night Football was highly unlikely is how to describe it best. How in the heck could that have happened? But it did! Don't ask me to explain it but know that you will see it thirty-five times in the reruns coming this week.

But the point is that it is never too late. Four seconds can change everything. Just be present, right? Look for opportunities. Being present is equal to not giving up. The things you learn on Monday Night Football.

December 2, 2015 / Caminoheads On The Horizon

Good friends of Annie's are coming for a few days to grace us here and walk Phil's Camino. They are coming from Salt Lake and probably at the airport now. I find myself scurrying around trying to catch up on things to make these guests comfortable and welcome.

It is comforting to me, as I have my first coffee of the morning contemplating all the undone details of welcome-ness on my "to do" list, when I think of something Annie said to me on her first visit here. Awaiting her, my little mind was stuck in the "Annie is coming, Annie is coming!" mode as I scurried preparing.

One of the items on my long list was to find some big flat rocks to put down in Raven Creek so Annie could get across gracefully when she came to walk the next day. Yea, got it done and was pretty proud of it. So, the next day when we were making our way around the first time in the typical rain of early March we came up to the stepping stones setting above of the flowing water and Annie complimented the engineering by saying, "Oh, how Camino!" I was flattered but followed by saying to be careful because I just placed the rocks and some of them may be a little shaky. And she quickly exclaimed, "Oh, how Camino!"

That's when I learned to relax and love Annie and better understand what being a Caminohead means. So, Caminoheads on the horizon, that's the way it is with us.

Ideally you will be reading this on the Wi-Fi on the plane. Know that we will charm each other "just because" of who we have become and therefore "we can't help ourselves" (another Annie) and my "to do" list will perhaps be little shaky. Welcome!

DECEMBER 3, 2015 / THE SALT LAKERS HAVE LANDED.

Caminoheads from afar have descended on Raven Ranch bringing buckets and piles of their lovely energy. Just when we thought we had a lull between Thanksgiving and Christmas in come this gang, Tracy, Loretta, Erin and Erin's husband Jeff. So we are walking and talking and partying hearty in between. Just alberguing down with cozy wood fires and tapas. Haven't had this much fun since Mary Margaret came through maybe a year ago.

The weather is beautiful for Northwest late Fall. But do these guys care anyway? All of us sat out at the picnic table last evening with Catherine y Dana tapas-ing in the dark and the drizzle with candles and twinkle lights. Are there any conditions in which Caminoheads can't tapas?

They all rented a beach cabin on the harbor for two nights. Could see Orcas out the front window. There were some bunk beds and Tracy claimed one of those for old time's sake. We will be there for dinner tonight. Maybe have a winter bonfire so can get them all smelling woodsmokey for the flight home.

It's pretty much an alperfect situation here. Will be out hiking today working the tapas off. There is a grove of giant cedars that we want to get to. Their giant roots go across the trail and you feel like a Hobbit scrambling over them. Feeling like a Hobbit, priceless.

OK, enough of this giddiness. Time for breakfast and getting ready for the Salt Lakers. They will be here at 0900. For my readers we will start our Advent celebration soon I promise. Thanks for being here readers, love you, Felipé.

DECEMBER 4, 2015 / SCARING AWAY THE FEAR

If you are going to walk one of the Caminos, foreign or domestic, Spain or in the backyard, fear not. The Way has been working for 1200 years, millions of people have walked before you, just start. Just start, St. Francis walked it 800 years ago, you will be walking in his footsteps. You will be walking in his footsteps so you can't really get lost because insights are everywhere, just follow the setting sun. No one accomplishes anything significant without the help of God, just ask. Your journey is an investment in your soul, rise to the occasion!

I will pray for your success, just start. Love, Felipé

DECEMBER 5, 2015 / A QUOTE FOR ADVENT

"The spiritual journey does not consist in arriving at a new destination where a person gains what he does not have, or becomes what he is not. It consists in the dissipation of one's own ignorance concerning one's self and life, and the gradual growth of that understanding which begins the spiritual awakening. The finding of God is a coming to one's self." Aldous Huxley.

There seems to be a lot of "out there" as Christmas approaches. Everything seems to be out there somewhere. Our job, get totally stressed trying to find all the required stuff and gather it in the time allotted. I haven't watched much news since back from Spain but did catch vital footage of folks fighting over Black Friday merchandise. Yea. Hmm.

Let's start the season here at Caminoheads with remembering what the basic story is and how each of us dovetails with God from way back before time. No fighting necessary. Just relax, the important stuff really is close at hand.

We are waiting on the Lord, love, Felipé.

DECEMBER 8, 2015 / THE PEACE . . .

The peace that passes all understanding. Have you ever dwelled on those words? I wasn't dwelling on those words in this early morn but got to that peace anyway. It was dark still, four o'clock maybe. Rain was coming down in buckets and a slight breeze was coming through the open window and touching my cheek. It was the right time for a face to face opportunity. For these formal meetings with my cancer I am flat on my back with my hands on my chest above my lungs, home of my tumors. Somehow it is important for my body to be straight and symmetrical as possible. Don't ask me why.

But we talk. I try and answer my questions and to find a way to relate to this renegade part of me. This has been going on for weeks, the talks. As time has gone on, I am more satisfied with not being able to understand everything. When does that happen anywhere anyway? Lately, I have been more into relating.

I think the process was started when I stopped looking for blame outside myself. My cancer could be caused by what kind of breakfast cereal I ate as a kid in 1958. Yea, maybe. Or the chemicals that we used in art school in 1970. Yea, maybe. It is endless and useless, this quest, for me anyway.

There was a point it became personal, "my" cancer not "the" cancer. Maybe first I saw my cancer as a wildfire that we were fighting. Then I saw my cancer as a loose cannon aboard the ship that is my body, that we were trying to get control of. Most lately it appears to be a sort of messenger, an agent sent to get my attention.

Anyway, this early morning, I reached the conclusion that it, my cancer, had a place and it was alperfect that it was with me. Whatever it was sent to tell me I would listen. So, this is all so personal I hope I am not weirding you out but I am trying to describe a process that may be helpful (vital) to someone. I've never heard this stuff talked about this way and I am in uncharted territory myself so stay with me.

As a kid I was fascinated by the idea of people whose job it was to disarm bombs, unexploded ordinance. Totally heroic activity. I knew that the process involved communication. As the person worked at taking apart the mechanism to get to the heart of it all, to understand it and ultimately to disarm it he described everything he was doing over the radio to his team members who were at a safe distance. This was especially important when dealing with something unfamiliar as there was always a learning curve ahead. There was a good chance that he would not survive the procedure but at some point the answer would come by repeating the process. So, I strangely feel like "that guy" all of a sudden. I am not trying to weird you out but I am communicating with you as I keep you at a safe distance. We are trying to learn something.

This morning is Mass, as today is a day of obligation, The Immaculate Conception of the Blessed Virgin Mary. Catherine and I are off to that. Then this evening we have a big Caminoheads dinner. Our Jennifer is cooking a big pork roast. So, thus it all goes on, love you, Felipé.

December 11, 2015 / Just A Few

Here we are in Advent, the few weeks before Christmas. A day doesn't go by that I don't think about the Camino and some of you that were there for me. That was in hotter than hot July and August. Maybe next time start May first or September first, right?

But that isn't where my thoughts are today. What about those few hundred hardy souls that walk every month throughout the winter. Thinking about them, praying for them now. Buen Camino from our armchairs!

Well, Our Jennifer and I are off to Seattle today. I have to get my driver's license renewed while she does some Christmas shopping. Then off to the hospital to get our pumps off. After that we have meeting with Sister Joyce to wrap things up. Then dash out to catch a ferry before rush hour. That's the plan and nice when things go uneventfully. But Commandos can handle the random hurdles anyway.

Yup, well, you have a good one. It's good though, uneventful or eventful, for God enjoys our personal stories. Give us strength Lord, that is what we pray for. See you tomorrow friends, love, Felipé.

December 12, 2015 / It Just Could Be Overwhelming

All of the time we live by the watchwords of "Don't get overwhelmed." This meaning don't let the bad stuff become too much. Keep in charge of the situation in other words. But this week has been exceptional in a little different way.

What do you think of a week that was so full of remarkably good things as to be on the verge of overwhelming? Not that everything was easy or unchallenging but it all was exceptional. Maybe I can power through this now and give you a rough idea.

Wednesday was my and Our Jennifer's big every other week big treatment day. This is such a hurdle to get over and it isn't always pretty but we did it once again. That was Wednesday and it is an all-day project.

Then Thursday morning we received a blessing from Father Marc at St. John Vianney's here on the Island. He is such a positive warm person and so supportive of our mission. This is so inspirational to have this kind of backup.

Then back to the hospital on Friday to complete our treatment. Sister Joyce saw us afterward for an hour at her office. She was on her A game for us, all guns firing, if I can say that about a Sister. After hearing what was new with us, she gave us a talk on the "thin moments" of life. These are moments when the distance between us and God is very close, when the veil is very thin. These are the moments that we would love to repeat, to experience again and again and again. Maybe specifically it would be the birth of a child or intense beauty or witnessing a heroic moment. We know it by our longing to get back there. These "thin moments" are glimpses of heaven according to Sister Joyce. Yes. This is rich juice to get us through the low times.

And then this morning I spent some time with friends talking with Art Kopecky who is president of Teleios. This is an organization that oversees over a hundred men's small group Bible classes in Western Washington. I have been going to one on the Island for ten years now. And my other great connection is that Art walked the Camino this last summer and I had a chance to help with his preparation. Also, a cool detail is that he took my walking sticks and used them and they went across again. Anyway, it a shot in the arm to be with him and just another good thing for me.

OK, just one more. I told you that I am overwhelmed. Then this early morning was one of my talks with the cancer messenger. He had me looking at a miniature scene like a diorama in a museum or interpretive center. It was a rectangular expanse of forest and we were looking down on the canopy. This was so thick that the ground could not be seen from our vantage point. It was clear to me, though implied, that there was a trail down there beneath somewhere to be walked and we were looking down on it in a bird's eye view. And he said, "This is the day that you have." Yes, simultaneously clear and obscure.

Well, there you have it. Have to go Skype with Angela in Australia. It's all happening, this is the day that we have, love, Felipé.

December 13, 2015 / The Lady Of Guadalupe

I was in Mexico in the early 1970's, on a December 12th when I first ran into her. Well, I ran into the celebration of her appearance which is pretty close to running into her. The enthusiasm that she inspires is over the top from what I observed.

Really don't remember the small stuff but the rowdiness after dark was a thing of beauty. Lots of fireworks were flying around the town square lighting up the night. I was ducking stuff and amazed at the scene when the bull showed up. This was a metal contraption in the shape of a bull with four human legs propelling it around. The whole outside was packed with rockets and the bull would charge the crowds and cause general panic. As it ran around the square it would dodge into various buildings and rockets were coming out doors and windows. Wild and crazy all around.

The meaning of all this was sort of a mystery to me until much later when I learned more about Our Lady and the history of Mexico. Great stuff, isn't it? I think it wouldn't hurt if we were a little more enthusiastic about our beliefs around here. Enthusiastic love, Felipé.

December 14, 2015 / It's Called "Sabbath Moment"

My breakfast eggs are on to boil, the fire is going strong, Aretha is singing Gospel in the background.

My neighbor Terry and I fly on the same Spiritual Blue Angels Flying Team. Flying wingtip to wingtip with Grace without a worry. Today he was talking of a Christmas battlefield truce that happened in World War One. A sort of wave of kindness in the middle of the opposite. And this very morning, minutes before, I was sending kindness into the war zone that is my chest. Mine being sort of a mini of what Terry was inspired by and writing about. Amazing.

OK, making chicken salad for lunch for Our Jennifer. Moving on to handle the day, love you all, Felipé.

December 16, 2015 / Nice Day Dawning, I Had A Dream

Vashon Island is actually two islands. At some point in the early twentieth century they were connected by a short land bridge. So, there is the larger Vashon and the smaller Maury that we talk about collectively as Vashon Island. We live on the larger island, Vashon. Why is this important? Well, it wasn't terribly except I had a dream last night about Maury that is somewhat revealing and I had to give you that background to help with what comes next.

So, the dream was that I motored over to Maury and got on a road that took me past a threatening raptor, along a thousand-foot gorge and into a dusty town above the timberline. I was looking for a place to buy supplies for an implied journey. None of that stuff exists on Maury except maybe a threatening raptor occasionally.

Upon pondering this dream, I recalled other dream trips to Maury Island where I drove up and up in elevation and crossed a pass, could have been in the Pyrenees. That happened on a small handful of occasions. Again, nothing like that exists on Maury Island here and now, so to speak.

And on pondering all this, it reminded me of dreams that I had in the innocence of childhood where I would walk out into our small backyard and go behind the garage and there would be a different world suddenly. It was a world of color that mimicked the palette of a children's book that I was familiar with. The colors were rich and bold and exciting.

I had never made the connection before between these dreams that are so far apart in time. They seem related and speaking of the same surprise though. There is a place around the corner from reality where other possibilities are present, exhibiting a more exciting palette. It is just a short journey with maybe an occasional threatening raptor to sidestep but possible and not that hard. Hmm.

Is this the place of sanctuary that Terry Hershey talks about? Is it a hint that reality is only so real? Is it a place to get supplies for a further journey? I don't know exactly but will ponder on. Thanks for being here for me, love you dreamily, Felipé.

December 24, 2015 / Christmas Eve

Before light here and Christmas Eve. A few words are better than a lot of words right now. Bless you, fellow pilgrims. Look for the star. Buen Camino! As always, love you all ways, Felipé.

December 26, 2015 / Boxing Day

While I am thinking about it, I want to tell you about something that happened the other day to the Cancer Commandos. We received a nice compliment from one of the nurses. You guys know that Our Jennifer and I travel together to our appointments and we get our treatment together, well adjacent to each other. All this sort of stretches the place's privacy policies. But we have everyone trained now to handle us together. This includes having a table right by our two chairs at the treatment center so we can unpack our table cloth, candle (battery power) and picnic lunch. There was a rumor that we were sneaking wine in but I don't know how true that is. Anyway, the staff is always checking in to see how the pumps are doing or if we are comfortable or just to hang out with the Commandos. This time we were done with soup and sandwich lunch and we were sort of lounging with the candle burning, me blogging probably and Jennifer reading a big glossy magazine with the general chaos of the hospital going on around us. One of the nurses walked in on our cozy scene and said, "You guys look like you are in your own living room." Somehow at that moment we were successful! Nice, Commando Caper completed in style.

See you tomorrow. but love in the present, Felipé.

December 28, 2015 / Finally

The toughest time of the year for me to get through is happening right now, the old bleak midwinter. I do find myself daydreaming of spring when the rains slack off and the sun dries out the soil and that magic medium starts warming up enough to germinate seeds. It is always such a miracle to watch those little seeds start that rampage of growth, amazing.

But this all is not stopping us from walking these days. I was out today with Cynthia, a new walking partner who has done the Camino Norte. And it looked pretty darn Norte out there with lots of rain/snow mixed. And she busted a hole in her rubber boots to boot. Always something. And there was mist between the dark green firs. And the alders were showing reddish and the willows a yellowish to complete the subtle palette. The beauty in winter is a subtle one for sure.

Yea, I am starting to realize that this here, this little Camino, is a pilgrimage for folks. They are coming to experience something different, something special.

OK, look at us, we got a blogpost hammered out on a dark evening in the bleak midwinter, no problemo. Thank you for being here.

No problemo loves, Felipé.

December 29, 2015 / Phil's Camino Walking Schedule 12/29/15.

Yup, the bleak mid-winter but we are still walking on Vashon. Areas of the trail are periodically flooded so rubber boots or pacs are apropos. We want to be fashionable, right?

So come please. Sometimes we have three or four pilgrims and sometimes I walk alone with the birds. I never know and that is the sort of beauty of it for me. And if you arrive late, hang out for a few minutes and we will be around.

And if you are coming from a distance and those times won't work, we can maybe get you a special time with some notice. It's really not all that complicated and it is achieving a life of its own, so no worry.

Buen Camino, Felipé.

December 30, 2015 / Breathe Easy

Nice phrase and it is sticking with me this morning. I feel like I am experiencing that more and more these days, not all the time but still noteworthy. Something has changed in the last month to calm me down in a very deep way. I'm reporting here and attempting to give myself and you a rough idea of what's going on.

This all started back at least a month ago when I started a meditation exercise that I came up with. A guy that can build his own Camino can come up with a reasonable mediation practice, right? So, to review, I am quietly flat on my back in the early morning hours practicing, putting to use, my times of sleeplessness. The idea is that I am inviting God in to the site of my cancer to bring some peace and harmony to that area, to that battlefield.

This led to me starting to pay attention to my lungs in a very intimate sort of way that had escaped me up until this point. It had been some obscure place that I couldn't access but now I was there seeing for myself the chaos, the damage, the disharmony of that area in the very core of my body. And going there with God to bring some relief was changing things for me, I was breathing easier, so to speak.

Here we are creeping up on New Year's Eve. It is cold here just like it is supposed to be, I guess. OK, enough of this loves, Felipé.

Part III

The Three C's

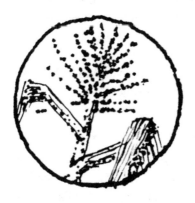

January 2, 2016 / The Second Walk

I started a map on a whiteboard at the rock pile on Phil's Camino to illustrate where we "are" in Spain on our second walk that we are on now. Then maybe in addition it would be good to have a regular report here on the blog about this, coming out say every Sunday. OK, let's try that mañana.

January 4, 2016 / Where Are We Felipé

I promised you a weekly report on our current location on Phil's Camino second walk "across Spain." It is not like we are moving quickly, for our weekly distance, six miles plus, is about the same as the distance that we walked before lunch each day in Spain.

So that equals 192.72 kilometers from St. Jean, the beginning. We are past the cities of Pamplona and Logrono with Burgos still a long way off. So, after Logrono are the towns of Navarrete, Ventosa. We are through those and we have Nájera less than a km ahead. Look, can you see it?

January 5, 2016 / A Hungry Heart

Somehow this Felipé coming out of the mud and the mist of grassroots life has been able to run into or bump into or stumble into some amazing situations, territory and relationships. How did that happen? How does that work? We could try to answer those questions but the real point is that Felipé is just an average guy, without degrees or money. And he stands for the idea that anyone could do this too, this isn't rocket surgery as they say. This is the real value of the Felipé story, that it is attainable.

Well, just reporting on life in the neighborhood. Remember Pilgrim Farmer John, our friend from Iowa, as he goes in for his new gleaming hip joint. Remember Our Jennifer and me as we go in for treatment tomorrow. Pray for us and pray for the thousands of stones on the pile a few feet from here, each has a story.

Always attainable love, Felipé.

January 6, 2016 / A Corner With a View

We are hunkered down at the treatment center with windows. We'll get through it but the trail has gotten rough here for now and it requires more care and the need to slow down.

Thank you for your many prayers. Thank you for your many thoughts. Some days are harder than others but we know that. Will be back to you tomorrow but for now I need to pay attention. Love you, Felipé.

January 7, 2016—Home Safe and Sound

All good now. Just want to let you know that Our Jennifer is home and I am home after a day with complications at the hospital. Can't be specific but because of excellent care, steely determination and a rosary we pulled out a victory.

Victoriously we love, Felipé.

January 10, 2016 / It Is Supposed to be a Challenge

Life is like that. We are constantly stressed by one thing or another as we walk on our Way. We groan and moan as we put another blistered foot down on the Walk. We see others that have greater challenges and we realize that we can do what we are supposed to do. We ask God for strength, clarity, peace.

Life is like that. Maybe someone along the trail sees us struggling and walks along with us 'til we stabilize and then they are gone. Who was that?

Life is like that. Semi mysterious, semi delirious we all go on. Look--there is a café and coffee up ahead! Man, it is going to feel good to just sit for a while. Can you join me? Love, Felipé.

January 11, 2016 / I'm no Expert But . . .

The Camino did start out as a religious pilgrimage and that is still there for the taking. It can be much more than an athletic event or a cultural tour or anything else.

Well, I know this blog wanders all over the landscape in terms of topic. It is not the place really to find the best brand and model of boot to wear or to find facts about availability of potable water or facts about bedbugs or anything else. But there is an amazing amount of info about walking this trail out there in other places. Our strong point or emphasis here has been integrating what the Camino teaches back into our everyday lives. And that has not been easy or very concise. I have been reporting for a year and a half about this topic and we have rambled all over hell and back in that process. But that's the way it is, you have to put up with it I guess.

Yea, but in the end it's alperfect, we have discovered that much and that's a biggie. So, we will continue to walk here at the blog and deal with issues as the trail dictates. Maybe tomorrow we will explore more Spain, or more Catholicism, or more cancer, or family, friends or the weather. It is a free-wheeling situation as life tends to be.

One thing at a time loves, Felipé.

JANUARY 13, 2016 / CANCER COMMANDOS FOR SURE

I lifted this book from the Treatment Center waiting room. Well, I did tell the receptionist on duty that I was going to bring it back in two weeks. Somehow I had missed seeing it before, hmmm, been in and out of that room for four years. Anyway, it was speaking to me and jumped into my hand.

It is entitled *Lilly Oncology On Canvas: Expressions of a Cancer Journey*. It is a selection of art works from a competition held in 2008.

Powerful stuff when you factor in all the upheaval, pain, unknowing, fear, sacrifice and loss that each and every one of those works represented. How many Van Gogh ears is that? The paintings or photographs are just final products built on mountains of other stuff.

OK, very moving, right? But have to regroup and get on with my morning life. That is the way it is with this cancer stuff. It is terribly sort of foreign and demanding but life goes on around it. A Commando has to keep one eye on it and one eye on life and look for opportunity to "paint a meaningful painting."

Thanks Commando Artists.

JANUARY 18, 2016 / SANTO DOMINGO DE LA CALZADA

I love this guy. He is St. Dominic of the Pavement. This is an actual historic figure and also the name of a town that we reached today on Phil's Camino. It is between Logrono and Burgos, closer to Burgos.

Saint Dominic is called the first engineer of the Camino. This was eleventh century when he made trails and bridges to help the pilgrims. Before that people walking filtered across the landscape and were easy pickings for the robbers. Being on a trail meant that there could have been safety in numbers. And he added bridges on top of that.

The church there is known for the live chickens that are inside the church proper. They are a reminder of the miracle that saved a young man's life. As the story goes a young man was traveling on pilgrimage with his parents and they stopped at the town where Dominic was. The young man became involved with a young lady of the town. He apparently promised her this and that and then tried to get down the road. She in the meantime hid some of the church's silverware in his duffel and alerted the authorities. In short order the young man is arrested, jailed and up for hanging. In steps Dominic, who goes to talk with the local magistrate in charge of the case. Dominic arrives as dinner is being served. The magistrate is perturbed and after having to listen to the pleas says something like, "If the man is innocent that rooster on the platter will get up and crow." and that is exactly what happened. The young man was set free and Dominic eventually went on to sainthood.

Only the best to you, love, Felipé.

JANUARY 19, 2016—BEEN BUSY

Been busy in the early morning wakeful moments bringing peace to the battlefield that is my body. Around four I was in my meditation position and invited the spirit of Mother Mary to be with me and my turmoil. Is there a way through this mess? Hmm. Not too long ago I came across a little card that had "Mary the untier of knots." Mary would help in your knotty life was the idea.

OK, I have to wrap this up and get to my day which looks like I will be here at the ranch playing catch up with projects that maybe should have been done last month. Projects needing attention, such as cleaning the chimney, cleaning the gutters and squirrel proofing my bird feeders on the Camino. I have been reading lately about how I should feel complete in my incompleteness. I'm busy with that too.

Alperfect in a very incomplete way, but very love, Felipé.

JANUARY 21, 2016 / JUST A HINT OF SUNSHINE

We will take it! Anytime we can see a shadow in Seattle it is a blessing. Well, it is kind of a hint of a shadow. It is a break from the ubiquitous overcast sky.

I'm hooked up to my chemicals and Our Jennifer is off to a meeting. Dr. Gold gave her a two week break so she could gain her strength back. Then she is going to get a new med to see if she can't make some more progress. Glad that is over for her today. One thing at a time and don't get overwhelmed, is the name of the game for us.

Here I am on Thursday morning and have a walk in half an hour. We had a challenging day yesterday but we are marching on. We have some practice getting through the sticky wickets so all in a day's work.

Our Jennifer asked me to talk to her tumors so I have been working on that. This is in regard to my new meditation where I meet with my tumors. It sounded a little strange to me at the time but I am onboard with the idea and am giving it my best shot. It is a form of prayer and that doesn't have a problem with time or space. So, I have started on that project. I am working that in to my wish to get Mother Mary involved with me, with us.

Thanks everyone for your thoughts and prayers. They are all important to us and buoy us up continually. You are important to us, you are our magic carpet ride. Thank you to our family of docs and nurses at Swedish Cancer Center. Thank you to our families and friends who check in on us and inspire us. Thanks to my church and the Bible Guys who are there for me, for us. Thanks to all my Camino buddies near and far, you guys glow in the dark! Miss all of you immensely. Love, Felipé.

JANUARY 22, 2016 / HEALING AND CURING

In one of the film clips for the Phil's Camino documentary, I was talking about the difference between being healed and being cured. I got started on that thinking by Dr. Robert Barnes just to credit him. But I was talking about healing being reconciled with God, our families and the bigger picture. Well that bigger picture is a big grab bag, right? And one of the important things in there is getting right with what has happened to us.

I am thinking that this has to be done one way or another. Can I tackle this and make it happen for myself? Can I forgive and forget? Can I be forgiven and forgotten? Can I concentrate on the Way or the big picture and perhaps see my past as crossing the river jumping quickly from one rock to another making those decisions quickly and with faith and nimbleness?

OK, enough to gnaw on for now.

Love again, Felipé.

JANUARY 28, 2016 / "I HATE CANCER!"

My Rebecca exclaimed that last evening at dinner after we were talking about several friends who were deep in their cancer challenges. And I said, "Well, there must be some reason for it." Like there is some reason for mosquitos, but who the heck knows on that one. A part of the web of life I guess, that you can't separate out.

At the Cancer Treatment Center parking lot there are a few bumper stickers and window decals that express nasty things that people want to do to cancer. Yea, totally understand the sentiment. Throw one at it for me!

But I was up at zero dark thirty meditating and getting in touch and a few ideas came to me then that are definitely blog material. I wrote down a few notes to remind me of the thread. Sometimes I don't write stuff down and lose it. I suppose not to worry as it goes into some brain bin somewhere for recovery later, maybe.

Yes, we can hate cancer, of course. Hate, hate, hate away, somebody has to do it I suppose. But suppose we were to take that energy and do something else with it. I guess I should speak for myself here. Personally, I realize that I have only so much energy. What to do with a finite amount becomes something to work out. Somehow I have chosen to try to observe it, cancer, to run reconnaissance on it. Somehow "battling cancer" is not my way or it is not what I am doing now, although we hear that phrase everywhere.

I was trying to explain this stance to Sister Joyce at our last meeting. She put the words "active resignation" on it. OK, that will do for now.

My present thought is that cancer is an expression of our own untidiness, our own chaos, our own craziness. It represents an incredible challenge to our sense of ourselves, personally and collectively. We/I have to admit a lot of stuff to get that.

To buoy me up I got a beautiful email form Gracie in Australia yesterday and another from another Camino buddy Mary Margaret this AM. Thanks guys, can't do without you, love, Felipé.

FEBRUARY 9, 2016 / JUST A TUESDAY

Somewhere along the line of Annie's and my friendship she gave me a rosary that belonged to one of her grandmothers. It has wooden beads and is from Jerusalem. Perhaps a souvenir from a friend returning from pilgrimage. Anyway, I like that it has history, either real or imagined. It lives out on top of the wooden post that marks the beginning and end of Phil's Camino. When I feel the need to say the rosary along a lap, it is there for me.

Well, I am off to my day. It is froggy foggy here. If the air could be any wetter we would be doing the backstroke. Have a good February 9th, love, Felipé.

FEBRUARY 10, 2016 / BIG NEWS FROM THE SOUTHWEST

Good morning! Annie, our intrepid producer (IP) of *Phil's Camino* documentary announced yesterday that our film was accepted at the prestigious South by Southwest Film Festival in Austin, Texas. This is great news for it was a biggie on her list of venues to show the film and to get it out for folks to see. So that is where the Grand Premier of "the little film that can" will be this spring. A big hurrah!

So Felipé, what is the basic idea of the film and what is the job that it is supposed to accomplish? Right, OK, let's tackle that while the coffee is still hot. Maybe it would be good to look at the genesis of the whole thing. The first that I can remember there was a conversation between myself and Dr. Zucker, my rehab doc at Swedish Cancer Center, and one of us said, "Wouldn't it be cool if we could document this." This being the upcoming trip to Spain to walk the Camino de Santiago which had just opened up as a reality for us. It just seemed like an innocent thing to say, "Wouldn't it be cool . . . ."

But that started the whole show right there. So the basic idea will have to be connected to that conversation and that sentiment. OK, it is the story of a cancer patient who used the opportunity of his disease to springboard into the understanding of life and love. Wow, I just came up with that! This is almost the kind of stuff that someone else should write about.

So what if we run with that for the moment, can we come up with an answer to the second question of what is the job the film is supposed to accomplish? In my view it should inspire, encourage and motivate a patient (hate that word) to get outside of his or her comfort zone and try things that maybe they were told they couldn't do or shouldn't even attempt. Maybe instead of walking across Spain they need to walk ten miles, or one mile or ten feet. And it is not about walking either, it is about reaching out in whatever manner. It's a lot about getting outside the disease even though OK you still have the disease, I get that, I'm trying to live that.

Thanks for following me here. I don't know if we got as concise as we should but we got a start on answering those questions. And additionally, perhaps we can set up some system to better inform you about movie news. I would love to talk Annie into a short once a week post here to give us the latest and greatest. Well, time marches on and things unfold in the place and time that they should, thank you St. James. And this seems like a most exciting spring coming up.

Love, Felipé.

FEBRUARY 11, 2016 / CHEESY GRITS

Also served over easy eggs and fruit salad this morning to complete our construction worker's breakfast.

Funny there in the previous sentence is the word served as in "served over easy eggs . . . ." That has never occurred to me before that use of the word. Christ calls us to serve, to be a servant. He demonstrates this to me most fully when he washes the feet of the disciples. I don't recall anywhere in the Bible where He cooks and serves food although the serving of the bread and wine at the first Eucharist was a serving for sure. Hmmm.

I came back from Spain a year and a half ago and was totally inspired to cook and to "serve", to serve tapas and wine and good simple foods for my fellow pilgrims here just as I had been served there along the Camino. All along the trail so many folks kept up that tradition that you couldn't help but catch it.

So now, just a reminder that Valentine's Day is coming up on Sunday. An opportunity to serve, to give something to those around us, wherever we find ourselves.

OK, off to Our Jennifer's to make some progress on the bathroom remodel. She has company coming in from out of town and I will probably get a few days off from that to work on stuff around the ranch. Rainy days I will be finishing up my books for taxes and dry days getting firewood in for next winter. Yup, that's what February means around here.

The best to you friends wherever you are today. Servant love, Felipé.

FEBRUARY 22, 2016 / I THOUGHT YOU KNEW WHERE WE WERE FELIPÉ

I know where we are, just a few kilometers west of Burgos. The cathedral was most beautiful but great to be out in the boonies again. Our next town is Villalbilla de Burgos coming up tomorrow.

Don't forget the rubber boots. Felipé.

FEBRUARY 22, 2016 / THE QUINCE

We had some new folks for the trail walk which is always good. But really it wasn't 'til tapas with my Rebecca and Catherine y Dana that I finally was able to take a breath and put the day in perspective. That's what tapa time is for, right?

Yes, and it was one of those tapa times that are so good and bountiful that it turns into the evening meal and Bob's your uncle after all. We had the standbys of smoked fish, salami, cheese, crackers, pickles and of course olives. But an addition to this that I must mention is the quince jelly. C y D had made this out of fresh quince last fall. Apparently there are areas along the Camino in Spain where it is quite common to serve this as a condiment.

But the quince is such a forgotten odd fruit that just because of that it may need a revival. I have seen half a dozen in my life, which would be like seeing something every ten years, rare really. So, just an idea to check out. It will definitely raise your grade on the next tapa spread you serve. Yum.

And maybe this odd little fruit has a lesson for us Caminoheads. We who walk ancient trails, search and commune, who are we really? We who walk at two or three miles an hour in the dirt but with the vapor trails of jets high overhead with folks traveling modern speeds. Maybe we are the almost forgotten odd little fruit. And maybe we are part of the revival?

Sweet quince loves, Felipé.

FEBRUARY 29, 2016 / I HEARD THE FIRST HUMMINGBIRD

Just in from my Monday AM walk. Nice morning here, partial cloudy, dry, no wind. Long ago I stopped writing in my log the comment "Alone", as in I am walking alone this morning, as in no other pilgrims. I am never alone and now when I am the only one walking, I write "not alone." Hope that makes some sense.

I heard the first hummingbird along Phil's Camino this morning. He buzzed me and I didn't see him, just heard him, the wing beat. They are attracted to red and I had my old standby red Camino cap on, although the sun has bleached it so. There are some Anna's hummingbirds that winter over. Our Jennifer's got them all over her house because of the feeders that she has out. But we don't feed them so they start being here when things are blooming. Spring gang!

OK, a life we have to live and today is important in that, let's go, love, Felipé.

MARCH 2, 2016 / EVERYDAY A PICNIC

Well, it's a goal. Traveling down the road that is life we pack some provisions, paying some attention to food groups, quantities, weight. Bringing along a little extra for someone we may meet. Having some sense of the balance between order and disorder, plan and chance.

I brought some chicken salad, a baguette and gummy bears for lunch here at the hospital. It's my treatment day. Also just had a powwow with my doc about my scan that happened yesterday. And that was good news! My tumors show no growth. My doc is doing a great job. No growth means that we can continue as we have been with treatment and life. Yes, good news!

Jennifer is here to go to appointments and to keep me on track. So yea, help us celebrate what is. I am going to take a little nap here in the comfy chair. The best to you, love, Felipé.

MARCH 4, 2016 / JUST THINKING ABOUT THE CAMINO . . .

I was doing my morning meditation and my mind was continually drifting to thoughts of the Camino. Is there something wrong with that? A big "NO"! I had the realization that thinking of the Camino or, better put, thinking things Camino will heal me or bring me farther down that healing road. It can't be helped, it just is. That was my realization this AM as I invited healing into my body, so embattled at this point.

If we consider God to be a gathering force, that certainly happened there, in Spain and France. People from all over the planet gathered to cheer each other on as we tromped through a gathering of history. The universe gathered starting with the sun beating on us to the "field of stars" ever present over our heads. The earth gathered to give us merciful clouds, to give us views of nature and agriculture to nurture our souls. The whole thing was a gathering!

If we consider God being a mix of truth, beauty and goodness, that could be found with being open to it. Beauty is perhaps the easiest road and a good one. Goodness seeps through in big and the littlest ways. Seeps is a good word for that. Truth is a concept that seems to be in short supply or our thinking has become muddled perhaps in the world as we know it. I think that the solitude that is truly a part of walking across the Meseta is where this truth comes out. Maybe you have slightly different thoughts or memories but I bet they aren't far off.

There comes a time when this thinking starts to imbed itself in our hearts and we are no longer simply thinking. I feel that coming. We are on a path, a trail, a road, a Camino to living this stuff, this gathering. Caminoheads on their way to becoming Caminohearts! It's all a healing force!

Simply Your Felipé. Love you.

March 7, 2016 / Couple of Items

This is totally hilarious! I don't know if this is a joke or real but either way. It was reported that someone at My Rebecca's church prayed, "Please let them be glamorous." A plea to the higher powers on our behalf as we prepare for Austin and the film festival. This is always a problem for Vashonites, presenting ourselves properly to the mainland. Haha.

Also, a friend had a question yesterday. It was quite innocent and to the point but it kind of opened up a little world for me and I thought that it was worth exploring. Of course, there is always the disclaimer that the following is the world according to Felipé. Of course.

The question is, "What do you serve at tapas?" Well, what would that be generally around here: olives (black and green), cheese, celery, bread (baguette is sexy) or crackers. That would be the basics. I like tomato, salami, peppers, green onions in addition, when available. When Catherine y Dana grace our environs they like some sort of pickle and the incomparable quince jelly. Our Cynthia adds lox. Our Jennifer adds an egg or chicken salad maybe.

Also, have to hydrate after a day's walk or a day's whatever. Water is handy, so is a red and white wine, nothing fancy which would confuse us. Beer is good for some who prefer that. When it's hot I like a wine cooler made with an Italian soda and white wine.

Well, those are the bricks that make the wall but really the most important part of this to remember is that this is a celebration. This is the mortar. We all did our best at our day's work and here we are gathered to enjoy each other and compare notes on the time since we saw each other last. Was that yesterday, last week, last year? Tapaing up with people can make sense of things that occurred for you that were backward or unfinished. Ah.

So, in that vein of tapa time being a celebration, the overall situation should be celebratory. Ambience is totally important whether it is a fancy place or the side of the road. How do we present this toast in the best possible way? Is it welcoming? Is it uncomplicated? Is it good to all the senses? Is it isolated from the hustle and bustle? Is our blood pressure going down? Is it that sanctuary that we need?

Yes, and not to mention the toast, the clinking of glasses, the wish, the prayer for one another. Maybe we say it in a couple of different languages, so much the better. This is when I realize that I/we are part of the bigger picture. Here we are huddled by the side of the road perhaps but we need to realize that this little ceremony admits us to something bigger.

Consider that anyone could show up for tapas with you. This is not a cult, a private club but an impromptu gathering that will be different tomorrow. Some different food, some different drink, some different folks, some different problems and some different joys will be there tomorrow. It is not a recipe or formula but a . . .

Always good, love, Felipé.

March 7, 2016 / Where Did You Say We Were Felipé?

The spring weather comes and goes and we make our way in between rainstorms. Since last Sunday we are moving west across the Meseta, the vast plain, the breadbasket of Spain. We've gone through Hornillos del Camino and Arroyo San Bol.

There is flooding here locally on Phil's Camino so rubber boots are necessary. And have rain gear close at hand.

March 9, 2016 / Moving Toward Austin

I am calling Austin, the screening of *Phil's Camino* at South by Southwest, our Cruz de Ferro. It is the point on the Camino where pilgrims leave tokens and prayers. It is a landmark that we all can be sure of. So much of the true work of this project has happened through the magic of modern communications and we haven't had as much real contact with each other as we should have and landmarks have been hazy. And that is why this gathering in Austin is important to me. Well, one reason.

March 17, 2016 / Our Jennifer And I Have A Gardening Project

When I described our project to Our Michelle, a knowledgeable horticulturalist, she said, "Yea, Guerilla Gardening!" Well yea, something like that I suppose. We have been working at it a month now since things are warming up around here.

A brief description would be that we discovered some viable patches of soil that need some love. They exist where thousands of people would see them every day if only they had a little color to show off. Right now they look like accidental piles of dirt that have built up over the years because of road dirt, bird poop and whatever has tended to collect due to natural forces. And the area is so busy with traffic that it would be a huge hassle to close the road to clean up these untidy little piles so there they live sort of invisible. We thought that there were three out of many that looked large enough to support flowers over the summer season.

This looks like a caper for Cancer Commandos if ever there was one. Our Michelle suggested Calendula since it is colorful and easy. I added California Poppy because they are colorful and thrive on neglect. So this is the blend. So how do we actually get the seed in the "soil"? We thought up this plan of mixing the seeds in water in a standard paper coffee cup like from Starbucks which are everywhere and attract zero attention. Then since our hopefully fertile piles exist so close to the car window and since most time the traffic slows us down to walking pace we thought that casually pitching the cup of liquid on a strategic area as we roll by would look like we were jettisoning some cold coffee.

February 19th I did the first cup and yesterday I did the last of six. And the piles are sort of rough with a lot of crevices so sowing with lots of seeds with no raking in should mean that we could expect maybe a 10 percent germination. That would work to bring some color to lots of folks from an unexpected place. Well, we have our fingers crossed.

Geographically this area is where the West Seattle Freeway enters I5 North and there is a ramp that curves down and to the left. There is a sign to Vancouver overhead and the three piles are the largest ones around that sign. So I got Wiley interested in the project and he could probably get all his friends to help water it over the dry of late summer. What family fun!

Yesterday while I was conversing with one of my lovely nurses this project came up. I am with these folks in the chemo treatment area for four hours so almost any new topic is appreciated and explored. I thought that this was a good one to mention. So I'm describing the situation like I just did for you and she was listening and forming a pic in her mind. And the dear came up with this great question that was a high point in my day. She said, "Well, how do you know that no one will come along and clean those up and destroy your project?" Actually I had been thinking of this so the answer came quickly. "That is the beauty of it! It is a metaphor for our lives here with our cancer, right? Get it? We don't know when we will be swept up from the living. But that shouldn't stop us from planting something for the future." Yea, nice interchange.

Off to walk this AM. Thursday morning is beautiful here with the rising barometer, rising love, Felipé.

MARCH 21, 2016 / "LA CONCHA"

Monday morning, light rain and cloudy. Crawling out from my funky chemo weekend. These Mondays are pretty good generally. We have been calling my every other weekend, laden with fatigue from my chemo treatment, my Pyrenees weekend. So you will know in the future.

We will be walking in a few moments here. Ah, that reminds me that I haven't put out my weekly Sunday post on the progress our walk locally. Will do. Yes, always more to do, keep walking loves, Felipé.

MARCH 21, 2016 / FELIPÉ, ARE YOU SURE YOU KNOW WHERE WE ARE?

We missed a few days of walking here because of the trip to Austin but we are back now. Yesterday, Sunday's afternoon walk, we got into the town of Castrojeriz which is 40 km out of Burgos. We are out on the Meseta now.

MARCH 24, 2016 / MAUNDY THURSDAY

There is Mass tonight, 1930, at our local Iglesia. I have to get in gear with Holy Week and be here now. Still reentering from the Austin trip. So, I will be at church tonight and won't be at work tomorrow, Good Friday. Well, at least I won't use my power tools. I am so distracted on Good Friday that I tend to be dangerous. We don't need that.

It would be interesting to be in Spain during Holy Week. I can only imagine the energy and the pageantry. Well, maybe that will have to wait for another year. But back to the here and now and Holy Week. Holy Week, the time to contemplate on Christ's Passion. What does it mean to the world? What does it mean for mankind? What did it mean for people then and people now? What does it mean for me here and now?

Yup, time to go for now. Hope that we all get some time to think about things in between all that seems to happen. Maundy Thursday loves, Felipé.

PS—so I nodded off with the iPad in my hands on the red couch. And Catherine, Dana and Cynthia show up to walk on Phil's Camino. They look in the window and think I am blogging and walk a lap without me. So, they come around again and this time I am awake because of a phone call. So, I hurriedly get myself together and walk the rest of the way with them. So, Phil's Camino has a life of its own and sometimes Phil has to catch up with it.

MARCH 25, 2016 / GOOD FRIDAY

Ah, a day to not use power tools, a day to contemplate. A day that so takes me over. A day that is a different day each year, that flits through our calendar like a summer butterfly. A day that affected me as a kid. A day as an adult where I cried in the middle of the service at a church that I was at for the first time. It's always a spring day but it doesn't feel like spring ever, sometimes. But ever a day to be caught up in a big cosmic drama. A day, just a day.

Yesterday, Father Marc washed my feet and today he will hold the cross for me to kiss. A tear now, today. It runs down my cheek now, today. A bird in the daylight, outside my window gathers up the perfect piece of debris to be an important part of her nest. Does she know about this day?

Or is most of it unsaid today? Is it some sort of underlying hum that loops up into my consciousness on a day where I am paying special attention? Days can go on for a long time without me paying this special attention, can't they? A day perhaps with more questions than answers.

Mayday, mayday, mayday! Doris Day, doomsday, worst day, business day, laundry day, Christmas Day, New Year's Day, Thanksgiving Day, Boxing Day, Doubleday, The Longest Day, Judgement Day, birthday, hump day, Sabbath Day, all day long, night and day, the Day of Reckoning, payday, heyday, yes but, ah ah ah, all of that too, but but, this is, ah ah, something different today.

The sun is out, right now, today. Underlying love, Felipé,

MARCH 28, 2016 / HAPPY EASTER

We had a walk today and tapas afterward. That was our Easter dinner. A little unorthodox but yummy. The trail is drying out which is a welcome change. Fruit trees are blooming and just hoping the bees can get moving.

Tired after all this partying, a tough problem. Off to work tomorrow so have to get some shuteye. Just want to say Happy Easter.

Joyful loves, Felipé.

MARCH 31, 2016 / THE BEST THING THAT EVER HAPPENED TO ME

I had a new nurse, new to me, yesterday at the treatment center. We were having some great conversation about the great state of Iowa since that is where he is from and where I am going in a few weeks for the Julian Dubuque Film Festival. Yea, that was good. And then we wandered over into some heavier cancer talk after that and I said to him, with the proper disclaimer that it may sound weird but, cancer may be the best thing that ever happened to me. This is a big picture idea and one that I don't often share. But he said that he had heard that before which was heartening for me to hear. I wasn't totally out on a limb, as they say.

The disruption that this disease causes in all its facets, details and deeper inner meaning is earth shaking to the individual and their family. Somehow I saw it as a catalyst for change. Somehow with the help of some key mentors I was able to discern a path that led to the positive. So what I was saying to my nurse was that it put me on a path to this change to the positive. And that led to a total revamp of my inner being. It's all a strange happening but totally worth it.

So according to one of my mentors, "In non-medical terms God is keeping you alive to complete your mission." Yes, I have had the luxury of having a very lazy form of cancer and some crazy good medical attention, granting me time. I have had time to work on the movie and do this blog which is so special to me. Thanks for being here.

Love you, Felipé.

APRIL 8, 2016 / THRESHOLDS

My Rebecca just pointed out that I could write about "being in the chair" last night. Yea, OK. She belongs to a singing group that is called the Threshold Choir and it is a small group of gals that sing for people that are really sick or dying. And when they practice they like to have someone in the chair and then they gather around and practice new material. It just makes it more real for them if they have someone and last night it was my turn to be that someone. So, I got to practice too.

What was that old truckers' saying about keeping the shiny side up and the greasy side down? Love, Felipé.

APRIL 11, 2016 / AH, A NEW WEEK.

From this viewpoint at the very beginning of Monday the week seems like a big blank canvas stretched out ahead of us. We want to make some progress down the trail. That would be good. We know things will come flying at us from various places. It would be good to be nimble and able to dodge some of those and take on the ones worthy of working with. And we need protection from some things that are too big to handle. Getting the week down to bite sized chunks would be a good thing. Will we have enough energy left over to inspire ourselves and maybe someone else? Will we be able to use our creativity to come up with ideas that will be helpful that maybe didn't exist yesterday?

Always good, love, Felipé.

APRIL 13, 2016 / DAMN THE ROBINS, FULL SPEED AHEAD

I was outside early this AM and an active little worm was making his way across the cement cobblestones as I hurried over him but he caught my attention. Sometimes we are very vulnerable in our travels and there is not much to do about it is the story.

I was out on the highway yesterday and at one point was following a landscape truck with a load of rock. It wasn't a dump truck but a flatbed with a wooden tailgate. The rocks were two-man ones and piled up and their weight seemed to provide a certain security as they nestled together. The truck is going at sixty miles per hour and I am traveling at the same speed. All of a sudden the whole vision turned into a physics problem in my mind. What sort of disruption in this funky inertia would cause one of those boulders to wind up in my lap? It seemed like there were a lot of random factors waiting to pounce on the situation. It had an eerie resemblance to my life with cancer.

Needless to say I switched lanes and got ahead of him. I mean if you don't have to be there then don't, right? Not that hard. But I guess the general theme of this post today is our vulnerability and the willingness to keep going in spite of it. Damn the torpedoes, the robins, the two-man rocks and all that stuff, full speed ahead.

At the hospital and about to get my chemo treatment. Just saw Our Jennifer a minute ago. We haven't been able to keep the same schedules so I see her here randomly. Any break in the Groundhog Day-ness of it all is a good thing though. OK, time to go. Love Phil.

APRIL 15, 2016 / NEXT VENUE

I have a really solid idea for what I want to have on my tombstone, that is, if I have a tombstone. What do people have these days? Anyway, how about, "Still walking!" I wanted to get rid of the finality and get more to the idea of a bridge to another venue.

I was inspired by this story on FB about this woman that wanted to be laid out in her casket with a fork in her hand. And viewers would obviously have to ask about the curious thing and receive her message. All during her life her favorite time was when at the end of dinner, the announcement would be made to "hang onto your fork!" Nice, huh? Remember the anticipation of the coming of something sweet and special.

I don't think about death too much maybe because I died ten thousand times playing army as a kid. That's what boys did post World War Two, well in between getting run over by cars. And I was pointing this death thing out to my tumors the other day, saying, "Guys, you know that when I die you go too." I was trying to point out the obvious benefit of getting together and dragging this thing out as long as possible.

Well, that's my life today. But starting to think of packing for the next big venue--the great state of Iowa. But first, this is the day that the Lord has made, let us be grateful and rejoice in it! Big loves! Felipé!

APRIL 28, 2016 / MY CAMINO WENT THROUGH DUBUQUE, IOWA

The Dubuque area is known for its energy due to the presence of ley lines that run through the location. Ley lines are mysterious lines of energy that define certain spots on the earth in terms of their energy. I wish I could say more on that but am new to the term and the knowledge. Google it I guess.

I ran into amazing people there and they will pop up here I am sure as the days go by. Yea, and Phil's Camino went there and was received well. Maybe we recognized each other's energy? Hate to get too woo-woo here but can't help it.

The movie has a way of connecting people to the real feelings and turmoil of the cancer experience. It may dredge up memories of hard past experience in their own lives. It's useful in that way. And it gives a glimpse of hope for positive outcomes. It shows a pathway, a Camino.

And that Camino just went through Dubuque, Iowa. As Annie always reminds me, "We can't help ourselves!" It's a scary and comforting zone to be in.

Make it happen today, energetic love, Felipé.

MAY 6, 2016 / JUST BECAUSE . . .

My neighbor has a problem that is serious, it's not cancer but something else life-changing. Anyway, early on in the process of dealing with this disease he and a friend who also had the same or similar problem were biking and making jokes with each other about how many other bikers they were passing. You know, like if those people only knew how screwed up we are and we are still passing them. But somewhere along the line they realized that perhaps there was more to it and maybe those people had problems too. It is the realization like on the Camino when you get outside yourself and understand that everyone walking has a story.

The sun is out, the sky is blue and off I go, love again, Felipé.

May 8, 2016 / A Tear

Yea, well, I can weep at the drop of a hat these days but this really affected me this morning. Our beloved Father Marc, the priest at St. John Vianney Parish, is leaving for a new assignment. I guess it has been seven years that he has been here. But he was my first priest. I gave him a hug and told him I would miss him.

I think it was General deGaulle who said on his retirement that no one is indispensable. That stands for us too, of course. What is the positive side of that? Well we, ego animals that we are, think that we have to do every darn thing all by ourselves. But in reality we are an important part of the Cloud of Believers, the Flow of Pilgrims, and the Communion of Saints and we don't have to do it all. We are not supposed to do it all. We are an indispensable part of but not indispensable. I think that makes sense.

Yup, time to go. Happy Mother's Day to All the Moms! indispensable love, Felipé.

May 9, 2016 / Ah, Blue Sky

It's been a really cool morning and I built a fire in the stove, which is unusual for May. It's been overcast but just this minute spotted some blue up there. It's the usual back and forth of spring weather. Was working on the corn yesterday and am ready to plant. A couple of more days for the soil to warm some more would be good. Farmer John in Iowa tells me that his corn is up there. Well, we'll catch up.

We have a morning walk here in a little over an hour. Maybe I'll have some company, feel like company today. Yesterday I dedicated the walk to a friend of Catalina's, Father Michael, OP who got a recent diagnosis. Ah. I did a rosary and put rocks on the pile for the dear man.

And yes, Catalina is coming up here over Memorial Day weekend to be with us. She is in the art history department at one of the Catholic colleges in Berkley. Anyway, she has been so interested in Phil's Camino the trail for a long time now. She has written a magazine article about it and now has plans for a book, pretty amazing. And that's why she is coming up, to walk the trail, meet the family and interview us for this project. I'm honored.

Little did I know when I built the trail back is 2013 that it would have the impact that it has had. Little did I know that there is historical precedent for the activity of building facsimiles of bigger things, far away things maybe. People in the past have made things to remind them of something bigger or have made things to participate in to get an idea of a larger experience. This is the reason for Phil's Camino in the first place. Sure it was to be an exercise program for my cancer rehabilitation but it was also a way for me to have an inspirational experience, simultaneously.

So, the freedom and downright joy of walking outside in Nature, with friends, with interesting conversation, with thoughts of St. James and the Spanish trail, with prayers being said is so astounding. Annie O'Neil helped me a lot at this point with her visit and with her book, *Everyday Camino with Annie*. It was a rich, heady mix of ingredients. I found something valuable and it worked for me, which was the important thing.

OK, glad you came. Come walk sometime soon. Love, Felipé.

May 11, 2016 / The Best Compliment Ever

It's my every other Wednesday treatment day at Swedish Cancer Institute. It's my 69th chemo treatment, gosh really? And the last few months I have been in this rut of thinking my visits here were looking like the repeating day in the movie *Groundhog Day*. Remember? Yea, it was my own little pitiful movie, "Treatment Day."

Anyway, walking through the parking lot this morning I decided that that had to go, go far away. I needed to remember that this was treatment for me, for my benefit and the alternative of not having treatment would bring radical changes to my well being. So, I made the old attitude adjustment, right there in the time that it took to walk across the lot, no muss no fuss.

Then inside shortly afterward a woman came up to me and asked, "How come you are so happy?" Like here you are with cancer and you're happy. Aren't you supposed to be glum? I was lost for words at first but realized that it was an incredible compliment. I was happy on the inside and it was spilling out. Nice. Thank you.

So, yea, life at the hospital, trying to make it fun. How can that be? Well, here for instance, I just absconded with an AARP mag from the waiting room and what does it say on the cover? It says, "Best Sex Ever! We Show You How Page 52." OK then, groovy, this could be better than the sixties.

And one nurse I just learned was an English Major so I am hitting her up for help with the blog, gramer and speeling stuff. And she has a great singing voice and we decided that there needs to be a musical called Cancer Treatment Center. Maybe the least likely place in the world where you think that there would be a musical, bursts into song! We need to work on this. This could be the next big project after *Phil's Camino*, the documentary. We have a vision!

So, life goes happily on and love you, Felipé.

May 13, 2016 / Fra Angelico

Our Catherine and I walked Phil's Camino yesterday morning. We did our usual three laps engrossed in our usual great conversation. Then we decided to say the rosary together as we walked another lap (.88 km) because the layout of one lap is in fact a giant rosary. We walk and say the prayer and know where we are by the six bird feeders which mark the six places that "Our Fathers" are said. Although sometimes I use the actual rosary as I walk, increasingly I am just using the walk as a rosary which has a great feel as long as I don't get distracted by too much along the way.

So, we said it out loud and I added a few explanations here and there, so our timing didn't always work out, but we got it done just the same. With a little more practice we will work though the prayer and there will be just the right amount of time and space to say it and that is with no frills, just the basics as I learned out of the Magnificat *Rosary Companion.*

This little beautiful book, the *Companion,* has reproductions of famous frescos (paintings done on wet plaster) mostly all by a man known to us as Fra Angelico. They mark various important places in the prayer. So my memory has captured these images and they appear to me at the right points "along the prayer." So, the trail, the six bird feeders and the mental images work together to give a beautiful new way to experience this age-old prayer. Works for me anyway.

So, I just wanted to bring you up on the current news on Fra Angelico (1387—1455), which needed doing. We need to dust him off here at Caminoheads and put him back to work. OK, got to get ready for my city trip and the rest of my day. Dusty loves, Felipé.

MAY 15, 2016 / FELIPÉ, WHERE ARE WE?

Yes, we are walking on Phil's Camino and yesterday we made the halfway mark on our second trek "across Spain." Since the coming of spring we have gotten more visitors and pilgrims from out of town. So, it is here for you when you get a chance to be in the neighborhood.

Physically the trail here is in good shape. The winter standing water is gone and most days it is warm and dry. Might need boots for a morning walk when the grass is wet from dew.

MAY 18, 2016 / STUFF HAPPENING

We know by now the feeling that we are on the right track when things around us turn synchronistic. It's the Camino feeling that we are in the groove with the flow of the universe, that everything is moving in the same direction and at the same speed and everything has a kinship. Things are all on the same page, including us. We know what that feels like, not that we are always there by any means but we know what that is.

So getting that far is significant. And it is not something that we can take credit for, like it is an accomplishment. Maybe we can take credit for being open, being outside ourselves, being willing to learn. But I'm just saying that it is something that we are gifted, more or less. We are sort of privileged to see.

So, I am identifying something else now that I would like to try and describe. It is to me a Camino/Cancer/Catholic happening. In my world it is showing up in all places, not often but I am just realizing that it is universal in my world. I first noticed it in the Camino area, then in the Catholic area and now yesterday in the Cancer area. It is something basic, something that operates below the point at where those things separate.

The basic concept as I see it is that I am this guy walking around in the mud who at some point starts doing something significant. What is the difference there? I always seem to start in the trenches but with enough time, effort and looking come across something that is significant but really just there for the finding. But somehow on my own I can't put it in perspective. I need someone with a broader knowledge to tell me, hey, that thing that you just found, that's something.

Maybe it is just how things work in the universe, hey? It has less to do with me and you and more to do with things as they are. We can't take credit for that. We are just privileged to see it.

So, after I had gotten Phil's Camino, the trail here on Vashon Island, up and running and I was walking "across Spain" and trying to have that experience who should show up but Annie O'Neil. And what does she say but "This really looks familiar." "Aren't I writing a book on this very thing?" And our ensuing conversation opens up to me that, yes this is something, something significant.

And Catalina Barush, the art historian, comes along and hears about how I am walking in the mud and trying to have an experience and says this is something that people have been doing for a long time. People build small replicas of situations or places to have the experience of the real time and place. In other words, you have something.

So those are two examples from the Camino sector. And sister Joyce, my spiritual advisor will do this in the Catholic realm. I will come across some "muddy idea" and she will clarify it for me and say yes that is something. Somehow it is almost like I have to learn it the hard way. I have to find that nugget by panning for it.

And yesterday this same thing started happening with Dr. Zucker, who I call my psychologist, but whose actual designation is Cancer Rehabilitation Specialist, which somehow feels too cumbersome to me to say. Well, maybe I was just starting to realize it and maybe it has been going on for a while. But somehow my observations from the mud about Cancer were having a great conversation with his knowledge on the subject. In other words I was starting to find interesting things that seemed useful to him. Stuff that I was exploring on this topic stimulated our conversation, brought maybe new ways to look at the same stuff. I don't know exactly what was going on but we were having a good time.

What I am trying to describe is perhaps synchronicity. Somehow all these examples are instances where we arrived at the same place at the same time but from different angles. And it seems exciting when that happens.

Thanks for bearing with me on this. Long and involved but perhaps important. As always, love,

MAY 19, 2016 / TERRI, SUSAN AND JACK

Our local newspaper the *Beachcomber* comes in to the ranch on Wednesday. This a.m. I opened our copy for a perusal of local happenings. The front page had two stories, one about the Japanese internment back in the 1940s and a story about health care on the Island. There was plenty of other stuff in there, sports, article about gray whales, upcoming music. Eventually I got to the obits.

I read Terri's obituary because I knew her. Our kids were on the same baseball teams and we had other connections, small island. She was a sweetheart, loved by all, mom, caterer, lunch lady, community volunteer. She succumbed to a "fast growing cancer."

Then I read Susan's. She was our daughter's Spanish teacher in high school. She had limited vision and had a guide dog named Sloan. I don't think I ever met her although I am sure Rebecca had, being a substitute teacher, probably taught her class on occasion. Yea, so she succumbed to carcinoid cancer. I don't know what that is exactly but a cancer.

Then Jack, don't think I ever met him, worked in the hospitality business. He looked like a fun guy, "He threw a party!" Jack was diagnosed with brain cancer in 2008 and died on May 8th this year.

That's it: three obituaries, three neighbors, three cancers, three deaths. Seems pretty grim. We will mourn and go on, as always. That's what we do. But at the same time cancer reinforces its hold on us, on our mind and spirit. A seeming juggernaut, incessantly coming at us, taking young and old.

I sit thinking about this and watching the clouds go by the window. Am I learning something from these clouds? They are broken letting the sun through occasionally. Is there room perhaps in all this cancer glum for something different, for some sunshine occasionally. I am thinking about "Cancer — the Musical!" Is there room for sunbreaks in our fear? Do we get to take a break? Can I make you smile in the midst of your "battle against cancer." Would it be like a USO show with Bob Hope for the shell-shocked troops, this musical?

Well, this is what I am up to this morning. We are walking in half an hour. I am putting the paper down. Love you, Felipé.

May 20, 2016 / We Will Survive Our Own Glitches

Yesterday I told My Rebecca that I "was beyond mistakes." I have been thinking about that since. What the heck did I mean by that? Was it just a casual remark or was it something substantial?

A friend just said that she was teetering on the verge of trying to do too much and making mistakes in the process. I know that feeling, that place. We all get there at times, juggling too many balls.

Then there is chemotherapy for me. Running gallons of "who knows what" through my brain can't be all that good for my memory, organizational skills and etc. I have to interject that my beloved docs at the hospital know exactly what the "who knows whats" are and are geniuses with my treatment. That I know and trust. It is I that am foggy on the topic. See, foggy is a good word for my seeing. I think that in some way it is a gift really. I give up the detail for the ability to see better the bigger picture. But, getting back to mistakes, now I am more apt to make mistakes in the details of things.

Yea, so? Well, there is age—that means that more mistakes of a certain kind are going to happen. I am just not as sharp as in years past. Right, true, but what about this statement that I "was beyond mistakes"? I am seeing it as an attitude that yes, I make mistakes but so what? They are in the minor category in the big scheme of things. I don't have the time or energy to dwell on them. I have to keep walking, metaphysically speaking, and guess what? Something is going to pop up soon to occupy me and I must get ready to do a good job with it.

So, I am looking on my own mistakes in a more loving manner. I am being more patient with myself. It won't be the end of the world, this mistake, this glitch. I will survive my own glitches in the end. And I think this is spilling over to include everyone that I am coming in contact with. I am more patient with others. I will survive their glitches and they will survive mine. We will survive our glitches together and maybe learn to thrive in the end. Let's work on that.

Time to go. Love, Felipé

MAY 23, 2016 / BLOG-O-MATIC

I remember coming back from Spain and everyone and their brother wanting to know how it went. Maybe the question is in the wrong tense. Instead of "How was your Camino?" or "How was Spain?" it should be "How is your Camino?" or maybe even "How is Spain?" The point is that it is ongoing, like the saying, "When you get to Santiago your Camino actually begins."

Oh look it's 0908 and I am late for my walk. Later, love, Felipé.

MAY 30, 2016 / WHERE ARE WE FELIPÉ?

We have been walking at the ranch and we are at the town of Calzadilla de los Hermanillos, a little west of Sahagún. Sahagún is the town that pilgrims think of as half way. So, the trail is in good shape with a dry surface and the grass is all mowed.

MAY 31, 2016 / BEAUTY ALTERS ME, ONCE MORE

Sort of lost in thought right now. I'm amazed at people. We meet each other as we travel down our individual paths, our individual direction. Sometime we are together for a while, sometimes we meet on occasion and sometimes maybe only once. But we observe each other and come away with a message.

I am noticing how some folks seem to move forward down the trail seemingly fearing everything that comes up or might possibly come up. What a burden that must be. Although perhaps it is not everything that they fear. Maybe there are areas that they feel comfortable in, I don't know.

And then there are other individuals that I marvel at that move through the environment with such ease, seemly fearing nothing. They are always ready for the next thing no matter what that might be. I'm inspired by them.

Off to my Tuesday. Paradise switch is on here on Vashon Island. Find the fearless, love, Felipé.

June 13, 2016 / Ah Felipé, Are You Sure?

Phil's Camino–the Trail just keeps on a-going. We had a nice walk and tapas today on a beautiful afternoon. We are doing our best to keep the Camino going in our hearts and minds.

So, we finished our 504th lap today logging in 444 km total. We are still on the Meseta, the wide open central plain of Spain, although near the end. Coming up is the town of Mansilla de las Mulas and beyond, the city of Léon.

June 23, 2016 / We have a flower!

I just wanted to report that one flower is growing in our guerrilla garden venture along the entrance ramp to I-5. Well, it's a flower plant to be precise and well, it doesn't look like a weed anyway, which isn't very precise. It doesn't look like California Poppy but must be the other flower which is Calendula. Anyway, I watered it this morning as I passed it, which is tricky. I had a choice of trying to photograph or water the new plant. So, I hit it with a bottled water. A big white truck waited behind me while I tended the little guy.

Maybe, Jennifer would be happy about that since she was in on the hatching of the idea to beautify that little part of the urban world. She has been in hospice, the dear. Prayers of peace for her.

So, this is Thursday and I am back at the ranch. I have learned that Our Jennifer passed away Tuesday evening. Bill, one our regular walkers, was with her about an hour before and I got the word from him. She almost made it to the Fourth of July. We had this thing about the Fourth. I remember we were all down on the beach in the dark watching the fireworks last year and she was happy to have been able to make it that far. So, we had almost another year to blow bubbles, plant flowers and sneak wine into the hospital.

Peace to you Jennifer. You are in our prayers. You are in our thoughts. Drink a glass of the heavenly wine for us and our travels. And we will drink a toast to you when we gather for tapas.

So, that's the way it is today. We will regroup and go on, having learned by the experience. Off to work, love you, Felipé.

June 24, 2016 / Pilgrim On

Our hearts and minds are with Jennifer these days. She was with us here for a little over a year. She walked the trail as long as she could, Phil's Camino–the trail. She has a cameo in Phil's Camino—the film as she walks the trail. She was my chemo buddy for numerous visits to Swedish Cancer Institute. We had fun with that, attacking the gloom with Cancer Commando bravery and élan. Yup.

Well, what to say. The only thing that makes sense to me at the moment is that we have a flower growing out of a pile of refuse in Seattle along the freeway wasteland that wouldn't be there except for the company of our *compañera*, Jennifer. Rest in Peace dear one.

Off to the hospital is coming up on my Camino this morning. Time to shower. Love you guys, Felipé. x

June 25, 2016 / A Western Tanager

Yea, a male bird sat on our lilac bush just outside the kitchen table. These are very pretty and maybe more so because they are rare here. Always refreshing to look upon beauty. And a break from other things.

The best to you, talk with you soon, love, Felipé.

June 26, 2016 / Father Marc's Last Day

Well, not his last day but his last day here on the Rock, on Vashon being our priest. I think it will be seven years for him. And I think that I have been there three years with him. The high point was when he came over to bless Phil's Camino way back when. Thank you, Father Marc, you were a part of it all here at this outpost.

I'm pretty deep in the fog of my chemo weekend. I expect it to be bad and here it is. Partly it is the side effect of the chemicals and partly this time it is the aftermath of Jennifer's death. I got it all wrapped together here at once. Your prayers of peace for us would be welcome.

OK, time to tidy up and get off to church. Hoping for swimmingly, although giddy would do just fine. Love you all, Felipé.

June 27, 2016 / It Is The Most Perfect Day

Right here, right now, it is the most perfect day. It is the day that we dream about for three quarters of the year. I think that I will skip all the words today and just be here.

Algood, alperfect, pass the sunscreen, love, Felipé.

June 28, 2016 / Monday Night

I know it's Tuesday morn but need to report on last evening. My Rebecca had the idea to have Wiley and Henna over every Monday for dinner. Well, tapas and dinner. It is brilliant really, like Monday Night Football brilliant. It is that extra five percent that can be squeezed out of the weekend that you are able to harvest, the last sweet glow.

It was so pretty yesterday and it went right on 'til dark. The mosquitos got a little thick but all the same. All the same it was a day that stopped everyone in their tracks around here, something to be thankful for.

Besides I was able to grab Henna to help me on my iPad. She seems to be able to navigate so swiftly through things where I feel like I have eight left feet. Thank you, Henna.

Then Wiley had in the last week heard about the apparition of Mother Mary in Guadalupe, Mexico and was all enthused by the story. And it is a huge story. I am searching for maybe a DVD on the story for us to watch.

Well, a nice memory to savor, our Monday evening. The best to you, Love, Felipé.

JULY 3, 2016 / SUNDAY ON VASHON

Earlier I was out in the driveway waiting for Catherine to come and pick me up in her pickup and transport me to church for eight o'clock Mass. I was a little early or she was a little late so I stood there in the quiet. I was appreciating the peace of the neighborhood and I could hear Catherine's truck from a long way off coming to get me. It wasn't traffic noise, it was one vehicle noise. How lucky am I/are we to have such a sanctuary as this?

Friday, when our lovely Chinese guests were here, they were saying that they lived there in Beijing on the twentieth floor of an apartment building. As I stood in the quiet I was trying to imagine what that would be like. Our lives are so horizontal here. All of our space that we are able to roam around in it seems so luxurious, I am going to stop taking that for granted.

Our new priest "came ashore" today, Father David. He seems so enthusiastic about being with us and being on Vashon. And Mass went well and I didn't have any trouble hearing him with his big voice. So, so far so good, swimmingly even! Father David, yea.

After Mass we went to town and did a little shopping for tapas later. Then we tailgated with our coffee and donut from the supermarket. Nobody does that in the busy parking lot except us. My insurance agent calls that lot the most dangerous place on Vashon. People rush in and rush out with their charcoal and meat but stop to say hi as they pass, or once in a while to dilly-dally with us as we sit and talk about the Sacrament of Reconciliation and what it will be like to be mano-a-mano with Father David. Catherine has named this Tailgate Theology, I'll take it, I like it. Suddenly it seems sort of luxurious even.

So, another great blog post wrapped up. Time to get out to the corn and get in the race with the weeds. Even that seems somewhat luxurious at the moment. Huh. Well, that's it here at Raven Ranch. Thinking of you, holding you in prayer, Love, Spacious Felipé. x

JULY 4, 2016 / A RED, WHITE AND BLUE HOLIDAY

Just got in from the 0900 walk, under an overcast sky. Could shower occasionally today which would please the fire department on this Fourth of July. This would have been a good day to walk in Spain, cloudy is merciful in July and August.

Had a nice visit from one of my old buddies yesterday. He was up here on a Seattle visit from Palm Springs. He caught *Phil's Camino* there at the recent festival. So he was pumped about it and had to make it over to walk with me. Thanks Eric.

Well, you Americans, keep it safe today, don't do anything goofy with those fireworks. We're not doing any personal explosives here at Raven Ranch, we got the horses which aren't big on booms. Off to the harbor tonight to watch the professional show with friends who live down there at the water. We will be missing Our Jennifer who almost made this far. She made it to last year's Fourth and was there with us. Happy Trails Jennifer.

God Bless America, as the song goes. And love you no matter where you are, Felipé.

July 6, 2016 / Small Starts

Today is my big treatment day and I made it to the waiting room with extra time. Never know how the traffic is going to go so I have to allow extra time. My Rebecca came in today with me.

The traffic being so light we didn't have the opportunity to dawdle at the flower project along the freeway entrance, we just caught a glimpse of THE flower. Yea, and the good news is it is 10-12 inches high and looking like something! In another two weeks maybe there will be a bloom. Until then it is getting sunshine and above average rainfall on its little head.

So, it's Jennifer's flower really. And it is a statement in its amazing singularity. We threw literally hundreds of flower seeds at those three mounds of soil. It is kind of a junkyard of gardens but stuff grows occasionally apparently. A little magic in the wasteland.

My name is going to be called any second now to go and talk to Dr. Gold. Have a great day, make the most of it! Love, Felipé.

July 7, 2016 / New Personality In The Mix

I am walking momentarily and I never know who will show up. Sometimes it's a crowd and sometimes I'm with Mother Mary alone.

Alperfect all the time, love you, Felipé

July 10, 2016 / Big Day At Phil's Camino

We will be walking under unsure skies later today at 1600. The Camino calls. Two small groups are coming to be with us. How great that we get to do this. How great that the Camino calls.

It was our second Sunday with Father David at the helm at St. John Vianney's this morning. The padre preached on the Good Samaritan theme. Who is our neighbor and how do we relate to him/her? He talked a lot about Mr. Rogers of TV fame. Maybe someone doesn't know who he was. He had a show for years and years geared toward kids that stressed respect toward one's self and one's neighbor. Matter of fact the show was called Mr. Rogers' Neighborhood. Fred Rogers was a Presbyterian Minister and this was his calling.

OK, need to keep moving. You are the best! Love, Felipé.

July 12, 2016 / Breakfast Outside

Well I didn't have to walk 5 km to get my café con leche this morning but sitting outside with my breakfast and coffee is bringing back memories of those times. There is not a day that goes by that I don't have some memory of my Camino in Spain come rushing back. Still think that it was a vision of heaven.

The overcast is breaking up and patches of blue sky are appearing overhead. I am off to archery camp again to make that happen. Wiley and I got things started yesterday; I'm always glad to be past that as there is always a lot of organizational stuff to get out of the way. Now we can get on to the fun stuff!

Well, have a splendid day. Let yourself be inspired, love, Felipé.

JULY 19, 2016 / THE CAMINO CALLS

"Men wanted for hazardous journey. Small wages. Bitter cold. Long months of complete darkness. Constant danger. Safe return doubtful. Honour and recognition in case of success."

Those were like magic words as five thousand guys answered that newspaper add. This was 1914 and Sir Ernest Shackleton was getting a crew together for an Antarctic expedition. What a wordsmith. I think I'll put that up on the fridge.

Well, the Camino is not quite that harrowing these days, hopefully. Could change the bitter cold to bitter heat though. But seriously, pilgrimage in the old days was sort of like that. I am reading some material that Catalina just sent to me on the topic. I am supposed to be on an interfaith panel on pilgrimage down in LA and I want to make sure that I am up to speed, so I have been studying.

One other little factoid that I uncovered was the number of old pilgrimage shells that have shown up in Europe. A cherished memento of the trip may be in the family archives. Is that species of shellfish which we know as the Camino shell common on the Atlantic coast of Spain and not the Mediterranean? There is something for someone to investigate. Do we have a clamologist on board?

We have a walk and tapas this afternoon, a party, a sendoff, before my treatment day tomorrow. But before that I have to get out to the corn and continue the weeding operation. I promised myself that I would get that slicked up before the trip to Southern California.

OK, constant danger loves, Felipé.

JULY 27, 2016 / A FOGGY MORNING

The film is doing fantastically well. To me the lovely thing has a life of its own as it does what it does to audiences hither and yon. If I am not wrong we started walking in France two years ago tomorrow. And Todd our videographer and Jessica our unit director and editor were there then, our newlyweds to be, documenting this great new adventure.

I think I will walk a lap around Phil's Camino and say my rosary for the world. We continue with confidence, love you, as always, Alperfect, SoBlessed, Felipé. x

JULY 30, 2016 / SATURDAY MORNING

Something really quite amazing happened yesterday at the Royal Theater. It was our second showing of *Phil's Camino* and was in a smaller venue at the Royal. The day before on our first day we pretty much filled the larger venue with maybe a hundred folks, maybe a few more. Anyway, this time as we got our eyes adjusted to the dark there was only one person there. One! Yea, right smack dab in the center seat was this one and only guy.

It was an Aaaarrrrgggghhhh moment but I got absorbed in the film as usual and forgot about it temporarily. So, the film got done and Annie and I came in close to our precious viewer to do the Q&A. But this one guy was totally on fire. Somehow surprisingly he filled the whole theater with his voice and personality. This seemed like a pilgrimage for him to be there to do this one thing, and nothing was going to get in his way.

He, and I don't have his name even, ran a hair salon and there played the movie, *The Way*, on a continuous loop for his clients. He said he probably watched it twelve hundred times. We had a copy of the Camino documentary for him to take with him to change things up. He had walked in Spain and was totally on fire about any and all things Camino. What a time we had fielding his questions. And somehow I have a feeling that we will see him again.

This was a real lesson for me and another case of one vibrant person having the ability to change a situation for the better. Hats off to you pilgrim, you taught us something important and brightened our day! Well, today hoping we will do better on attendance. Also, I am to meet Dr. Asher who is our good friend Dr. Zucker's Californian counterpart. We are scheduled to both be on a panel about cancer and exercise. OK, more fun, right?

So the trail goes on here in the Southland. I get my chance to do my own freeway driving today and looking forward to the Padres game tonight! OK, off we go, love you as always, Felipé.

JULY 31, 2016 / BEFORE THE WEDDING

At Sherie's in San Diego for the night. Just getting up to get the day going. First a shower then the quest for coffee. It's that marine overcast sky out, I recognize it.

We are off to ten o'clock Mass at Mission Basilica San Diego de Alcalá, I think the original mission in SD. Then we are off to the wedding which is late afternoon.

But the catch up on yesterday is that the Padres got a walk-off homer last night and we watched that with all of Todd and Jess's family and friends in attendance, as part of the wedding celebrations.

The screening went fabulous with maybe thirty in the small venue. The panel discussion was amazing with Dr. Arash Asher from Cedars Sinai Hospital. What a great addition to our group of pilgrims and artists. Here is the main idea that he brought to the table: connectivity equals wellbeing. And that is what he was seeing in our film. He cited a study comparing data from 1980 to now in which people were asked if they felt isolated. In other words, do you have anyone to confide in? So, earlier it was one in ten that didn't and now it is one in four. In terms of cancer rehab, connectivity is important and perhaps one of the major factors in my success.

Just got back from the mission which had a truly amazing service. I wept at communion and after communion there was a quirky occurrence where people applauded because it was so beautiful. It seemed perfectly appropriate but I'd never seen it before.

Well, we are driving to La Jolla in a few minutes. Todd and Jessica getting married after falling in love on the Camino when we walked in 2014. Yea, connectivity in action.

See you tomorrow, love, San Diego Felipé.

August 1, 2016 / The Wedding

The big day was yesterday in the late afternoon and twilight of lovely La Jolla, California. Todd and Jessica were married in a beautiful service. It was their day. In a few words of explanation, they were on the Camino with Kelly, Rick and myself in 2014. Todd the videographer and Jessica the unit director fell in love there somewhere along the Way. It is wonderful that somehow Phil's Camino played a part in this as we put them in the same place at the same time. And it was a beautiful place and a beautiful time. Buen Camino to them as they go onward!

My Rebecca and I drove last night back to Burbank after the celebration. I didn't have anything but water at the wedding, which was tough. But I was prepping for the journey. We made it in two and a half hours as opposed to four and a half on Saturday. So that was good. But at one point I mistakenly took an exit instead of staying on the Five. Off into the unknown. We didn't have any GPS gizmos on and was worried as I had no idea where this "the" was going to lead. Feeling totally lost in the wilderness I had that sinking feeling, when all of a sudden here is Quint and Annie alongside of us waving to follow them. What?? Where the heck did they come from?

It was the Freeway Angels appearing when we were in need, we strangers in a strange land. They led us all the way back to where we needed to be to get to Burbank, and Bob's your uncle. Little did we know that they had been following us for an hour and a half. So, there you go.

Well, that's it as of the moment. Goodbye to California!

As always, Monday love, Felipé.

August 3, 2016 / The Cancer Commandos And The Connectivity Machine

Sounds like an exciting thing, maybe a book for teens. But it is us the Cancer Commandos rocking the boat again. Couldn't we just be satisfied being plain old cancer patients like normal folks?

Actually I need to credit Dana with the title, which came out of our walk yesterday on Phil's Camino. We were talking about the notion that being well connected with others seems to be vital to one's wellbeing. And this came from the panel discussion with Dr. Asher in LA. But to back up even more, Erica from Austin has been beating this drum for a while now. So, somewhere on our walk yesterday we talked about Phil's Camino being a connectivity machine, being a way to really be with folks. Of course the Camino in Spain does the same.

At the treatment center right now practicing on connectivity with a chemo machine. I have two more hours to go, then back to Vashon.

Good to be connected to you all, Felipé.

AUGUST 9, 2016 / THIRD TRY

Sometimes when I write this blog things are clear and other times I need several starts to make it happen. Today we have a little shaky start but let's see what happens. It would be nice if we had it all figured out all the time.

Early this morning I was doing my meditation, my brand of it. At one point I was visualizing a warm toasty sweet spirituality seeping into my body cell by cell like my all too well-known chemotherapy. I was being saturated by the good stuff in a way that I couldn't ignore. It wasn't just an intellectual knowing it was an inside-out knowing, an every-cell knowing.

Chemotherapy seems like such a cruel and unusual place. It is always so hard to relate to it. Yes, it is keeping me alive. Yes, it is the state of the art. Yes and yes and yes but what a beast. What a strange bed partner. Hopefully twenty years from now we can throw it all away for something better and more humane. But for now we are stuck with it, with him, with her. I need you but baby you are sooo weird!

Ah. But this morning I was using the idea of chemo in a new and unusual way to bring me some other good, some additional good. So, that's a good thing right? But also what occurs to me with this conversation about internalizing the Spirit is that really it has two parts. One is so extremely basic that I miss it, and that is that it is already there. No matter what my consciousness believes or is aware of, the Spirit already saturates everything everywhere at every time no problem. Two, it is really the awareness of the Spirit that I had saturating every one of my cells this morning. They are two different things but related.

Well, ever onward down the road we go. The Camino, the Soul Train is bound for glory, love you, Felipé.x

AUGUST 10, 2016 / THE TAPAS TABLE

Twenty-seven years ago Rebecca went away for a three-day weekend to a retreat or workshop, can't remember which. Tesia, a nine-year-old, and Dad were here tending to things. We had a great idea to build a picnic table to surprise Mom on her return. We got out the drawing board that I used at forestry school with the T-square and pencils and stuff and drew up a plan. It was going to be big and solid, no dinky tippy thing.

And off we went to the lumber yard to pick out the Western Red Cedar planks, a hundred dollars' worth. And we built it, just her and me, daughter and father, no distractions. And it looked exactly just like the plan, thirty inches tall with the seats eighteen and a generous ten feet long. Yes, there it is!

And now twenty-seven years later, after being out all those winters in the rain and all those summers in the sun the table needs help. It needs its relay partner to take the baton. So, this time Wiley and I got to build the table with the same plans that somehow I still had. Wiley got to participate this time when last time he was busy growing inside Mom and gone for the weekend.

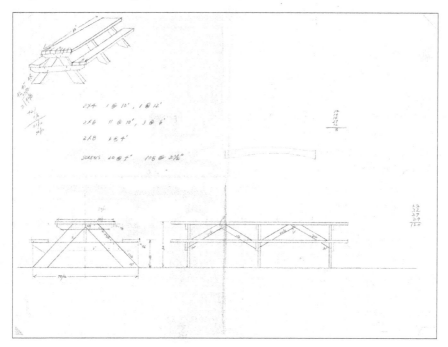

Yea, the story of the tapas table, somehow not two tables but always one. Not old and new but one taking over for the other. Not just death and birth but a certain continuation. The idea of the tapas table with connectivity at its heart being one thing going on into the future.

Yea, and yesterday Patty was here to walk and after to have tapas and wine on the new Western Red Cedar planks. Tapas go on. She is such a dear and a great new friend for us here at Phil's Camino. We were celebrating life yesterday in the warmth of the afternoon knowing that she was to be off to cancer surgery today. We are grateful for our times of lightness in all this. If the table was built for this one event then it would have been worth it. We laughed, we cried, we found out we talked the same language.

OK then. You are all beautiful, love, Felipé.x

AUGUST 13, 2016 / WAS READING

If you say that I started the Camino in Saint Jean Pied de Port you are saying it simply, basically, this is where my boots first hit the ground. When I watch *Phil's Camino* I am always moved by the scene of Kelly and myself on our first day. "OK, boys and girls, up an over the Pyrenees." Yea, we all have a survival story about the first day. And that gives us a way to look at the Camino. To me that was mostly about conquering or overcoming.

And if I think about my Camino starting when I got to St. James with all that conquering and overcoming it is different. And when I got that far it was the Camino that actually conquered me, that overcame me. And it was acknowledging that fact and now the question of what do I do with that? That was the beginning of the whole reentry phase which was a definite journey. And I am still on that journey.

But what happens when I think that it started with my intention to walk? I don't remember an exact moment on that. But maybe three things were in place. One, I had seen *The Way* and that was fermenting in there somewhere. Two, I was already walking some as I said my daily rosary. Three, I needed an exercise program that I could live with for my cancer rehab. And that had requirements of being compatible with my rehab program, being outdoors, being close by and having no machines. Somewhere in there was the intention.

But it was more at that point than "just wanting to exercise" as I said in the film. There I think I was answering the question, "Did you think that this was training for going to Spain?" Obviously, there was more going on here at Phil's Camino the trail than exercise. I was out to try and capture the experience somehow or at least to taste it.

Yup, that's the way it seems. I like all three of those ways of looking at it. It all encourages some thinking and soul searching.

OK, here I go to get on with Saturday. Always good to be with you, Camino loves, Felipé.x

AUGUST 17, 2016 / GETTING THROUGH THE DOOR

One of the things that make it easier are all the people that I have fun with here. Doctors, nurses, assistants, receptionists are my friends and fellow walkers on this trail. We have great conversations and buoy each other up. If it weren't for that I would be in trouble.

Best to you today, love, Felipé.x

AUGUST 22, 2016 / IN THE COOL OF THE MORN

"The first man who actually measured the earth was a poet. The very idea of any man going out and taking the girth of the planet he lives on (and sometimes gets lost on) is in itself poetic. Wherever did he get the notion it could even be done? And just how did he do it? Didn't it take a lot of apparatus, higher mathematics, and celestial engineering? Here if anywhere, scientific curiosity mixes with poetic wonderment and they become the same thing."

I remember vividly browsing in a secondhand store and opening a book randomly to that paragraph. How in the world could one guy be so lucky as to stumble across something like that? It doesn't say much but it says a lot.

This is the way chapter three opens in *Mapping* by David Greenhood. He is writing about Eratosthenes who was a resident of the ancient city of Alexandria. He got it in his head that he could do this thing, measure the diameter of the earth and he did it with amazing accuracy, sort of in his backyard, well in 500 miles anyway. The book goes on to explain the method and calculations but we aren't going there, fascinating as that is; read the book.

What is important here is the idea, the fact that an individual can have a vision and act on it and accomplish something quite amazing. And not really an ego sort of thing but maybe closer to a contribution sort of thing. How do we rise above all the commotion of our lives and neighborhoods, so full of drama, to find a vision that is creative, different, helpful, inspiring? Are we capable of coming up with things on our own? Doesn't it take organizations with resources, facilities and backing?

This whole notion of this possibility has been immensely inspirational to me. It is the sort of spirit of how Phil's Camino came to be perhaps. There is a line in a Mary Chapin Carpenter song, "Couldn't it happen?" Well, couldn't it?

All this really got started this morning with reading *Sabbath Moments* blog by Terry Hershey my neighbor and buddy. Last week he had a story about a young Iraqi woman who competed in an Olympic swimming event and came in 28th. Yea? Well, she recently escaped from Turkey across to one of the Greek islands with a group in a small motor boat. Along the way the motor conks out and she and a few others jump in and swim the boat to Greece. And this week he had a story about an Iraqi man, a cellist who came out on the street and played shortly after a car bomb went off and killed a bunch of innocents. The swimming to Greece to deliver the boat and the playing the cello even while the dust settled were beautiful examples of this ability to envision and act.

OK, 471 words, long winded. Thanks Terry, thanks David, thanks Eratosthenes, thanks Iraqis for inspiring us. Love you all out there in the big world, Felipé.

AUGUST 23, 2016 / AHH

I find it very freeing to be out in nature to be able to be outside myself there. That is what I am feeling right now sitting here listening and looking out. So great to be able to give myself a break.

A bevy of cars go by, ferry traffic. But what I am seeing out here in the distance is the fecundity in the plant world right now. The hawthorn, pear and apple trees are so loaded with fruit that they are sagging and look distorted. This is the time of year when main branches break and whole trees can be destroyed by their own success. A lesson here maybe.

Be good to one another, love, Felipé.

AUGUST 24, 2016 / OUR GROUP

We had an historic walk and tapa time yesterday here at Phil's Camino. All the old Camino walkers showed up: Kelly, Rick and Maryka. Rick's wife Carole Lynn was here too. The only addition I could think of is Mary Margaret, but that will have to wait for now.

Maryka was last here I don't know when, it would have to be at least a year. It was so great to have her again. We did all the usual stuff plus watched the film; it was the first time she had seen it. She put her stamp of approval on the film and our whole Phil's Camino scene.

I so want to get Maryka together with Catalina our official unofficial art historian of the situation here. They both bring so much to the table. I'll have to have her be the official unofficial head of something.

Just thinking of our group, of all the folks that come and walk and eat tapas. What a fantastic world-wide community. This is our group, pilgrims from all over the place, what could be better?

Bye for now. Love, Felipé.

AUGUST 25, 2016 / 58 DEGREES F.

I have a walk in a few minutes. Never quite know who will show up. The morning walks are good for contemplating and talking and saying the rosary. Afternoons are rowdier with visitors and tapas. Today somehow, I have both. This morning is scheduled and this afternoon have pilgrims from out of town so we are having a special walk. My Rebecca asked where these folks were coming from and I have to admit I don't know. It is always interesting where folks hear about the trail. We will find out over wine in the shade later today.

Love as always, Felipé.

AUGUST 29, 2016 / WHERE ARE WE FELIPÉ?

We are moving along toward Ponferrada. It is about twenty km away. We are currently in the town of Manjarín. Plenty of blackberries still for foraging as we walk.

SEPTEMBER 1, 2016 / A HELPFUL REALIZATION

I'm in that few days where my steroids keep me awake. We have been tweaking the dosage lately to get the best of all worlds but still have some sleep loss. But actually I get some of my best work done now. I started at 3 something in the morning with my meditation. Out of that came an idea for helping my caregiver's fatigue that has been plaguing me lately.

To back up a little you know that I have complained about not being able to summon up enough energy in my "work" with cancer patients. People come to me with their own situations or the situations of relatives and neighbors. And I want to listen and maybe try to add something helpful. But I am a beginner and things can overwhelm me, sometimes don't have enough energy to go around.

But it came to me what I say to my archery students would be applicable to this also. First at every stage of development, you are only capable of achieving so much, whether it is number of arrows shot or number of people talked to. As time goes on, we become stronger and we learn how to be more efficient so that we can handle more. The important part is to be able to see our limitation at any given point so that we know when to back off and renew.

So, I am going to work with that model and see what happens. Hoping that these posts lately don't scare people away. I am open to them but have to work at my pace is all. That makes sense, right?

Working around the ranch today. Change of season always brings work that is necessary for future conditions. Alperfect, love, Felipé.

September 2, 2016 / Raisin Bread Toast

It feels good to have learned how to be a country mouse. It seems that little gifts and smiles amongst us suffice for a lot of the glitz and glamor of the city. Not that the city isn't important but our country sanctuary seems to us to become more important as time goes on.

The raisin bread was a hand-built loaf given to us by a pair of my archery students. They are a grandmother and granddaughter combo, nice. They just finished up ten lessons yesterday. But back to the raisin bread which I just had toasted for breakfast. Cream cheese and homemade peach jam on top. The jam was a nice gift left by one of our out-of-town pilgrims who visited recently. And fresh eggs come in from a neighbor whose daughters have been here shooting bow and arrow. And those are a great breakfast ingredient, obviously.

And Our Catherine and Dana just started archery lessons and are excited by that. They are great students. And they are here a lot for walks and tapas. They are involved with the local farmers here on The Island and are always treating us to the local produce and cheeses or sometimes smoked fish.

Early in the mornings like this morning I clean up the dishes and pots and pans from the previous evening. This time of year lots of buttery plates, the evidence of corn on the cob which we are picking from our patch trying to beat the deer and the raccoons to it. I enjoy the clean-up from friendly dinners and friendly tapas. Just part of the process.

Many people have come and gone this summer. The season is starting to wind down now as we slip into back-to-school mode. But our visitors have been lovely, leaving gifts and smiles. They email pics in so we all can remember the occasion. And they take something away, hard to say what that is exactly but none the less they are smiling.

So the riches of us country mice are simple but wholesome. We smile because that is a country monetary unit, a sort of hard-earned gift to one another. It's a "Buen Camino" on our trail here. Hope that you can stop by sometime.

Well, just a simple little blog post celebrating some of the subtleties of life. Thanks for being here, love, Felipé.

September 3, 2016 / If You Go There, They Will Come

OK, it's Saturday and my escape from Seattle and treatment is complete. That was my seventy-seventh treatment. I'm not going to dwell on that but I want to write about another aspect.

I often write about how the personnel at the hospital are such dear friends and good companions and just treasured people. If I have no other reason to be happy about a hospital visit then I will always be buoyed up by them and our interaction. It shifts the equation. And yesterday was not an exception and actually was totally amazing how many people I was able to touch base with. I wasn't keeping track but after a while it became definitely noticeable. "If you go there, they will come."

People are assigned to me and of course we converse. Then people are walking by on their own assignments and say hi and have a minute for an update. Then other folks are off duty and they are coming and going and they stop to talk and maybe they have more time and we share a coffee. It seemed like the day was wall to wall folks.

I wound up my day sitting on a bench outside with one of my hospital chums and we were deep in thought and conversation. And I look up and who is walking by but the Archbishop of Western Washington, J. Peter Sartain. I jump to attention and give him my best Buddhist bow and he stops and we are off talking with him.

That's how the day went. Finally I get to escape Seattle and am the last car on the 5 o'clock boat to Vashon. So, glad to be loved but have to go.

All right have to get to work here at the ranch. Take care, hope to see you soon, love, Felipé.

September 5, 2016 / Folks Coming And Going

We had a beautiful day yesterday for our walk. Nancy from Kansas City came with two friends and we did the whole Phil's Camino routine. It was fun. We picked corn and had it fresh for tapas and had Trader Joe's Spanish wine. They had time to watch the film, which I never seem to tire of.

Nancy had seen *Phil's Camino* in St. Louis this summer at the Gathering. That is the annual meeting of American Pilgrims on the Camino, the national pilgrim organization. I should have gotten more info from her about that but she did talk about one important thing. And that was the showing of the film there which Annie had brought. Nancy said that two hundred people attended and that there wasn't a dry eye in the place. I had never thought about that particular showing but it must have been amazing with all those Camino veterans there.

Another fine person coming and going around here is Jeff who whittled out a Torta de Santiago for Burton Church coffee hour yesterday. Well actually have to mention that Jeff's wife had a part in the production of that tasty treat. Thank you both. My Rebecca brought me a piece from church and I had my first taste of the cake of St. James. This is the cake from the Middle Ages made with almond flour, sugar and eggs. Jeff had been here and walked Phil's Camino last weekend and saw the film and was all inspired.

Wednesday some pilgrims from Southern CA are going to show up. They are from the Santiago de Compostela Church. We met them in July down in Santa Monica. More great folks coming and going.

OK, have to go. Walking this morning and got an invite to go to a Mariner's ball game this afternoon. OK, that's it. Thanks for all you bring, love, Felipé

SEPTEMBER 8, 2016 / I MET MY MATCH

One of my favorite memories, one of my favorite life lessons, was the one about the hummingbird on the windowsill.

I spent some time yesterday with someone who left a big impression on me. And I cannot talk about what happened directly but I met my match in terms of ability as a cancer commando. It was such a powerful encounter that I am still reeling. I did some heavy duty praying for everyone involved afterward. I am thankful and honored to have been a part of that, and somehow I feel on a higher level, even though breathless.

But the hummingbird is anxious for me to tell his story. So, I was on a job in Seattle, it was a rather extensive remodel of an old home. Lots of nice features were going in with lots of money being spent. And that translates to lots of time being spent by the contractor and workers. I was working as a carpenter there for the duration and since the work was more than a few weeks we had taken over the big garage as a work area.

It was hot out, say July maybe, and the inside of the garage was busy and the sawdust filled the air at times and it settled on everything in there. And I was coming and going in between what I was working on in the house and the machinery out there. One time on my travels I came across the most beautiful hummingbird motionless on the dusty window sill. A motionless hummingbird is not right. It looked like it had died trying to get out, exhausting itself up against the glass. I remember how beautiful the colors of its feathers looked lying there in the dust. It's dead right? Ah, too bad.

But something told me to try something, anything. There was a warm bottle of coke there and I found a metal bottle cap and poured it full of the sugary caffeinated stuff and slid that carefully under the beak of the lifeless bird. I went on my way doing what I was doing and returned in fifteen minutes and guess what? That beautiful creature was long gone! Never saw it again and didn't have to.

I love thinking about that story, just how I love thinking about yesterday with all its particular details. It was different but similar. We all flew away better creatures.

OK, walking time, Felipé.

SEPTEMBER 12, 2016 / SOMEWHERE OVER (THE RAINBOW)

Just wondering how to start this morning, searching for a title and Eva Cassidy starts singing "Somewhere Over the Rainbow," hey the Camino provides. I changed up the title a little so people looking for Dorothy don't show up here by mistake. Dorothy's not here. Well at least I haven't seen her this morning yet.

So how are you? Things to do, people to see? Wiley was here for the construction worker's breakfast: bacon, eggs, fried corn with salsa and toasted baguette. We were making a plan to try and get things organized for all the pilgrims descending on us for the upcoming Port Townsend Film Festival. The full meal deal for them includes being here and walking at Phil's Camino the trail.

Quiet right now here. Time to praise God and know that everything that needs to get done today will. The sun is breaking through the trees, not a cloud in the forecast. Walking in a moment. Maybe I will be alone or maybe someone interesting will show up to walk with me, maybe Dorothy, I never know. It's all a blessing!

Let it happen today (as in we just have to get out of the way). Dorothy says hi, love, Felipé.

September 13, 2016 / "Look At You . . . "

People don't usually bring up my cancer situation. It's hard for some folks to talk about or even relate to. But if they do it is usually with a kind of sadness, concern or obliqueness. Yesterday I was at one of the Island businesses that a friend of mine owns. It's the end of the day and we are all tired and a little giddy maybe. And he spots me from a distance and yells, "Look at you all alive and stuff!" It cracked me up. I had to yell back, "It's a miracle!" How fun.

I love giddy, we do some of our best work when we are giddy. OK, it's Tuesday. Have a scan at the hospital today to check on my insides. See you tomorrow, look at you all alive and stuff, love, Felipé.

September 14, 2016 / My Scan Results Are In!

Hey, looking good on the inside according to yesterday's scan. My tumors showing slight growth but we are staying the course with my treatments. So far so good. Always an anxious time waiting for the results but things good. Next scan in four months, January.

Now just cruising along on the chemicals for another hour and then I can start packing up for my escape back to the Island. Man, hoping the traffic is better this PM, bad, bad this morning.

Just had a talk with one of the nurses that I have become closest to. We had a talk about Jennifer's passing. Sort of a catch up on the whole year of the Phil and Jennifer Show here at the Treatment Center. My takeaway is that we were doing great work in lessening the fear of the treatment itself, of the chemotherapy.

It is an interesting process to be fighting cancer and fighting the treatment at the same time, kind of a two headed monster. The cancer is bad and the treatment is bad. The fear of the cancer is bad and the fear of the treatment is bad. How do we get a handle on that? So apparently the folks in the know gave us high marks in lowering the fear level for both of those. Cancer Commandos on the job!

That's very rewarding to get some positive feedback on our work. We all need that. More to come, of course. Love you guys, Felipé.

September 16, 2016 / I'm Back And TGIF!

Friday morning and I got some sleep last night, hurray. Off to the big city today to get Pancho, my portable pump, off at the hospital. So while I am in the city I am doing a big Trader Joe's shop for the oncoming pilgrim influx.

Next Thursday all kinds of folks are showing up here on Vashon to check out the scene on the way to Port Townsend for the film festival. We will be walking and having tapas and networking of course, fun fun!

I feel so lucky to be a part of all this commotion. So fantastic to know and work with so many wonderful and alive people. They are all stellar in their uniqueness. They are all leaning forward in the saddle like pony express riders of old getting their particular mail though. But they fit together in a certain way that is wonderful to see, like pilgrims on the trail. I just want to applaud you group, you are something special, individually and together.

Who knows where this will all wind up? Maybe this is only the start? Let's keep the band together and push it forward, see what happens. All we have to do is do the next good thing. Off to Friday, love you to bits, Felipé.

SEPTEMBER 20, 20162 / MORE ABOUT CANCER

Maybe I don't write about it often enough but the battle against cancer is almost always on my mind. Dealing with the disease itself is hard, but if that weren't enough. what I became aware of at some point was the other battle against the fear of the disease which seems in some ways to be worse than the disease itself. That fear can be a highly personal thing but it is also a collective cultural thing that influences thinking on a big scale.

The concept of cancer hangs in our collective consciousness like some giant monolithic boogie man. When I or anyone gets branded with the cancer brand, that boogie man descends on us to cloud the view of every one of us. We are seen through the lens of "too bad." It so complicates things. We have to fight for our individuality, our particular song in all this. We are not our disease!

The presumptions go on an and on. Even people I know well get caught up in this and don't really see me. But these presumptions can be even more dangerous if I would start mirroring them as my reality. Instead of taking a really close look at my situation as it exists for me, it would be bad if I accept what it is I am "supposed" to see.

Ah, books have been written on this I am sure and I am out of time for now. Have to go to work. Thanks for taking the time to be with me. Love, Felipé.

SEPTEMBER 21, 2016 / LET'S PROVE THEM WRONG

Anyway, I am still stuck on the thread of the last few days where I was writing about the "fight against cancer." Now is the time to get it out there as tomorrow guests arrive for the beginning of the big weekend and I will be lost in trying to give you the report on that.

When cancer was sitting before me like some giant monolithic boogie man, I had to move on it. Yelled at it and watched and saw what happened. Talked to it and watched. Drove wedges into it and watched. Prayed about it and watched. And over time I realized that it wasn't as scary as it first seemed, that it had cracks that could be exploited, that it was slow and could be outmaneuvered in some ways. What came to me was that there was wiggle room for me.

Not all cancers are the same, not all doctors are the same, not all treatments are the same, not all patients are the same, not all support systems are the same, not all . . . It goes on. The important thing is to find out the nature of the threat and see exactly what it is for you. Try and strip away the fear of the threat. Try to strip away the general cultural ideas about what cancer is or isn't.

Pit your strengths against its weaknesses and exploit anything that presents itself. You are looking for wiggle room. Shoot it full of holes and move into it, move through it. Think about it differently. Get help. Talk about it. Laugh at it, laugh with it.

Be creative with your own personal situation, it's a do-it-yourself deal. Looking for wiggle room? Can you go around it? Can you go over it? Probe and watch. What will I try next? And ultimately you could say that I made my life in the wiggle room that I was able to find. Good, I like that.

Well, I hope there is some sense in all that. I remember telling Dr. Gold my oncologist early on, "Let's prove them wrong Doc."

OK, time to go. Make it happen, love, Felipé.

SEPTEMBER 22, 2016 / PERFECT MORNING

In a moment is a walk which I need terribly to ground myself. It's misty and foggy out. The perfect morning to see the mysterious cougar that has been roaming around. The trees are all laden with fruit and there are apples and pears all over the ground. The deer are fat and happy and the cougar is grabbing an occasional one, Wild Kingdom.

Wish you were here with us for the weekend. All the best, love, Felipé.

SEPTEMBER 27, 2016 / BACK IN THE SADDLE

Here we are regrouping after an incredible weekend adventure at the Port Townsend Film Festival 2016. Time to get back to the adventures of Ordinary Phil here at Raven Ranch, writing blog posts and such.

I might share some of the high points on PTFF for me. One was the birthday dinner for My Rebecca on Sunday evening; she had so much fun after not getting into a movie that she really wanted to see. Sometimes Plan B's can be better than Plan A's.

The Q and A's after the screenings are always special. Talking with audiences is precious. They come up with so many great questions and we do our best to answer them, to honor them. We are always with the people from other short docs so it is interesting to see how they operate. This time we were "thrown" in with Coffin, the yoyo master, with the film *Throw*. I will have to say that I enjoyed him immensely after getting to know him.

I think that I wrote about this before but I got a kick out of how many people recognized me and My Rebecca on the street. We had numerous great conversations continually. It was hard to get to anywhere on time for everyone saying hello and wanting to ask a question.

Then hanging with our Camino buddies is always special. Every evening we had a get together to tell stories and laugh. Well, you already know if you have been reading this blog that hanging with Camino people is pretty much my vision of heaven.

OK, Erica is coming here today so that will be special. And I have a couple of jobs to take care of before that. Time to go for now, cool hanging with you, Love, Felipé.

September 30 / Under the Spell of Hildegard

It's true, Hildegard of Bingen. She is reaching across the centuries to hold my hand as I walk my Camino. This is the role of saints to help us and in my case she is definitely present at this time and place.

I'm out of time today, sorry, have to run to Seattle and the hospital. Things are good, fall is here, blessings abound, love you, miss you, Felipé.

October 3, 2016 / An Afternoon Palaver

I am still deep in my Pyrenees weekend when the chemotherapy side effects are the worst. But it is after nightfall now and Sunday Night Football is happening so what the heck, things are OK, things are manageable. So, manage on!

Well, let's see what trouble we can get into tomorrow, stay tuned. In the meantime there are miles to walk, wine to drink and palavering to be found. Lovin' you guys, Felipé. x

October 3, 2016 / Patchy Sky And 51 Degrees F

Thinking that it is a pretty decent day outside. Looking forward to being out there soon after my blogging and numerous coffees. I am feeling better also but want to not overdo it today 'til I get up to speed. Pacing, so much has to do with pacing, right?

The weekend has concluded and the Seahawks won and the Mariners lost. I missed Mass but had an hour with Sister Joyce. The chemo kicked me pretty hard but it is subsiding now. The whole thing kind of matches the sky outside, patchy.

OK, let's get the week rolling. This is our precious time that we have been given. Alperfect even if patchy loves, Felipé. x

October 5, 2016 / Visitors

It is such a blessing having people come to the ranch to check in on us. As the rainy season progresses I would guess that their numbers will decrease. It has been a truly busy summer with company coming and going.

People come to talk about the Camino as in Spain or the other Camino, our everyday journey. They come to talk about cancer and curing and healing. They come to talk about spirituality, religion, being a Catholic or being something else. They come to talk about gardening and farming, hunting and fishing.

I am always referencing my doctors, lawyers and Indian chiefs which is what I call the hyper-talented group of people that supports me. We are heavy on doctors, good on lawyers and so far a little light on Indian chiefs. But yesterday a new visitor, Randall, showed up to fill us in on Native American spirituality, and although not a chief he is an adopted member of the Lakota tribe. So, we are getting closer on that. Thanks Randall.

Then I heard from a little bird that we may receive a royal visit in the near future. One of my three Angels from Spain is putting together a plan to come. This is

Anamaria, the Princess of Viana, the one and only. I will have to get out my sword and armor and shine them up as she knighted me Sir Felipé of Viana. I haven't seen her for two years and she just got back from a year in Madrid so we will have plenty to catch up on.

I am a lucky guy to be in such company. Sometimes it is a challenge to match their energy but I have fun trying. Thanks so much for everyone that has come this past season, it was wonderful. You keep me going and energized with our walking, talking and tapas.

Time to go as I have a full list of things to accomplish today. Light rain and overcast today, rapidly closing the door on summer here. The best to you all, love, Felipé.

OCTOBER 10, 2016 / AT HOT SPRINGS

Somehow at the dinner table I got on the topic of the old Zen saying that "First there is a mountain, then there is no mountain and then there is." I think this was in a Donovan song at some point in the day. I need to mention that it is four in the morning here and I can't sleep so I am up writing to you.

But it occurred to me that maybe this is the key to my question. Before the Camino I have a mountain, a reality, my personal reality part of our collective reality. Then on the trail I am separated from my normal life, my reality, my mountain and I learn to like that. Someone has said that the Camino is a drug. Was that what they were talking about? Then I come back because I ran out of time and/or money. And then what? And the mountain reappears. My reality is still there. And the only way to deal with it and keep my Camino dream is to have a changed perception. To find a way to look at the mountain in a new way, a way that works now. Funny that I am using the word way so much. The Camino is a way. I am seeing that it is a way of physical movement but also a way of perceiving, a way of dealing.

Later, love, Felipé.

OCTOBER 18, 2016 / WHAT IS THE MOST POWERFUL THING I CAN DO AT THE MOMENT

What is the most powerful thing I can do at the moment? Well for me that would be writing to you, of course. And that is what is going to happen.

OK, how about a story right now. This may fit in nicely. It is a memory of just an hour spent at the local Dairy Queen when we had a DQ on our little island. It was probably a fall day, the season we are most prone to wind storms and the resulting power outages. I was there having lunch and the place was crowded at usual. It was then owned by a great couple and was in some ways the center of the community. Joan, the wife was there on duty when the lights went off and she had some funky temporary lighting rigged up and proceeded to star in a fashion show with all the odds and ends in the lost and found box. Hilarious, right? I don't know, maybe you had to be there but what a great way to respond to what the day throws at you.

Jump into the arena and do the do the fashion show, big loves, Felipé.

OCTOBER 19, 2016 / THE BAROMETER IS BACK UP

Back in ninth grade Earth Science we learned about barometers in the weather section of the course. An instrument to measure atmospheric pressure and helpful in predicting weather. When the pressure drops it means stormy weather is approaching and when it rises it means that fair weather will reign. So, finally my trusty barometer is back in the "Change" part of the dial where it usually resides. During the height of the recent storm it was way down and pointing to the "M" in "Stormy." Just thought you needed to be let in on that.

We are on an earth topic today I guess. I start these posts most of the time not knowing where they will go or end up. But way back around 1961 when I was a student in that Earth Science class, I remember the course had three distinct sections. The semester started with Geology, moved to Meteorology and finally wound up in Astronomy. In that way it moved from something we were used to something more unknown. This was the beginning of the space race with Russia launching Sputnik in 1958 I think. When we were kids everyone knew that the moon was made of green cheese. Generally we had no idea of much beyond our atmosphere here on earth.

Not long ago I was looking at the materials of a recent Earth Science course taught by a friend and noticed that the order of the sections had been reversed, indicating some shift, I think. Now they start with Astronomy, go to Meteorology and end with the apparently lesser known Geology. Interesting, I think. Have we in the last fifty years gotten away from our roots so? Now are we more at home with digitized photos from outer space telescopes then we are with the rocks and soil in our yards? Just an observation.

Very earthy, right? That's what we are up to today. We generally got it under our fingernails around here. Off we go, love, Felipé.

OCTOBER 21, 2016 / THE WHALES HAVE RETURNED

The orca whales, used to be known as killer whales, are back in the vicinity of Vashon Island.

Time for a little story. I was fresh here on the Island and to the Pacific Northwest and it was 1972. My first job as a carpenter was working on a beach house on the westside of the island. I was getting two dollars an hour and I could stay there at the site. We had all the windows out of the old house which we were moving and remodeling. The house is right on the water I remember being woken by the sound of the whales breathing as they came up the channel. The sound of the half a dozen animals was echoing back and forth in the calm of the early morn. What an exotic way to wake and what a welcome to my new neighborhood!

I don't know what this going to mean this year as the salmon season is closed due to the poor return of fish from the ocean and the orcas eat a lot of salmon. So will they still hang around? I guess they still have seals. Wild Kingdom out here, up to our armpits in nature.

Planting my cover crop on the corn field today, after getting it tilled yesterday. It's not going to rain this AM, better get out there. Well, go get 'em today whatever you are up to. Big whale loves, Felipé.

OCTOBER 24, 2016 / WHERE THE HECK ARE WE FELIPÉ?

Bill and I walked this morning and made it to Laguna de Castilla just before O' Cebreiro. We are getting there slowly but surely, little over 7/9ths the way.

Come walk with us, Felipé.

OCTOBER 25, 2016 / A CERTAIN LIGHTNESS

Maybe it is nimbleness, maybe it appears slightly naive, maybe a certain knowingness, sort of a bit of happy go lucky. Just trying to figure out what all pilgrims have in common, well when they are in the zone anyway. I have Catherine y Dana for archery lessons this afternoon and I am always shepherding them into the archery zone. There is a place to be that gives you a bull's eye.

And as a pilgrim there is a place to be that gives you the Way, the learning of how to be on that different plane. Kind of feel like I am walking around in circles. Perhaps I can try again. In order to get the big lesson, one must be open to it which means a certain amount of trust in the process. One must say yes, I am ready to be the clay to be molded.

I have met people who have been on the Camino and said that they just didn't get it. Yea, I can see that happening. There is a difference between a traveler and a pilgrim. And being a pilgrim is being on the quest to get "it." You know there is an "it" and you work toward that. And you have to have the trust that if I am the clay good things will happen as the kilometers go by, as the church bells ring, as the snorers snore, as your pack gets lighter, as you get lighter.

There it is again, the lightness. Well, perhaps I can tackle this on another day, got a start anyway. I like the part about being in the zone gives you a bullseye. OK.

Started *Don Quixote* yesterday. Well, I am fighting my way through two introductions anyway to finally hopefully get to the "greatest novel ever written" here soon. Trying to catch up on my classics is one reason for reading it but also because my "battle" against cancer has been described as "quixotic" and I want to know what that means.

Yup, that's it for today. Get in that love zone and get a bullseye, Felipé.

OCTOBER 26, 2016 / SO FAR SO GOOD!

That's a punch line to a joke that Bill my cancer commando buddy told me. And it has turned into a greeting that we use with each other. I need to tell you the joke so that you will be in on it.

So, this guy jumps off the roof of a five-story building. As he is falling past the fifth-floor windows someone yells out," How you doing?" The guy yells back, "So far so good!" And he falls past the fourth-floor windows and there someone yells out,

"How you doing?" And the guy yells back, "So far so good! And he falls past the third-floor windows . . . Well, you see where this is going.

So, that is our big joke, it's a cancer joke really, kind of gallows humor. This is part of how we cope with the uncertainty of it all. "So far so good!" Thanks Bill, your company is priceless.

This is my big day at the hospital for treatment. Bill just dropped by to visit me for a half hour while he was here for another appointment. Again, thanks Bill.

Time for a coffee, have about an hour to go and I have to get up to speed for the drive home. Take care for now, love, Felipé.

OCTOBER 28, 2016 / LOOKING GOOD IN MY NEW RED HAT

Yesterday in the mail comes a new hat from the Mazama Store, Mazama, Washington. A new one just like the old original one used to be, used to look like but really hard to remember. So, the old one, the real one, the one that made it across Spain in the sun of July and August will be retired except for special occasions. But the important thing is to thank the mystery person that ordered that for me. Thank you, whoever you are!

So, Cubbies game tonight after I get back from the hospital in Seattle. The commute on Wednesday was a bear and hoping today's will be easier. Might even be some sun breaks. Do weathermen use that term in other places? In Seattle it means that it has been gray for far too long and then the sun "breaks" through the clouds for four seconds and everyone goes, "What's that?" Yea, really.

We had a tremendous party last night. It revolved around Jan, William and Starr's visit to walk Phil's Camino. They were in from California and Oregon. Then Bill my cancer commando buddy showed up. Then Kate Munger with Barb and Ken came in. Kate is the founder of The Threshold Choir, which is a world-wide movement to have little choirs bring comforting song to folks on their deathbeds. My Rebecca is in that, in Barb's group. So we had a walk, tapas and watched Phil's Camino. A great afternoon and evening!

OK, have to go for now. And thanks for everything to so many people that make my life richer. On the lookout for sun breaks, whatever they are. New red hat love, Felipé.

OCTOBER 30, 2016 / WHERE THE HECK R WE FELIPÉ?

We are here on Phil's Camino clawing our way "across Spain." I know it has been over a year to do this but I guess we don't care at this point. Anyway, we have walked 723 laps for 636 kilometers. We are at the town of Hospital da Condesa just west of O Cebreiro. So that's 152 kilometers to go.

Come walk with me,

OCTOBER 30TH, 2016 / 1000TH BLOG

Poem by Rebecca:

What if?
One thousand blogs.
More than ten times the number of chemo treatments,
And more than the number of walking days.
More than the times of tapas and friends coming by,
More than the film festivals you've been to.
Of course it's the chemo and walking that keeps you alive,
But what if it's the blog instead?
What if?

November 1, 2016 / Day of the Dead

Day of the Dead, or All Saints Day in the Catholic Church, is here, when the veil between the living and the dead is very thin. It is a day of obligation, so Catherine and I will be there at St John Vianney's this evening. We are supposed to take photos of our loved ones that have gone on. I have a nice framed shot of my folks on their honeymoon at Niagara Falls in 1946 to take.

OK, I have a long list of things to accomplish today, time to go. Love is greater than death, Felipé.

November 2, 2016 / The Seventh Game!

It has almost a sacred feel about it. The seventh game coming up, the Armageddon, the last possible . . . The Cubbies did it right last night, winning game six by a decisive margin. What was it 9 to 2, something like that? Catherine and I were off to church last evening and we were juggling that with the game. Maybe we didn't do either well but it was fun trying. They both seemed like obligations.

Catherine said something interesting about the situation of the Cubbies forcing game seven. She said something like, "No matter what happens their fans will love them." I've been thinking about that since. That's true right? And really how could it be otherwise? They have such heart that they are going to push it as far as they are able and perhaps won't win the ultimate prize. But as long as the fans think that the team did everything that they could and sacrificed everything along the way, they will be loved.

And doesn't that go for us with the major life-threatening diseases? Chances are most all of us will get overwhelmed but pushing it to the seventh game and then getting overwhelmed is all one can do. Then it becomes sort of how do we do that best with what we got, with the most style, the most verve. The cards are stacked against us but realizing that and continuing on in spite of it and doing the best one can with that is the goal in my mind. And doing that for as long as possible is the winning. Maybe that is why Maryjane calls my Camino, my life, quixotic. I'm still thinking about that.

The best to you on your trail, whatever that might be. Game seven loves, Felipé. Go Cubbies!!

NOVEMBER 7, 2016 / MY FRIEND THAT I NEVER MET, BEING WITH YOU IN HOSPICE

Dear Caton ~ I know that I am two thousand miles away from you and your family, me being here in Seattle. It was last month, October, that I was there in Hot Springs. It was warmer than Seattle and the trees hadn't started to wear their fall colors. Annie and I were there for the film festival. Your lovely Mother drove us from the hotel door in Hot Springs to the airport in Little Rock on our way back home. As we drove east into the most magnificent sunrise we got to know Lisa and learned of your story.

It sounded grueling then, all the procedures that you had been through in your ordeal with your cancer. And I know that you have been through more since then. Please if you don't mind, I would like to salute your bravery. I have cancer too but mine even though it sounds bad in the language of the doctors is something less bad in my reality. Somehow it is lazy enough to be out maneuvered, or porous enough for its strength to be diluted or maybe disorganized enough to be stalled. I am trying to put it in terms that we use every day instead of doctor language. Anyway, I have been successful in eking out some years of life from my stage four. Sorry, doctor language there, from my dire straits maybe.

That's my story these days. I have been granted some time, some precious time. And I feel a need to be with you now, to let you know that you are loved and being held by thousands of pairs of hands that are not visible. All is well even though things in general have seemed strange since you left your familiar basketball court and your friends there. We all are holding the Universe steady for you in some inexplicable way. We all expect things to go well for you. You be steady just as the Universe is steady for you.

I am off to do the things that my day requires. Later this afternoon I am meeting with my spiritual advisor, Sister Joyce. She is a very wise person that always understands and always makes things right. We will speak of your bravery. Thank you Caton for letting me know you, we all make each other's lives richer. Only love to you and your family and friends always, Phil Volker.

NOVEMBER 10, 2016 / A CALL FROM DOCTOR JIM

I grew up with Doctor Jim in Buffalo, NY. Of course that was long before he was a doctor, but his Dad was one and we hung around with him and I guess it rubbed off on one of us anyway. He and my father were good friends as was my mom and Jim's. I used to call his mom Aunt Marion although we weren't really related.

Doctor Jim called me on the phone this morning and we talked for 52 minutes. That's a long time for two guys to talk but it had been a while. It was good and I got a lot of good pointers from him about things that I am up to now. You know I talk to a lot of folks these days and they are doctors or nurses or patients or people in hospice. So, he was helping me with that.

Going back in time my dad was also involved in the medical field. He was an Army medic in World War Two in the Pacific Theater. He was in four major battles 'til he was wounded on Okinawa. I can't even imagine what that was like but he helped a lot of guys survive and he did himself. Dad got back to Buffalo in 1946 after his stay in the hospital and married Mom, and I came along in 47.

So, Jim's Dad and my Dad used to talk a lot about things and healing was a big topic with them whenever they got together. I guess some of that rubbed off on me. I have a feel for healing it seems, in a sort of medieval way. I'm not a professional by any reach of the imagination but things come to me from the depths of my experience.

Later, love, Felipé.

NOVEMBER 15, 2016 / LITTLE TINY BEACH CHAIRS

I've been waking up at four in the morning lately. There must have been some cosmic shift out there that I am reacting to. Anyway, I had time to check in with my tumors early today. If you are new to the blog I may have to explain that I have tried to create some sort of positive relationship with my cancer, with my tumors. This has been going on for a while and I have blogged about it. Well OK, and this morning they seemed their usual selves, sort of quiet and shy when I saw them.

> "Apprehend God in all things, for God is in all things.
> Every single creature is full of God and is a book about God.
> Every creature is a word of God.
> If I spent enough time with the tiniest creature—even a caterpillar—
> I would never have to prepare a sermon.
> So full of God is every creature."
> — Meister Eckhart (13th-14th-century German theologian and mystic)

So, mix together this expansive state where we search for God in everything, with my mood to invite and celebrate, with my visit to my tumors and what do you get? What I got was the question, "Am I supposed to find God there?" Is God there in those little guys like he is in you and me and a caterpillar? This is I admit, a strange thought given our mindset of fighting cancer but worth exploring nevertheless.

So I decided to try and invite them on an outing. I started thinking about a day at the beach maybe. That's where the little tiny beach chairs come in as they will need somewhere to loll around. Maybe little tiny drinks with parasols for the guys. I know, all this sounds totally crazy. Yes, yes I am thinking that myself but . . .

Looking for common ground, trying to find the positive, love you, Felipé.

NOVEMBER 16, 2016 / BEEN MUSING ON THE UNEXPECTED OR THE OUT OF PLACE

We wound up suspending the butt end of a romaine heart that was being thrown away in some little bit of moisture. It was just an experiment and look what is happening, new growth, some new life. Major fun to see this in November when the whole outdoor world is shrinking and packing up its tent. And here it is right in front of me as I eat my meals. I know that it will not last long but neither will I. Just a little miracle produced out of the stuff we were throwing away.

A couple of days ago I was driving on the back roads of the Island going to a job site and came around a corner close to a bluff overlooking the water. The afternoon precious sun was pouring in and the wind was blasting in over the bluff and the wind picked up a quality of the golden leaves that littering the ground and swirled them in a whirlwind. Like a dust devil but it was a leaf devil. What a sight! And it was crossing the road and I drive through it and it rocked my little pickup, this golden whirlwind which lasted a few dozen heartbeats.

I have been thinking about my tumors lately in sort of the best terms that I can come up with. What energy they have. What tenacity they have. The conditions that we put them in week after week, month after month means they are just hanging on to the cliff face with their finger nails, so to speak. Sometimes the scan shows no growth, sometimes small growth and one tumor got smaller and smaller and disappeared over time. Overall they are sort of amazing little guys if I can look at them objectively.

There is so much we don't understand. There is so much to see and be rocked by. There is so much to wonder about. Energy seems to pop up out of nowhere and cause happenings that are miracles or catastrophes, depending.

November love, Felipé.

November 20, 2016 / Fun Day at the Old Camino

Great and fun day today, for Sister Joyce was here to "walk" Phil's Camino. I say "walk" because she drove the riding mower around the trail and we stopped every so often to talk and laugh.

We are walking this afternoon and tomorrow morning and by then we will be in Sarria. And we all know what that means—that there is 100 km to go. So, we are getting there.

November 20, 2016 / Just Where Are We Felipé?

We have a little standing water on the trail so wear some rubber boots and you may need a rain jacket depending. Felipé. x

November 23, 2016 / Wednesday at the Hospital

Bill my Cancer Commando buddy and I were talking recently and he was expressing his feeling about his cancer, how he was fighting it tooth and nail. He really hates it and is totally all out fighting it. And he reads my blog and he wonders what I am up to. He has a hard time relating to my approach. The only thing I can think of to say to him is that I am trying to learn something. Is that what you are doing Felipé?

What are you doing exactly Felipé? I have always had trouble with the concept of "battling" or "fighting" cancer. It never seemed to fit my perception of the situation. Maybe looking at it as if cancer were pirates boarding their vessel is helpful to some, it doesn't fit with me. I am more at home looking at it as part of me that is off-kilter. Believe me I am thinking and thinking about this. In that light, yes, I am trying to learn something.

My fighting is more involved with working on myself and my relationship with others and with God. It is more about making me stronger or more integrated than repelling invaders. Somehow this fits my personality better or fits with what I can do with the tools in my tool kit perhaps.

I had a meeting with Sister Joyce recently and she was talking about the difference between reacting and responding. It was about the answer that one gives to a change. Are we reacting from a highly emotional place? Or are we moved to respond to the change in a different way, perhaps a more constructive way? Maybe one blends into the other over time.

Anyway, this is the stuff I grapple with day to day. Somehow, I am more apt to ask "why are you here?" to my cancer than "why me?" I am always looking for the message that I should be receiving. I have fully accepted the "why me" part. Maybe this all comes from dealing with it for so long now. Anyway, maybe this is helpful for someone out there. It is an alternate way to look at things.

In *Don Quixote* I am on page 308 out of 940. I just renewed it for another month and the librarian said that I could do that again. Grueling journey, this book, similar to my 909 laps on Phil's Camino.

I will blog tomorrow from home, We Never Close! Hope your turkey day is coming together, hot gravy loves, Felipé.

NOVEMBER 28, 2016 / TOO MANY IDEAS

Is the trail the new church? I know from my wanderings that there are different sorts of ways to belief that exist, as one based on knowledge and one based on experience, say. My stay at the Catholic Church has been brief but what I appreciate most is the experiential quality of it. So much that I take in is gained by my physical doing. This is different from knowledge where I read and study and try and reach an understanding. I am so much of a kinesthetic learner maybe but I get so much more out of putting my whole body into something. Now that is just me, but the trail has that aspect, you have to admit.

As one walks long enough and hard enough part of us actually becomes the trail. We sort of donate it. We give it away. We don't need it any more. And that sudden empty space in us is where God moves into. It's holy implant. He isn't an idea any more. This is the trail, the new church.

Wow, and on a morning when I didn't have any ideas. Bless you all as we get back to work on this Monday morn. Blue sky is appearing for our walk here at 0900.

love, Don Felipé.

NOVEMBER 29, 2016 / MOSTLY ABOUT JESUS

This morning I saw a pic of the "Jesus Barn," a landmark here on the Island. It was beloved, if sort of taken for granted, by everyone. I say taken for granted because I think that we all thought it would last forever but no, it collapsed, I think in the nineties. My Rebecca and I remember it in its heyday during the seventies and eighties. I don't know the history of it. Maybe it just dropped out of heaven.

But the pic is gorgeous! Heyday shot if I ever saw one. You are looking directly north and the afternoon sun is over your left shoulder. The grass is all dried, so it must be late July or later, high summer or better. It speaks of sustained sun and the heat it brings when we locals finally are able to uncurl our bodies locked in position still from the long winter.

Sometime ago the county came along and imposed its will on us and laid a grid down on the landscape and gave it all numbers of streets and avenues. I still don't know the numbers, refusing to learn. It's oppressive, like the Romans rolling into ancient Israel. But some of the original names have persisted like, "Bank Road" which is the road the savings bank is on. And there is a pond on Bank Road and the pond's name is, you guessed it, Bank Road Pond. See, easy-peasy.

But what is really interesting is that if a landmark somehow disappears as in the case of the Jesus Barn you still call that spot or even area the "Jesus Barn." This is why outsider city people tend to look at us funny. Well, there are other reasons too I hear. Anyway, just thought I would bring this to you this Tuesday morn.

Maybe all us old timey Island carpenters could get some kind of fancy grant to raise it, to reconstruct it again. You know I didn't even write of the quality of the calligraphy. Someone really busted butt on that. Thank you, whoever you were. And thank you Jesus Barn in totality, teaching us that you are there just like Jesus even though we can't always see you.

OK, have to go, miss you, love you, Felipé.

DECEMBER 5, 2016 / MONTERREY TODAY

What a full day today. It started out with Esther giving us a tour of Cannery Row, remember the Steinbeck novels? Yea, she used to be a professional tour guide there so we got the full meal deal. Then off to Mass with Padre Tomas at 1100. What a nice job he did. This was at the Chapel at Fort Ord. Then lunch with the Knights of Columbus.

So, our work began at 1300 with a showing of *Phil's Camino* and an almost hour-long question and answer session. This audience was really great and had all sorts of questions mostly of the religious kind. Annie said it well when she said that she was way more comfortable when she could talk to an audience where she could mention God. I am with her on that, and she drove home the point with the folks there how important it was for my success that I had not only assembled a great medical support team but also a great spiritual support team as well. True, true.

It was such a great day to be with the Padre today, not only to see him serve Mass but also to receive some of the Church's major blessings. Of course Mass includes participating in the Eucharist which was my first Sacrament of the day. Then in the privacy of Padre's office I had the privilege of participating in the second Sacrament by receiving Reconciliation which used to be called Confession. And if that wasn't enough Father Tom Anointed me with Oil at the end of the Q and A, me being held up by one of the parishioners on one side and a major Caminohead Dave on the other just in case I swooned. It will be a very memorable day for Felipé.

A funny thing happened after we left the church that is worth relating. Since we couldn't sell anything at the church due to federal government regulations, we met with all the folks that wanted to purchase the new DVD and other gear down the road off of the property. There was a big empty parking lot next to an abandoned burger joint that we pulled into. We were selling stuff out of the truck of the rental car with all these buyers coming and going. It looked like some kind of big drug deal going down. We were all laughing waiting to be surrounded by the local cops. But in the end we escaped with the money and were on our way down the highway to Berkeley.

After an hour and a half drive we got to the Jesuit housing and got settled in before meeting Catalina and her family for dinner. They treated us to a hearty Mexican feed and we played with Electra, their three-year-old daughter, and hammered out the details for tomorrow's work. And that is being with Catalina's class on Pilgrimage Art that she teaches at the Jesuit School of Theology.

Pretty darn heady day, and I at this very moment am exhausted. And on top of that the Seahawks are winning with a few minutes to go. OK, enough, time to curl up with my fat book. Thanks so much for being here with us, love, Felipé and company.

December 9 / Back Again

At the hospital early and I have a little time to complete my earlier thoughts. Yes, a tremendous article came in that I read this morning. And it is not newly written, 2009. It's been hanging around waiting for me to find it. But the basic idea is that increasing numbers of cancer patients are surviving as compared to years past and many of those folks are experiencing extra special quality of life due to their brush with death. But by golly we already sort of discovered that in our little corner of the world right here. Neat to have it seconded by another source.

It's not all fun and games because folks die here. We have to acknowledge that obvious fact while we go on our merry way. But so far so good as we say around here. Might be our turn next, never know and actually don't care. It's all in God's capable hands anyway.

When I tell someone that I have something really weird to tell them and then I say that cancer is the best thing that ever happened to me, it is what this article is talking about. Strange but true as they say. This is part of what we have been wrestling with here at Caminoheads for almost three years now. And I guess we have more to go.

Yup, well that enough for now. You guys are super, love, Felipé of the North.

December 10, 2016 / A Troika

If I remember right this is a bit of Russian history. A troika is the three-horse setup used to pull vehicles where the three are abreast. We don't have anything like that here in the States.

I have a troika going with my three "C's." My Cancer, Catholicism and Camino is a team that pulls me along. Each one of those three has a whole world around it. For example, the horse Cancer is the whole world of that for me which includes my family, friends, doctors and nurses. It is that world that the disease cancer brought together.

And Catholicism has its own world, a spiritual place with its many moving parts. And likewise the Camino isn't just a physical trail it is a Way, a spiritual world of the hearts and minds of pilgrims past, present and future.

These three strong horses work together to get me through the snow or down the road or wherever I need to go or is worth going. They are a team. That is the way I see things at present.

You are the best, love, Felipé.

DECEMBER 12, 2016 / HUMMINGBIRDS AND A MARIACHI BAND

The hummingbirds are a joy and we have been seeing them regularly since Catherine came by and installed a feeder outside a kitchen window. A "build it and they will come" sort of thing. They are just so small and delicate and they manage to survive these nasty ass winters of ours, a miracle. They should be in some place with blue sky overhead and mariachi band music in the breeze. But glory be—they are here to keep me company, super!

Speaking of mariachi bands, today is the Lady of Guadalupe feast day. We are having a big afternoon and into the evening celebration at our parish here on Vashon Island. We will be at part of it for sure. What a marvelous holy day. North Americans are just not as familiar as they should be with the Lady of Guadalupe story. It is mucho powerful and equally fascinating. Please Google it for a knowledge update. She waits for you.

Off to walk in a moment. Gray but dry out, and there is some standing water on the trail. It is definitely rubber boot territory. Come join us when you can, we walk and talk, easy-peasy.

Monday loves, Felipé.

DECEMBER 14, 2016 / YOU KNOW . . .

You know, once in a while I fall off the end of the spectrum of my own consciousness. I am having thoughts that are way bigger than I can really deal with. So, just hanging out with one at the moment and will try and explain.

Julian of Norwich had a vision one night, she called it a showing, and she spent twenty years trying to communicate it afterward. She was a Christian mystic of the 1300s. Well, I can scale that back to 1 percent and go from there. Not trying to compare myself to J of N but in some realms we are all equal. But hanging out with the words of someone like her can definitely expand one's boundaries, a lot.

So, back to my thought and I won't go into how I got there but it was sort of a logical progression from one flat rock to the next as I crossed the river. In other words, I didn't think of it in its final form on my own but was led there step by step. And on having the thought, it felt so different, so unusual that at first it was hard to grasp.

Let me quit dinking around. The idea is that in our eternal life you and I are going to learn the story of everyone that ever lived. We will have the time and luxury to commune with everyone, as in everyone that ever was or will be. Anything less would really be unsatisfactory, incomplete, unfinished. There, that's it in a nutshell. What do you think? I know it's terribly out there but hey who said we always had to dwell in the mundane, the little, the usual? With God all things are possible, I'm going with that this morning.

Yup, have to go be a carpenter and bend nails this morning. Then this PM have to go work on the plumbing at the rental house. How can I be so lucky? This is the kind of stuff our days are made of now here on this planet. Time to go, Felipé.

December 15, 2016 / A Couple of Things

I had a meeting with the universe these small hours of the morning. As usual my tumors were there but were pretty low keyed which is good, considering I have a scan in less than a week and it would be good if they were as meek and mild as could be for that. And I put in some thought on them as I usually try to do and this is what I came up with. I am thankful for the fact that they are so slow moving and come to me more like Marley's Ghost than Attila the Hun. I am appreciative and have always considered them messengers, if dangerous ones.

Yes, a gray sky morning and lots on today's dance card. Hope that you are keeping things under control and not getting stressed. We have a walk in a few minutes, who will show up? Miss you, love you, Felipé.

December 17, 2016 / Beauty As A Pathway

What a tremendous morning. The barometer was off the charts high, the thermometer lower than usual and a glorious sunrise happened. Mount Rainier just a little south of where the sun was coming up. And the mountain had the lens shaped clouds encircling the peak, in other words it was making its own weather. Mist was coming up off the water in the harbor and a huge flock of ducks was in there forced south by the colder weather up north.

I was at my Bible Guys class at a private home on the harbor. The sun streaming in was too much for us and we had to evacuate to a different location. Life's a bitch, right? Too much sunshine, not complaining. We studied the 16th chapter of John's Gospel. It's all Jesus's prayer asking his Father's help for himself, the disciples and the future world. We got through it in an hour but could spend a year of classes on it equally.

Aleppo, Syria is in our prayers. Civilians caught in the space between two opposing forces is a hard one to not get moved by. Let's please consider opening our wallets and helping out some relief outfit. This is a horrendous thing to happen at Christmas time, well, or anytime. But we are in the giving mood and what better thing to do?

Well I'm sorry sort that I don't have a pic of all that glorious landscape/seascape this morning. But in my world everything can't be documented. There are times we must stand in awe and dampen the urge to click a photo, we owe it to ourselves. It's too precious to be distracted from the beauty that is one of the pathways to God. Anon, love, Felipé.

December 18, 2016 / No Chipmunks Yet

Last evening as we sang the old favorite Christmas songs, I was struck by all the great lyrics. There are some beautiful lines in the old hymns. As a kid I always wanted to write a great hymn that folks would sing in years to come. A sort of immortality. I still like the idea but I don't think that is where my talent lies. Advent loves, Felipé.

December 21, 2016 / Starting Over

We are getting close to being in Santiago. Just passed Portomarín. I guess we will be starting all over again here soon.

December 25, 2016 / You Don't Need No Ticket, You Just Thank The Lord!

Here it is—the mother of all holidays! On the red leather couch watching the "yule log" on TV. We have the house all tidied up and Henna and Wiley will be over soon to tackle the presents.

Now there is the Seahawks Football team reading the "Night Before Christmas." They are so cute in their Christmas sweaters. Oh, back to the "yule log" with Nat King Cole singing. He is the smoothest dude that ever was.

That's what it is all looking like here at Raven Ranch. My Rebecca and I and Wiley and Henna wishing you the Bestest Christmas ever! of course.

December 27, 2016 / Tell Me That You Are Terribly Interested In My Cancer

I need help with this. Just your thoughts of encouragement for Felipé. Early this morning I was hanging out with my tumors and I was telling them the story of God, the whole thing from beginning to end, well as much as I am aware of and can remember. It was an attempt for us to see how we all fit into the bigger picture.

Somewhere along the line I thought it would be nice to have little white dinner jackets made for them. It would be quite a project as they are of varying sizes, custom job. Well, they were thought jackets really, obviously they couldn't be real jackets. It would be cool for them to do the James Bond thing: "Cancer, Colon Cancer" in their little white jackets. Is that too goofy?

Well, this is how I spend my time, some of it anyway. It is kind of an exploration. Going where no man has dared to tread. This all might be significant or I may get lost in the jungle, who knows? Your thoughts of encouragement anyway for this seeker.

The sky is looking promising out there. A break from the rain here in the lowlands. There was supposed to be two feet of new snow up in the mountains for the skiers and snowboarders.

OK, off to the city for materials and fuel. Things looking good, love you always and abundantly, Felipé.

December 30, 2016 / We Came, We Partook, We Gave Thanks.

I started looking at the seed catalogs at breakfast a few minutes ago and realized that there is unfinished business for us. Here I am thinking about spring and planting corn and we have just two days left to wrap up our present 2016.

It takes one kind of hope to show up and another kind to partake. I don't think we are supposed to be casual observers here with our precious time. Hope turns to faith that we will be okay no matter what happens. Everything should be on our bucket list: be interested in every moment, every baby, beetle, ear of corn and hummingbird. Let's slather it with butter and sprinkle it with salt and enjoy! And of course, that is after we have toasted each other.

And now "We Give Thanks." Maybe the most important step in the process. We showed up with hope, we developed faith and now looking back, we have gratitude, piles of it. This is at the same time that we remember the deaths of friends and celebrities, of elections won or lost, of our own personal failures, shortcomings and quandaries. In spite of that we are thankful.

Time to welcome the new year! Back to the seed catalog. Love you in big year-long chunks, Felipé.

Part IV

Radical Hospitality

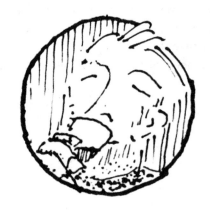

January 5, 2017 / Best Venison Roast Ever

My Rebecca went off the charts yesterday with a big venison roast she cooked all day long in the old crock pot. It was max juicy, falling apart tender and had great flavor. Venison isn't beef, it has a wild taste and it is harder to cook due to the lack of fat. The challenge is to get the meat tender without drying it out. Her secret was she cooked it with some coffee and red wine. That sounds like a possible safety violation, trust she checked with the fire marshal on that combination.

I hear of folks escaping to Palm Springs and other destinations southerly but we are pretty happy hunkered down in the twenty-degree weather here. This is cold for us but so far so good. The cougar has been around, the neighbor saw it a few days ago across the road. I'll have to say that the wild kitties put a bit of spice in our walks.

Inside the house and driving I have been listening to my new love in music, the ensemble Pink Martini out of Portland Oregon. They have an international feel with a big band sound. I got the OK to hang with Pink Martini for a while in our afterlife from my Rebecca. She agreed that we wouldn't always have to be together. She agreed pretty strongly on that actually. Guess that is one of the benefits of almost forty years of marriage.

Hanging out with the band may be on the wilder side of heaven. Kind of fun to think about that, what is the wilder side of heaven? I'm thinking the harps and little puffy clouds are a rather unimaginative view really, good start but still. I can do better than that on a bad day.

Walking this morning in a few moments, sunny but cold. We'll see who the hard-core guys are. So happy that you came along for the blog. fun to be in contact with you, Southern or Northern Hemisphere, East or West, coastal or heartland. We got it all loves, Felipé.

JANUARY 8, 2017 / THE MANGER OF OUR HEARTS

The cold snap has broken, it's raining and the barometer is in a tailspin. There is still lingering snow along Phil's Camino but it may be gone by the walk this afternoon. People coming for the walk, some local some from Seattle. I am going to try and make some cornbread for tapas. I'm happy.

Father David's homily was about how is God showing up in our lives. Or to me how well are we paying attention. And he brought up the phrase, "the manger of our hearts." How magnificent is that little combination of words. The image of our hearts being a manger as a place to welcome and maybe shelter God who presents himself as a defenseless baby. It knocked me over. I'm happy.

I'm here on the red leather couch writing you and drinking water out of a wine glass. I am trying to fool myself which isn't hard really. Always feel like I am not drinking enough water, everyone is always on my case. So yea, the wine glass is making it way more fun. I'm so easy. I'm happy some more.

Yup, Sunday in the rain in Seattle WA, we know how to do this. So, find some reason to be happy today. I guess fool yourself if necessary, get the job done. Thanks for being with me, love you in a wine glass, Felipé.

JANUARY 9, 2017 / FIVE O'CLOCK IN THE MORNING OR PAGE 642

Reading *Don Quixote* is definitely a Camino. This edition being 940 pages long reminds me of Phil's Camino at 909 laps. It goes on and on into the distance and patience is always needed, no quick fixes here. It isn't drudgery but I learn to do it just to do it whether feeling good or otherwise. It calls.

Being in the book in Spain in the 1500s and 1600s is most interesting. I have been spending part of each day there for the last almost three months. There is a vast amount of information there about the culture of the times. And it doesn't appear all that ancient to me. This seems to be a symptom of getting older, the ability to relate to older and older times. Anyway, I feel at home there in the book.

And here on Phil's Camino in the rain of January we are in Pontecampaña with 66 kilometers to go to get to our goal. With our pace of 10km per week we should be there, God willing, toward the end of February. And then what are we going to do? I don't know, maybe out to the coast? Come and help us out. The more the merrier on the trail as always.

Time for lunch here. Time to get to work after that. This is my good week, my time of the least side effects, time to get things done. You are on my mind, love you, Felipé.

January 13, 2017 / Fact-Finding Mission

I had a fact-finding mission to my insides this morning, a talk with my tumors. Sort of like a scan but different. With the scan we are after one sort of information and with my personal investigations something else. Again I get a picture of my tumors as resolute and uncaring for their own future. They have a job to do and they are doing it. I talk to them to find some place of entry but they seem unconcerned. It is almost like talking to myself in some strange way. Or like talking to the negative space that I take up or like the positive end of the magnet talking to the negative end. What to say? It is basically just a very basic primitive grunt of recognition.

Still I am operating with the idea that my cancer is a manifestation of disharmony and not some invasion of weird industrial gunk. I am striving for harmony now. How to be integrated, all parts working together.

It's what I am thinking about and dealing with this morning, certain ideas are appearing out of the mist. I am going to chew on this today and maybe write more tomorrow. But the day is happening with breaks in the clouds and some sunlight on the trees. Cold here and the wood stove is going nonstop. Alperfect, love, Felipé.

February 5, 2017 / The Big Day, Walking Schedule

Super Bowl 2017 today. We're going to be there with Lady Gaga this afternoon. A big day is unfolding. But we are here to report where Felipé and his merry troupe is along Phil's Camino. We have left Arzúa and currently are within 38 km of the Cathedral at Santiago. They are remarkably slow but remarkably happy, they don't seem to care that it is taking forever. There is some talk of where to go next and it looks like they will walk out to the ocean and back. So, come along when you get a chance.

Wear your rubber boots and have your raingear handy. We travel in all sorts of weather and laughter seems to be rain resistant. So come and join us. Loved you yesterday and it should be the same today, Felipé.

February 6, 2017 / Snow Day!

We got four inches of wet snow here at the ranch. Finally daylight. The power is out because of the weight of the snow breaking limbs and those falling on the power lines. Just the kind of day that we delighted in as kids but now not quite as much. We got the generator going and the gas stove is working. The woodstove is cranked up and pumping out heat.

So, we are in good shape here at Raven Ranch and time to work on communicating with you. I have half an hour before our Monday morning walk. So, we made it through Super Bowl weekend pretty gracefully. Time now to forge ahead through the last of the winter. It won't be that long before we feel the warmth of the sun starting to make a difference.

Will be outside walking in the snow and will be looking for lion tracks. It would be fun to show you some. Cat tracks are round and the claws don't show. The tracks that I have seen up in the mountains were the size of a large orange.

There is such a strange parallel for me with this cat showing up here that we could meet any day and my cancer. Both potentially deadly and here in place along my Camino. Hmm. Interesting living with this stuff. Oh well, all in a day's work.

Got to put on my boots and gloves and get out there. The best to you. Love, Felipé.

FEBRUARY 10, 2017 / THINKING THE STORM IS OVER

I have been with a men's Bible study group for something like twelve years now, that beginning seems lost in the mists of the past. Anyway we meet once a week for study and fellowship. There are a bunch of these classes all over Western Washington and these guys are getting together for this retreat over on Bainbridge Island. I had coffee with Art the main guy on Friday a week ago. He previewed our film and if we have the time I will be able to show them *Phil's Camino* on one of the evenings.

This will be a good way for me to loosen up these guys. Protestant guys tend to not get pilgrimage is my experience. It seems their spiritual quest is more intellectual, more bookish. Pilgrimage is mainly experiential in my thinking and, well, experience. I talked with this group last year about my Camino and the response was lukewarm. This year I'll let the movie do the talking.

One of the big pluses is that Art walked the Camino Francés the year after I did and maybe you remember that he took my walking sticks across Spain again. So we are trying, both he and I, to introduce these guys to something new. We here at Caminoheads all know the value of pilgrimage quite well.

Oh, that wind is picking up again, maybe this storm isn't over. Well, we will march on. Stay well, love you, Felipé.

FEBRUARY 13, 2017 / TRANSFIGURATION/TRANSFORMATION

The Transfiguration is described in at least two places in the Gospels. It is where Jesus appears to three of the Apostles, Peter, John and James in his heavenly form where "His appearance changed from inside to out."

As the days of the week go by and I say my rosary I've noticed that I have the easiest time remembering the sorrowful part where Christ carries the cross and the hardest time with the luminous part where Christ is Transfigured. Thinking on that I realized that I have carried an endless amount of wooden timbers on my back in my day as a carpenter. I knew exactly what that feels like. But the opposite was apparently happening with the Transfiguration, the Fourth Luminous Mystery, which seemed like I could never bring forth. What was going on there? Could I change that?

So, this last weekend I spent at a retreat with a bunch of Bible scholars and I thought perfect, I'll corral one of those guys and he will fill me in and that's all I'll need. But there is a flaw in that. To have one of the scholars fill me in would give me a better intellectual understanding maybe but I already had that to some degree and would that help me to remember any better? See the difference between that and hauling heavy timbers on my back as that relates to carrying the cross?

We all get injured in more ways than one as we hang around this life. We can be so used to thinking that our bodies totally represent who we are or who Christ is but that is not so. As important as our bodies are to each of us we always have to remind ourselves that it is only a vessel for our spirit, for Christ's Spirit. And that is what will conquer our injuries and in the end even our deaths. Love, Felipé.

FEBRUARY 15, 2017 / TREATMENT DAY

St. James Cathedral is just a few blocks away from the hospital and I got a window seat here so I can see it. Two guys in bright orange rain gear are crawling around on one of the two towers doing some kind of work. I prayed for their safety.

Bye for now, That's it for another treatment day blog. Thinking of you, love, Felipé.

FEBRUARY 18, 2017 / SUMMIT MEETING

One of my doctors, David, Dr. Zucker, we use the call sign "Danger Zone" for him, wanted us to meet with both our spiritual advisors. And we did that with one more person present, a friend. This was at Sister Joyce's office, she being my spiritual advisor, a Roman Catholic sister. DZ practices Buddhism and had his advisor along, a Buddhist nun, a lovely woman named Dhammadina.

Great conversation ensued for or hour and we agreed to meet again soon. Maybe I can get everyone out here to walk the trail. And maybe we could meet at the Buddhist Center another time. We didn't really have any trouble finding common ground, I will say that to very briefly describe our meeting.

Yea so, all interesting stuff. Weather continues to be an issue here and down into California with all the rain. We have landslides here and there which aren't fun. Well Spring can't come too early for this guy, I'm totally ready.

OK, ever onward, love you immensely, Felipé.

FEBRUARY 19, 2017 / GETTING CLOSE

We have a walk later today and we are on the last few kilometers of our trek across Spain. It's been a long walk but we are still smiling. It's soggy winter but we are still joking. It is unsettled times in the news but we have a certain stability. We have no money but the Camino provides. We buoy each other up when we need it. We walk maybe when we don't feel like it and it always ends up good. We invite people to come and very few do but that's OK, I know they are thinking about us. We tell stories that need telling. We ask questions that need asking.

So, here we are with nothing else to do but be together. It's not a holiday; we don't have to get prepared or have to cook a big meal. It's not snowing or raining heavily, nothing to worry about from the weather. The Super Bowl nor the Stanley Cup nor the World Series are happening. If there is a meteor shower coming it will probably be cloudy and go unseen. Nothing much is going on right now anywhere near here in time or space to distract us.

Alone we might feel lonely. Together we will fill our time together no problem and pledge to meet again. We will walk and not notice the discomforts. Miles and kilometers will fly by like a brisk wind. We won't have time for the small stuff and life will seem good.

Come walk, love, Felipé.

FEBRUARY 20, 2017 / THINKING OF ANNIE O'NEIL

Annie and I were on the phone on the 18th of February and she reminded me that that was the date I had sent my first letter to her three years ago asking whether she could come and walk with me. I had just gotten to San Juan de Ortega on Phil's Camino, about a third of the way across. And it seemed like a few hours afterward that she wrote back, "How about March 2nd?"

Here is the notation in the logbook in Annie's writing for March 2nd: Buen Camino (Heart Symbol) Annie O'Neil. Yea, it was raining like a son of a gun that day. The day before was nice and the day after was nice but the 2nd was a downpour. But we walked and talked and hit it off. And really that was the start of our whole relationship and the whole film project. It just wasn't going to happen without Annie but we all didn't know that yet. We were still walking in the mud, a phrase I am fond of.

That was three years ago and a whole lot has happened since. I have to mention that Saint James is the Executive Producer of this whole shebang because really we didn't do it on our own. So much fell together as if by magic. In the end it is all good and we are all the richer for it. But surely it couldn't have been done without Annie. Thank you so, so much and Happy Anniversary. Love is squishing out all over, Don Felipé de Viana.

FEBRUARY 23, 2017 / EVERYTHING IS POSSIBLE

"Everything is possible" is from *Don Quixote* which I just finished recently. The first time I saw it in the book I had to do a double take. I said to myself, I say that. But that's not quite true. I would say, "Anything is possible." For weeks now, off and on, I have been racking my brain trying to see the difference. Help me out, is there a difference?

The words may mean roughly the same but the feel of them is different to me. Maybe it is in the context of how and when I would use the "anything" phrase. I would use it like a Hail Mary pass is used in football, sort of a last resort.

"Everything is possible" has so much more meat on its bones. It is not tentative. Maybe I am connecting it with the Bible quote, "With God everything is possible." I like the feel of the "everything" much better and I am going to retrain myself to switch over.

I hope that I am not boring you to death this morning but had get that one out of the way. And speaking of "everything", little patches of blue are appearing in the sky. Things are brightening up for our walk in half an hour, how nice. Maybe some folks will show up. My two morning walks of the week are most times solitary for me on these winter days.

A couple of days ago I was writing about the "How about March 2nd?" quote of Annie's. It has grabbed me like "Everything is possible." Maybe starting March 2nd things will be totally different. Possible!

Hey, thanks for sticking with me. Have to jump up here and get my walking attire on. We will be out there searching for signs of spring. Come join us if you get a chance. It's all possible loves, Felipé.

February 24, 2017 / I got nothin'

In art school there was this period where everyone was into crafting all this stuff out of these expensive materials that took a great effort to get a hold of. The products were beautiful but my point would be, yes but can we pull a bunch of stuff out of that trash can there and make something good out of that? Can we?

Sawdusty loves, Felipé.

March 2, 2017 / Everything Could Happen!

This is the third anniversary of Annie O'Neil's first visit to Phil's Camino the trail. It was a life changing day for me, my family, for all of us. It was a life changing day for Annie. There was a bolt of Camino energy that day that we are still living off of. And as Sancho said, "Everything is Possible on March 2nd!" Well he did say the everything is possible part, I had to help him with the rest.

I have been working on my Spanish language in my own Felipé way these daze. At the new shop I generally have the local Mexican AM station on the funky radio. It is fun to try and decode the talk. I am not quite that far to get meaning but am working on picking out individual words. And sometimes I need help. Yesterday there was a Spanish speaking couple getting chemo in the next comfy chair over and I started a conversation with them by asking what the Spanish word "también" meant. They were more than happy to help me out. Now I know that it means "also." And I got "punto" hammered out, which means "point."

Everything is possible loves, Felipé.

March 9, 2017 / Lifelines

At one point I had a vision that I had three lifelines that I was relying on to get me through my cancer situation. And part of my vision was that I was braiding them together to make a strong cord. But the three were, one all my doctors, nurses, family members and friends; two my spiritual connection through church and my Bible class and three the Camino. Sister Joyce quickly filled me in that this corresponds to the three pillars of Christian life, community, faith and service. Ahh, said Felipé.

So, that is pretty important to me to see my way a little more clearly and I will be more effective in the future. It's time for me to pack my saddlebags and get ready to go. It's a long road but it is bearable if we have each other and we can make it easy on ourselves.

Thanks, love you, Felipé.

MARCH 10, 2017 / EARLY MORNING HERE AT THE WESTON HOTEL, SAN FRANCISCO

This whole trip is focused around a luncheon showing of *Phil's Camino* at the maker of one of my chemo drugs.

Yesterday we were talking about the meeting with the group of doctors in Seattle.

I did my best to answer questions that were sparked by the film. One was to tell us more about the difference between healing and curing. Then questions about the walk itself in Spain and on Vashon. But mostly it was about attitude and motivation, mine and their patients' in general. I gave them a little song and dance about Hildegard and medieval medicine and the book *God's Hotel*. I related the story of the power outage in Seattle and the Treatment Center running on 10 percent electrical power when things went medieval for an afternoon. The lights were low, the chemo pumps ran but without all their noises and alarms and buzzes. The computers were down so the nurses actually spent the majority of their time with the patients. It was a temporary shift that gave us all a different view, a view that favored quality for the patient and not the efficiency of the hospital.

When one is a patient and maybe a patient for an extended period, things at the hospital start to be seen "through the patient's eyes." It is hard to do that for others, doctors included. This is where I have heard that cancer doctors that get cancer actually learn a lot about the whole process. A different view appears.

I have to go and search for breakfast and coffee. My Rebecca said maybe we should get room service to bring it up but that seems too weird to me. Alperfect, love, Felipé.

MARCH 14 / CELEBRATION TIME!

This PM the Phil's Camino gang will be at the Cathedral of St. James having completed 909 laps of Vashon countryside.

Wiley said recently, "What's next?" Well we thought that walking out to the Spanish coast and back would be good. I didn't have a chance to do that in 2014 when I was there. But we will do it in the backyard like always. In my hand is the Brierley "Camino Finisterre" so we can't get too lost. So come join us.

Alright, have a good day there, Santiago loves, Felipé.

MARCH 15, 2017 / WEAR YOUR RUBBER BOOTS!

If you by chance are coming to Phil's Camino in the next month wear your rubber boots. Or if you come anywhere near the Great Pacific Northwest wear your rubber boots. It is crazy wet and we aren't supposed to see the sun 'til Sunday. That seems appropriate.

Despite that we were out there in the elements yesterday to finish our second walk across Spain. We had seven walkers and three big Rhodesian Ridgeback dogs tearing up the trail. Yea, the end of 909 laps, seems impossible sometimes. Of course then we had to have tapas and wine to wash those down.

What strikes me is the realization how much effort goes into a Camino walk that last forty days. That is the time the average walker does it in. Compare that to six months for the first Phil's Camino here and a year and a half for the second. I am just blown away when I think about how much we did in Spain in such a short period. But what we do here is good, it is appropriate.

So please come by when you get a chance. You probably need a break from doing your taxes about now, right? Rubber boot loves, Felipé.

March 17, 2017 / St. Patrick's Day

I am reading *Regina Coeli: Art and Essays on the Blessed Virgin Mary* by Father Michael Morris, OP. It was a gift from Our Catalina, our art historian. Lucky me. It might be the most beautiful book that I have ever had in my hands. In my mind there is nothing that compares with Christian art. *Regina Coeli* translated from the Latin means Heaven's Queen.

I remember vividly sitting in dark classrooms watching art history slides and being some impressed and mesmerized by Christian art. What were those artists on anyway? I want to be one of those guys when I grow up.

Well, I have a late lunch date after my treatment and then back to the ranch for a big St. Patty's Day corned beef and cabbage feed. Catherine y Dana, Wiley y Hanna and My Rebecca will be there. Mr. Guinness will probably show up.

See you tomorrow, greenish loves, Felipé.

March 21, 2017 / The Cupboard Was Bare

We were out of bread this morning and first thing I made a batch of cornbread. I noticed that the date on the package of corn meal was '14. This is our meal that we make from our corn and that package was from the crop that is in the film. Nice. This goodness that I am enjoying, that will fuel me, is in that shot of the corn with Wiley and me picking.

The film, what a lovely and powerful instrument. I am so close to it and have seen it so many times that I don't appreciate it as the audience does perhaps. But it travels on to places that I will never get to and to be seen by people I will never meet. It is all an interesting phenomenon. Corny loves, Felipé.

March 27, 2017 / Pilgrimage-in-Place

Just saw an email from Annie saying that she had a talk called "Pilgrimage in Place" at the gathering in Atlanta. I think that was the title. Yes, this is something that we both have been working on for years now. We are making progress. It is tricky.

There was a National Geographic that I blogged about not too long ago about the part faith plays in healing. They went from religious pilgrimage to the placebo effect. So much of who we are and how we do things is invisible and not able to be quantified. How much of a pilgrimage (the effect) is a result of place and how much is a result of spiritual homework? And how much is from rubbing up against pilgrims from other cultures, places and climes? And what else?

We are in this together, that I know for sure. Muddy boot loves, Felipé.

MARCH 30, 2017 / THURSDAY

Sister Joyce is at Swedish Hospital. She is recovering from hip surgery but somehow had a complication and is in ICU. I will try and see her tomorrow PM if they let me after I get out of treatment. A prayer, a thought sent her way would be appreciated. She is such a vital part of this whole lash-up (cowboy slang for organization)

Love again and again, Felipé.

APRIL 1ST, 2017 / FALLING OFF OUR HORSE

Just got back from my Bible Guys class. We always have a good and productive time. It's a steady group. We generally try to cover one chapter out of the New Testament each week. Someone different studies up beforehand and leads every time. Next week I volunteered to lead because it is a really dramatic if not important story. It is Acts 9, the conversion of Saul to Paul, the great evangelist and writer of half of the Christian Bible.

This story is often called the Road to Damascus because that is where it took place. Saul, a heavy in the old paradigm, meets Christ while he is traveling alone on his horse. Saul has been persecuting members of the new paradigm and he is traveling north to continue his work in surrounding area. He is knocked off his horse and temporarily blinded by this encounter with Christ, the new paradigm. The experience is so powerful and instructive that Saul changes direction in his inner life 180 degrees, which is what conversion means, to change direction.

His inner life changes and then his outer life changes. Saul becomes Paul the exporter of Christianity to the gentile world. In other words he embraces wholeheartedly the new paradigm and becomes its biggest salesman to the known world.

We can't hang around this life without getting thrown from our own horses sooner or later. It's how I view my encounter with cancer. It could just as easily be a divorce, or death in the family or other major catastrophe. But is that the end of the story for us? Somehow we have to come up with a valuable ending, that's one of our major challenges really.

OK, off to split firewood. I have some hours before the big Gonzaga game this afternoon. Talk to you tomorrow, love, Felipé.

April 6, 2017/ Still Beaming From The Dinner Party

We had the pleasure of dining with Catherine and Dana last evening. Roast chicken, mashed potatoes, asparagus, kale and I made some cornbread. I love seeing a whole golden-brown roast chicken, it has got to be a celebration. What a great occasion but at the same time a simple meal. So great eating over there, a form of sanctuary really. The hospitality is so thick and wide that it makes up for all the chaos and clutter of the day.

We need a constant reminder to hold that space for someone coming. Maybe we don't know who that is but that doesn't really matter. We offer hospitality because that is who we are or who we are trying to be. Maybe this blog is a form of hospitality. We organize the space to offer you a place to rest and recharge away from the chaos and clutter. Yea, I like it.

Short and sweet today. I start my day out by having a 9 o'clock walk and have to find my boots. We are back to the mud and the puddles after all the latest few rainy days.

OK, you are the best. Keep smiling. Love, Felipé.

April 7, 2017 / Madroño

This Sunday is the start of Holy Week, Palm Sunday. And Easter will be my Fourth anniversary of entering the Church. I am so happy with that. I am really floating along on their support. I am a patient in God's Hotel and finding that a happy end in itself.

Yup, time to get out of my jammies and face the world. Time to tackle the firewood project. Two more trees to fell and split up (madrona here or madrone in California, Arbutus menziesli, madroño in Spanish). It is an important task of the calendar as the wood has to dry for most of a year to be ready to burn well next winter. OK, you are my favorites, love, Felipé of the North.

April 8, 2017 / Hospitality

We have been batting this topic of hospitality around for a few posts. So, if our short-term topic is hospitality and our long-term topic is about how our Camino really starts in Santiago, let's put them together maybe. So, the Way has taught us to love God and our fellow man, to be trusting and open, to risk, to share, to be present to all situations and to be grateful for what we have. So, if we are grateful then we are likely to be relaxed enough to be generous. If we are present to all situations we will notice when someone needs something, food, drink, shelter, acknowledgement, encouragement. So maybe we will feel moved to share what we have in time and treasure. We will make ourselves vulnerable. We will risk because we have learned to see Christ in others.

This isn't always easy but we are working on it. And we will need help and hospitality ourselves as we go down the trail. It's all a two-way street, the give and the take.

OK, make it happen, always in love, Felipé. x

APRIL 10, 2017 / HOSPITALERO

The hospitalero from the albergue in Rabanal said it: "the little we think we can do for the other may just be all the other needs." We were so materially poor on the trail but we provided for each other what the Camino itself didn't. We learned to help the other. Let's see what do I have, four-day old sausage, a liter of water, a Band-Aid and a head full of poetry. Will any of that help?

Sometimes we felt like the other. How can that be? How can I be the other? The lines blurred. We learned. Bless you this day.

Love, Felipé.

APRIL 17, 2017 / HOSTILITY TO PILGRIMAGES?

A few days ago our lovely art historian Catalina sent in this article on the Church of Scotland being asked to reverse centuries-old hostility toward pilgrimage and it piqued my interest. I have seen indifference and ignorance of the process and the power of pilgrimage. Always it seemed a more or less passive activity. Even that seems amazing since we at Caminoheads consider pilgrimage up there with sliced bread. But the word hostility came up. What?

They are seeing the light there in Scotland. With all the interest in pilgrimage worldwide it seems it is finally coming up on radar. What is this phenomenon and why is it appealing when interest in churchy church seems at an all-time low? Something is going on.

Speaking of pilgrimage we have a walk here in a few moments. Phil's Camino, maybe the world's smallest pilgrimage, is a going concern. Time to find my rubber boots and logbook. The trail is still wet but the grass is starting to grow and trees are blooming. Come and walk with me when you get a chance. Love on the move, Felipé.

APRIL 19, 2017 / BACKYARD CAMINO

It is nice to see routes opening up to give people more opportunities and opportunities closer to home. Maybe this will take some of the pressure off major routes like the Camino Francés. And maybe this will bring some income to the country places that always seem starved for cash.

Maybe if you hear of something of interest along these lines you could put a link in the comments and we could chat it up. It would be good to encourage this sort of thing and especially if they are in our own backyard. Wait there is one in my backyard! Hehe.

Yea, it's all Camino if you can get Camino feelings, or experience or friendship from it. Right? Blisters are not enough. Mileage is not enough. But it has to be that transformative thing. That's what we are looking for gang, that transformative thing.

Love, Felipé.

April 20, 2017 / 'Making Pilgrimage a Life Style'

Can one have a life style of a pilgrim? What would that look like? Do you have to walk to have it? It is a quest; something with deeper levels than the physical walking.

But I know that this whole idea of pilgrimage in the largest sense is something amazing. My mind is jumping back to the book *Pilgrim's Progress* which closely matches the ideas in this conversation. It was a major book in the Western world, read second most to the Bible. It is kind of out of vogue now. Maybe I need to reread it.

Ok, love as a lifestyle, Felipé.

April 21, 2017 / Your Camino right here

Well, yesterday it was about 3:30 and I was thinking that I pretty much had a wrap on the day. The landline phone rings which has been infested with junk calls lately and I am tempted to disregard it. But I do look and it is a number but no name but it is a Vashon number so I answer. It was a good friend from church and walking who wants me to take her to the nearest emergency room. You drop everything and go, right? This is your Camino right here right now. Just because you didn't see it coming becomes unimportant.

We were so synchronized that we just drove right on board the next ferry to Tacoma without a wait. So, in the end it all worked out. It was a panic over pains but the tests came up good. So a referral was generated to see a specialist and we were on our way for late evening teriyaki. Back on a late ferry and all is well.

Just a reminder to me how our well thought out and sacred schedules are sort of made to be broken like rules. If your fellow pilgrim needs help that is what you do right then. You don't call back later and say that you have a slot next Tuesday. Well, and I was kind of honored that I was chosen for the task also.

OK, sort of life as it happens around here. That's the report for today.

All good, love, Felipé.

April 24, 2017 / Radical Hospitality

Radical hospitality, where did I hear that phrase? It was sometime over the weekend. I keep saying it over and over to myself since I heard it.

Is this what we experienced on the Camino de Santiago? Eternal hospitality, on-going, repeat it over and over again 'til you get it hospitality? Could be, right? At times it was funky. Maybe they were overwhelmed and had been for days and weeks? But I don't think that you can ever say that it wasn't heartfelt.

We as pilgrims learned lessons great and small continuously day after day. We had an amazing experience. But is there equal reward or knowledge gained from being the folks that serve the pilgrims? Is extending this radical hospitality a journey or discipline in itself? All kinds of pilgrims train and go back to do this. What is that like?

Maybe we could corral some of those folks and ask them. It is an interesting twist to the story. We have been so concentrated on the pilgrim side.

Hey, it's Monday, the start of a new week. What kind of hospitality can we cause? See you tomorrow, love, Felipé.

APRIL 28, 2017 / ENFORCED DOWNTIME

Here at the hospital with nothing I have to do for the next two hours. It's enforced downtime while I hydrate. A whole liter of saline is going in to my body. My we could have used this treatment in the Spanish August. OK, see you tomorrow, love, Felipé.

APRIL 30, 2017 / ALL THAT I AM GOOD FOR

This is my bad weekend in the chemo cycle, my Pyrenees weekend. Yea, that's it. All I have been good for today is watching baseball and hockey so far. But I did have an incredible meeting and walk this AM with Art and Marvin who came from the mainland to play. Marvin is an African American who is a little younger than I am, and he runs an outfit called Dads. His wife is with him in this endeavor. Dads puts Black families back together, that's as easy as I can put it. We are both serious believers and are both on our own Caminos. What we realized is our own personal ministries have so much in common even though on the surface they look worlds apart. That brought us together.

Art, the Bible Guys leader, brought Marvin and a group of Black guys to a *Phil's Camino* screening. There is something very authentic happening with Phil's Camino that resonates with people even if they have no evident connection to Spain, or Camino, or other surface details.

Marvin had a great way of expressing the plight of us when we are so involved with a project that we can't see what it is that we are really doing. We are so wrapped up that we can't what outsiders see. He called it, "When we are in the can and can't see the label." Yea, I get it.

That's it folks, love you immensely, Felipé.

MAY 7, 2017 / REINVENTION

Sunday morning and just back from Mass. Catherine and I were out at Thriftway after Mass to do our tailgate ministry. It was nice and sunny and warm enough to sit out and have our coffee and doughnut and talk to folks. We did have to pat ourselves on the back for surviving the winter one more time. We had a lot of business to cover since we were apart last week.

Oh, at church our Father David was away on retreat. A cousin of his filled in, also a priest. He was fun, a real personality. At the blessing with the holy water he drenched everyone after saying he believed in being generous. At the passing of the peace he got out and shook hands with everyone that had come. Nothing stodgy about this guy.

So, our day is off to a tremendous start. Now I need to mow like the wind with my time today. Everything is nice and dry out there, perfect for the mower. Well, that is my plan. First though we have to get to reinvention.

I was watching a Seattle Mariners baseball game yesterday and they had Gaylord Perry on who was a longtime pitcher with the team. He has been retired for years but he was with the team for many years back in like the 60s through the 80s maybe. I don't know, I wasn't interested in baseball back then. But the commentators said something interesting about him after he had taken off from the broadcast booth. They said that anyone who pitches for that long has to have the ability to reinvent themselves numerous times. The body gives out, not allowing him to pitch a certain pitch so he changes and develops a new way of doing things. Or maybe the game even changes over time and a new response is needed. Anyway the importance of adapting was brought up. If you don't adapt you won't be able to continue long term is the lesson.

This brings to mind the old Marine Corps motto of improvise, adapt, overcome. This is all as I grapple with issues in my own life, trying to make my life continue to "work." Nothing for you to worry about but just sort of constantly readjusting on my part.

Yup, time for lunch and then riding the mower. Make it happen today. Love you, Felipé.

May 8, 2017 / More on Reinvention

I know about reinventing through my own life. At least one-time reinventing. But I have never given it the thought it deserves really. And what if I or we just had it in mind that maybe that is a continuing process not just a response to a specific onetime happening. Perry seems to have used it as a strategy not just a stop gap measure.

I hear such amazing stories these days of people I come in contact with who have made a break with jobs, careers or life styles and have fashioned new more effective situations. All this is very creative and brave. Sort of dancing with the "hands we are dealt."

Just thinking that this reinvention ought to be something that is celebrated not just observed. And maybe the process of continuing reinvention ought to be celebrated. It is sort of hopping across the river on the rocks not exactly sure of what is next but trusting in our ability to be nimble.

Yea, time to gear up to walk. We are getting close to the salt water "in Spain" here at Phil's Camino. After reaching Santiago for the second time we are on the side trip to the coast, to Finisterre and Muxía. After while crocodile, love, Felipé.

May 10, 2017 / Lunch on Annie

To have a real lunch at the treatment center one needs a tablecloth, size doesn't matter but a tablecloth. It is the idea of it really that counts. And we have this nice brown and white one that Annie sent this last week. And there was other stuff as well, sort of box-o-tapas. Let's see, what else was in there: Spanish olives, cheesy crackers and dolmas. And I added a ginger ale from the cantina here. Nice classy lunch, right? Thank you Annie.

David, one of my nurses, is off on the Camino Francés now as we speak. I think he is around Pamplona. I am writing him to slow down. As Kelly used to say, " It's not a race people!" David posted a pic of a spot where Kelly and I had a photo taken. See you tomorrow, love, Felipé.

MAY 15, 2017 / CANCER, IT CHANGES EVERYTHING

I was just merrily cruising through my morning when I got this notification that one of my associate's wives has been diagnosed with colon cancer. They are in that early stage of recognition. It was a crazy whirlwind for me back five and some years ago. Prayers for Shawn and Anna please.

I know that we don't talk about cancer often but it is part of this blog: Cancer, Catholicism and Camino are our center around which we revolve.

Thoughts on cancer are woven into the three years of this blog, sort of imbedded. It would be hard to pull them out if you just wanted that separate from the other two. But maybe that is the point. Maybe my relative success has been because I embrace it and keep it close to the other two.

Well, it is all part of the big picture somehow. 99 percent of us must deal with the big picture at some point in our lives and we get drug kicking and screaming into it by some cause. This cancer that we curse and battle against is underneath it all a catalyst for change. Working with that idea is the art of this whole deal.

OK, off to walk Phil's Camino. I will be thinking more about this as I go I will guarantee you. I will say a rosary for Our Shawn and Anna.

You are the best, love as always, Felipé.

MAY 16, 2017 / A SUMMER OF VISITORS

Travelers, pilgrims really, are starting to come to Phil's Camino for a walk. The season is upon us. We have made it through the rain and the snow, the flooding and the wind storms.

On to my day, love, Felipé.

MAY 17, 2017 / FROM AUSTRALIA

I just got a message from Gracie all the way from Sidney. She finally got a chance to view *Phil's Camino* after all these months. So glad that she liked it, heck she was in it too. What a great person and wonderful walking companion.

I associate Gracie with the sunflowers. To see millions of sunflower blooms in the Spanish sunshine did make us giddy. Most of my fondest memories of the Camino were these moments of pure elation mixed with pure exhaustion. Giddy is our closest word to that.

This all was definitely an adventure in God's playpen. Gracie was next to me in the film where I pass out in church and she prevented me from injuring myself on the stone floor. Catalina and my African American friends say that power was the Holy Ghost getting my attention. And it was the occasion of my big claim to fame of me surrendering and falling into the arms of Grace. God's playpen, right?

Ah, can't make this stuff up in a hundred years, that's the beauty of it. And so glad that Jessica captured that on video. She dropped the camera in the process of trying to catch me and then picked it up and continued filming. Crazy scene that one.

Well, all major fun. Off today on more adventures. We are home but that doesn't mean that adventures are not possible. They are hidden there somewhere. Love, Felipé.

May 18, 2017 / Don't You Think It's Weird?

My Rebecca came up with that yesterday. We were talking about all the people that were going to come to walk at Phil's Camino this summer. This conversation that we were having was doing me good because I have been grappling with this for a while. Rebecca was saying don't you think it weird that all these folks are coming to see you. Well, I replied that I don't think that they are coming to see me but they are coming to see what I have discovered. Or maybe more accurately what we have discovered.

If you are not a Caminohead maybe it is hard to put your finger on what it is. But people that have partaken of the essence of pilgrimage know what that essence is. They/we probably can't put words on it but it resides in us just the same. But it seems to be somewhat fragile and can get overwhelmed or eroded by the concerns of life in general. I think the way to look at Phil's Camino the trail is to understand that it is a sort of laboratory for the nurturing and keeping of that flame.

This blog is part of that effort. For three years I have been writing this journal of my journey with "The Way." It is not always pretty but it is definitely what it is. It is all here somewhere. All of this is in the neighborhood of being as long as the novel *Don Quixote*. It may not have the literary value of that great work but it has value as a log of everything that has happened in three years, the ups and downs and the in-betweens.

Here is a sidebar to this. I just heard that there was a woman visiting our neighborhood that had the ability to read the landscape and tell if good or bad things had happened in places. She reportedly said that this stretch of road where we are located had some lingering signs of something bad that had happened in the past. Well, OK, maybe we are here to rectify stuff like that. We have power, we could do that. Just a little side job.

OK, I have a walk in ten minutes, time to dress for the occasion.

Love you most certainly, Felipé.

May 28, 2017 / A Thing of Beauty

Anyway have to give you the corn update. Got it all planted and the irrigation system set up yesterday, a small miracle. Yesterday evening I sat out under a tree and drank a couple of beers and watched the sprinklers go around, a thing of beauty. Ah, life in the fast lane.

All good here at Caminoheads. We have a walk this afternoon at 4, tapas at 5. Hope that everything is well in your hemisphere. Love, Felipé.

MAY 30, 2017 / HIKING THE CAMINO

Hiking the Camino: 500 Miles With Jesus is a book by Father Dave Pivonka. When a priest or a nun writes a book about the Camino different things come up. They may start with the same beginning point or stimulus but they wind up going further or to different places than me or you. I suppose that is to be expected. But it is fun and productive to read their thoughts on daily walking.

There was a whole chapter on the daily clothes washing ritual. And that turns into a thoughtful commentary on the Sacrament of Confession or Reconciliation as it is known today. I learned something in that chapter and it is the thing that is salient so far in the book.

This priest, Father Dave helped celebrate Mass in churches as he went along. See right there the word "celebrate" in conjunction with the word Mass is a good thing that I am learning from him. Felipé just goes to Mass, at least he did in the past. I get "celebrate" and I will use it in the future. But back to Father Dave and him choosing to go with all his gear to function on the trail as he did at home. I have heard of some priests who go under cover, just traveling anonymously or privately maybe.

Ah, then there is Nurse Dave. This is one of my nurses from the treatment center that just finished in Santiago. He had a pic of his Compostela or Camino diploma on FB. I am so proud of him for doing it. I wrote "thank you" to him. Can't wait to see him in person.

OK, have to go and move some wood before the rain comes. Chilly morning here. Take care dear ones, love Felipé.

MAY 31, 2017 / CORN, FELIPÉ STYLE

It is going to rain this evening. I have been watering the corn for the past few days but maybe can hold off on that today. Next thing to do is plant a row of sunflowers. They are a nice addition to the plot and to the roadside stand coming in July. The goldfinches will be happy too. Nothing better than happy goldfinches. Love, Felipé.

JUNE 9, 2017 / DOWN THE ROAD

This morning I had a glimpse of something extraordinary. I was just driving on the Island and suddenly it was like a veil was lifted and I was viewing a bigger picture than normal. I know, pretty woo-woo. It didn't last for long but was definitely there. I remember thinking can I function safely here. I was driving and was doing well at that so I concluded yes I could.

It wasn't as though I didn't have my own thoughts but they were joined to a larger vision that's all. I don't know what else to say about that but it didn't seem so complicated or impossible a place to get to. Maybe it is a deal like prayer or contemplation where you practice spending longer and longer times there. Yea.

You know, this is a journal of my journey and things come up and I report on them. It is partly cloudy out right now and that would be a report. In the present everything sort of has the same value, it all seems equally important. But somethings are more important in retrospect for seeing patterns or trajectory say. So, just reporting.

A book that I read about the Korean War written by a young Marine officer who later became a famous writer left a big impression on me. At one point he listed all the things that were in his pockets that day. Seems very mundane, as in why bother, but it put flesh on the bones of his story. Things that we take for granted in the present may just be important to someone down the road so I continue.

I think that I will read a few poems from my Brian Doyle book.

See you tomorrow, love, Felipé.

June 19, 2017 / Happy Monday, or Do You Call This Summer?

Man, I am hunkered down under my Camino sleeping bag and on the red leather couch trying to stay warm. It's a couple of days from the solstice and it still feels like soggy spring around here. I am going to walk in a few minutes. I need to look around out there for the summer mojo. It must be huddled out there under a tree somewhere sheltering itself like I am.

buen camino, love, Felipé.

June 21, 2017 / It's The Perfectest

Perfectest, a totally new word that I thought of this AM. I was inspired by one of my nurses.

In Camino terms perfectest would mean what? It would mean that one is moving forward, experiencing things so to speak. Or if not moving forward at least healing up or regrouping so one could get going soon, just a temporary state. Perfect is another word for whatever comes up on the trail next. Deal with it gracefully and that's it, we have bigger fish to fry down the road.

In terms of perfectest in the ordinary world, it would mean something else. The ordinary world is the world governed by ordinary thinking. It is full of right and wrong and them and us and super full of expectations. We feel like all sorts of things are due us. We expect things to happen in a certain way, in a certain perfect way.

Ironically, today I got the news from my scan that happened yesterday. In layman's terms it didn't look great. My little guys were rowdy and have grown more than the usual pace. Yea, and the result of that is my oncologist, code named Nugget, put me on a stronger chemo that I am not looking forward to. We have always known that I would probably need to do this and all of a sudden the time is now. Yea, stronger chemo means stronger side effects and that is the worry.

So, do you see the ironical (I know that's not a real word but it's fun also)? This is far from the perfectest news or this is not what I expected today. But in terms of Caminothink (oh, is THAT a new word) I am supposed to deal with it gracefully and move on, right? And that is what I am going to do to the best of my ability. I've got bigger fish to fry down the road might be the key to the whole deal.

I am sure glad that you guys let me make up stuff as I go along. I am blessed. And you know that no matter what happens with my rowdy friends in my lungs the blog will go on. This is a description of the trail that this blog is. So if the trail gets rougher it doesn't mean that the blog will end. There are more new words that need making so I'll be here.

OK, time to order some lunch here at the treatment center. Caminothinking about you, love, Felipé.

June 24, 2017 / Along the Way

Well, we are finding out that being a pilgrim involves more than just getting down the road. It also involves paying attention to each other along the way.

> "Always, everywhere, people have walked, veining the earth with paths, visible and invisible, symmetrical and meandering." —Thomas Clark

All good, alperfect, as always, love, Felipé.

June 26, 2017 / Archery in the Morning

Monday morning before our 9 o'clock walk and before our first ever Women's Archery Retreat convenes for its final session. This has been grueling and a complete success. Sounds like the Camino. And yes, we covered a lot of ground in a very short time and have a few sore spots but we are still smiling.

So Felipé, what does this archery thing have to do with the Camino thing anyway? Why are we talking about it on Caminoheads? Well, excellent question and I have been thinking about that. They both seem to offer a gateway to things deeper not only in our past but in our basic makeup. Things that are hard to get to from our high-tech world of speed and progress.

We seem to live our lives in the thin layer of the uppermost layer of the body of water called life. We live in those fast-moving reflections of other things. Taking the time and effort to dive down to the depths is refreshing, fulfilling, vital. That's what we were trying to achieve this last weekend. I'm pretty sure everyone felt that.

OK, the walk here in a few minutes. We are on our way back from Muxía to Santiago on our "walk in Spain." Here I go, love, Felipé.

June 29, 2017 / Up to My Neck

Yup, I'm deep in the race with the weeds. All options are being considered. I am going to leave you early so I can get out there in the corn. Thanks for your long-term loyalty.

Walk at 0900 today. Love, Felipé.

June 30, 2017 / About the Weeds

Here is a quote my good buddy Pilgrim Farmer John sent from his home in Iowa. I mean if there is ever a guy or a place that knows about corn and weeds he does/ they do for sure. And he quotes his wife's grandfather, going back even further for this:

"I feel your pain! Forty or so years ago when I first started farming here on 'the prairie,' Cathy's wise grandfather said: 'You'll work all your life at it, and the weeds will still be here when you're gone.'"

I'm feeling part of that long proud tradition for better or worse. Geez, talking about pushing the rock up the hill. There is something I am supposed to learn here somewhere.

OK, off to the corn to get some lick in on it before work. Work before work, get it? It will all be worth it when we sit down to a platter of the fresh stuff in August I am sure. Love, Felipé. x

JULY 1, 2017 / OVERCAST WITH A LITTLE MIST

Oh what a perfect day to not get burnt by the sun. Looking forward to weed patrol again. I am making some headway on this project. Pilgrim Farmer John calling me the Weed Warrior. That has nothing to do with smoking anything.

"There are things that we never see, unless we walk to them." —Thomas Clark.

Love, Felipé.

JULY 2, 2017 / YOUR LUCKY SHIRT

The thing that is really trying to get out of me is the idea that if I come back to this world I want to come back as your lucky shirt. I realize that would mean being in a lot of different places at once and looking like a lot of different things but maybe that won't be a problem. Anyway, I want to be that shirt/blouse that you have had for a long time and it fits you perfectly and comfortably always. It never seems to be too thick or too thin, too warm or too cool, too dark or too light. It always makes you look good, not too dressy, not too casual. You want to say that you are welcoming and warm at the same time that you project a certain sense of decorum but well short of fussiness.

Whoever made me sewed the buttons on like they should and my whole being is functional although you just now noticed a little fray around one of the cuffs and oh there is the small spot on the collar that is slightly worn. Just enough to know that you have to pamper me and know that my time needs to be drawn out and savored.

And then one day tragically I won't survive the washing machine and you will have to prepare me for burial at sea or your equivalent. You will be torn (nice pun), your feelings will be mixed. And in the end we will have a long drawn out goodbye. Yea, love, Felipé.

JULY 3, 2017 / HOSPITALITY, WHAT A CONCEPT

Father David had a homily about hospitality yesterday. He brought up aspects of welcoming that I hadn't considered before. Great homily. Maybe if you had to boil down the Camino into one word that would be a really good candidate.

The word hospitality must come from the same root as hospital. Maybe I should look that up in the big fat paper dictionary. Yea, it's connected to hospital, hospice, hospitable and hospitaler. The Knights of St. John, also known as the Knights of Malta, are also known as the Knights Hospitaler. They opened the first hospitals which served pilgrims traveling to Jerusalem way back when.

Hospitality the bigger concept seems to be the opposite of isolation and insulation. It is opening up rather than boarding up. It is opening up to God also. It is becoming part of that "flow of pilgrims" or that "cloud of believers" or the "communion of saints." I think all of those are the same ultimately. So far so good loves, Felipé.

July 5, 2017 / 99th Treatment

Here I am in the comfy chair. There is a man next to me that plays a Peruvian flute for his wife. It is a very soothing sound. The hospital could employ him to play. Or maybe we could all chip in. Love, Felipé.

July 6, 2017 / Survivor Guilt

I had lunch with a friend that I hadn't talked to in a long time and after catching up he started talking about how he was caring for his brother who lived an isolated life because he was missing his lower jaw due to his run in with cancer. Definitely sent a shudder up through me.

I feel the need to make sure to acknowledge those who are suffering the most. I feel some sort of survivor guilt. I am out walking, partying and giving talks. It is hard to reconcile for me when I run into this conflict. Cancer obviously brings some bad stuff into people's lives, big time.

Before I started my blogpost I was waffling about writing about cancer and I read a FB post by one of my favorite people that has just written a book about her exploits. This is Edie Littlefield Sundby who wrote *Mission Walker*. It is about her walk along the Camino Real the trail connecting all the missions though the Baja and up through New California. She had a quote: "I knew that in order to survive, I had to help my doctors believe they could save me." That is so powerful.

People have such different experiences confronting their obstacles. Thanks, I feel better having talked through some of this stuff. Ever onward my friends, love, Felipé.

July 8, 2017 / We Walk Together

We meet, we walk together, no big deal. We converse and maybe work out something that has been bothering us. We see something new in the randomness of nature that reminds us of where we came from or where we are going. We get wet or cold or get a blister but it's not the end of the world, just a badge of courage. No big deal.

No big deal, that's just the way we want to keep things, right? Just get there however you can, in whatever shape you are in. Come as you are, as it were. The important thing is to get there to be with us, to be together or alone if that is the best thing.

But to be moving and letting the environment work on us, massage us, teach us.

You are really the reason this is all here now. OK?

Alperfect, love you, Felipé.

JULY 9, 2017 / TRUCK SAILING

A story came up after our Tailgate Theology session today. Catherine and I had been to Mass and the supermarket and she was driving me home. We stopped at my job site to grab some tools and I said, "Hey, push the button so the hatchback flips up so I can throw this junk in." And she replied, "Lift the lever back there, this Prius is groovy but not that groovy." Anyway this started this conversation about cars and conveniences.

Somehow this led to my Truck Sailing story. Catherine liked it so I will try it on you. I have this old black panel truck that sits in the weeds here. It used to be a going concern and, as a matter of fact, I drove it across country at least a dozen times give or take. It was pretty primitive compared to things these days. It had no radio (early sound system) but I used to turn the heater on for some distraction for instance. Anyway on one of my trips going from west to east I was trying to make it on fifty dollars for food and gas which could be done. At some point the battery gave out and I was running without it which involved getting some jump starts now and then from strangers.

So, that is the background. And on this trip I was being chased by this storm going through Wyoming. The wind was howling behind me as I pulled into one of those Little America places with a hundred gas pumps. I had to shut down the engine before the attendant would pump my fuel (33 cents a gallon). So, I thought that's cool I will just ask for a jump. Well the jump cost a dollar. A dollar!

So I paid the guy five dollars for the gas and jumped in the rig and then a little light bulb came on and I opened the front doors, started rolling and sailed out of there. Popped the clutch and off I went. I caught the attendant in the rear-view mirror with his mouth open. Yea, the old mother of invention thing. And I made it all the way to New York on my budget but I never had to do that again.

Just goes to show you something, I not exactly sure what at the moment. OK, have to take off for now. Love you, and remember when you get into trouble open your doors and things will come together for you, Felipé.

JULY 14, 2017 / A MERRY BAND VISITS

Yesterday Loretta and her merry band showed up from Southern California. We walked Phil's Camino and tapaed afterward in the shade of the cherry tree. Then we cleaned up our mess and moved down to the beach to continue the party. These guys are hard to keep up with.

This morning in a little over an hour this gang will reappear here at the ranch for more walking and I promised them an archery lesson. This is my life now entertaining pilgrims. Some folks ask whether I am going back to Spain and the Camino but it is right here in our backyard.

Let me say that Loretta's group is pretty special and we feel pretty special having them here on our little island. Loretta just got back form Medjugorje. They all have visited various of the world's significant holy places and here they show up at Phil's Camino like somehow we are on the worldwide circuit now. That's just what it feels like.

Here is something special: every day at eight something in the morning the 39 students in Loretta's fourth grade class all pray for Phil and Phil's Camino. Huh, I didn't know that. I wasn't even close to knowing that but I am so moved. This is the kind of stuff that gets me through 100 chemo treatments I am sure. Amazing. Just another example of community being a healing tool. Thank you all.

Well, have to go and prepare for the merry band. It is all quite amazing. Amazing love coming at you, Felipé.

JULY 21, 2017 / A NEW ONE ON ME

Friday morning and this afternoon I will be jetting off to California. Here I am going to a church's mini-Camino to celebrate the Feast of St. James and I find that My Rebecca has ordered a wheelchair for me at the airport. What, wait a minute, new one on me. All of a sudden I am feeling like the Velveteen Rabbit thing where the poor guys eyes pop out and his joints are all wiggly but he is being loved. Geez, really, is this what it takes?

This last chemo round has been really hard on me and I am all beat up. I don't know if I am going to walk at all down there but do have walking sticks from Catherine in my luggage. What a deal. I heard that we are having three showings of *Phil's Camino* there with Q and A's after each. It's been a while since I did one of those.

Well, I had better get back to packing and make sure I have all my essential stuff. Trying to make it all good all the time. That sounds pretty improbable at the moment but trying none the less.

Love you, Felipé.

JULY 25, 2017 / ST. JAMES DAY

Feast of St. James today, wherever you are around the world. Can't get away from him although I don't know why you would want to. So us going from here to Spain to walk was all St. James. He is the patron saint of Western Washington and Spain and pilgrims in general you see.

In the Bible he is James the Apostle, brother of John, both sons of Zebedee. They were fishermen known as the "sons of thunder." It gets a little confusing because there is another apostle with the same name but he is known as James the Lesser. Then there is the "brother" of Jesus who wrote the beautiful book of James. He is a whole other character.

We do know the James the Apostle was the first of the Apostles to be martyred. The story goes that his body was whisked away and he was taken to the "end of the earth" which we know as the west coast of Spain. His body was buried a long time unbothered. Then somewhere in the 800s it was discovered and the first church was built.

Then for 1200 years we have been tramping through the dust and mud of our beloved Spain to get near him and his energy.

We at *Phil's Camino* the documentary film know him well in his role as Executive Producer. No one worked as hard as he did to make sure that movie was made. And now we are thankful.

Happy St. James Day all you Caminoheads out there! Love, Felipé.

JULY 29, 2017 / WHAT ARE WE DOING HERE?

After coming back from Spain this whole endeavor began to be fueled by the notion, "When you get to Santiago your Camino begins." I now take that to mean, yes, you have been trained and now what are you going to do with it? Or perhaps, you are still walking, can you feel it? Anyway, it has been a place to talk about this phenomenon and more exactly what my personal walk looks like.

In my Bible Guys class we are reading the Acts of the Apostles. And that whole book was written by Luke as a view into the walk of St. Paul and his fellow travelers as they rough and tumbled their way around the eastern Mediterranean spreading the news about the Gospel. Interestingly enough we do know that before the word "Christian" those who followed Christ were called people of "the Way."

What are you getting at Felipé? Well, I think there is still value in this sort of journaling that we have been up to but also I am starting to see something new emerging. This is with the help of Cris from Buenos Aires. She is grateful that we provide space where the Camino "exists." It is a place where we talk about it in such a way that it is here and now. It doesn't exist just in Spain or just on the way to Rome or Jerusalem. It doesn't exist three years ago but now in the here and now.

One of my Angels that I walked with in the early part of my trek across Spain was Laura from Barcelona. She runs a place there that provides a space for performing arts. The name of the storefront is translated Island in the Sky. It is a space, a chance, an inspiration, an acknowledgement, an environment for growth. This is what I see anyway. Maybe it is more than that but you get the general idea. That is what I am seeing in the Caminoheads blog now with the help of Chris looking at us from thousands of miles away. It is serving that purpose for her there where apparently fellow pilgrims are few and far between.

Buen Camino! Felipé. x

AUGUST 12, 2017 / ST. CLARE

So today is St. Clare day, the 11th of August. I vividly remember this day on the trail in Spain. I was walking with a teacher from Assisi, Italy whose name was Clare and she celebrated all day long. She was celebrating her name day which was a new one on me. She could have been St. Clare in modern clothing there just for me. The old magic moment on the Camino.

Enjoy it, love, Felipé.

AUGUST 21, 2017 / ECLIPSE

Eclipse morning here at Raven Ranch, actually it has started according to all the news. Funny, I don't feel any different yet. The sky here is totally clear so we are good to go, talking the lingo.

1017. OK, Tesia, my daughter, got the cereal box viewer going. I was just fumbling with punching a hole through my pie plate. OK, this is it! 1021. Well, I don't know about the glow emanating from Phil's Camino. Our equipment may not have been sensitive enough to pick it up. 1024. OK, that was it sports fans. 1028. The shadows still have the funny crescent shapes though.

OK, a good time was had by all. See you tomorrow for another excited adventure. 1030 and love, Felipé.

AUGUST 31, 2017 / FUTURAMA

I salvaged this word from my daily cleaning of spam from the blog. FUTURAMA! That's just what I needed, a glimpse of better things to come. I have a few minutes before my morning walk and just wanted to report in to you. Yesterday's mood was pretty gloomy after a scan showing minor growth. In itself it was a pretty good scan but we got caught up in the expectation thing, wishing and hoping for better, for a reversal after two months of hard work.

Well, I should practice what I preach at this point. The road to improvement is never a straight line or even grade, there are ups and down and even reversals along the way. But the overall trend in upward. That's what I say to students in archery. Don't let the memory of your last arrow affect your next arrow.

Last year I walked a labyrinth for the first time. That was at Grace Cathedral with Annie and Padre Tomas. I had never done one because I mistakenly thought that it was a maze. A maze has dead ends where a labyrinth has none, big difference. You go and you go and you go on the labyrinth. You can see your goal at the center but as you move forward on this trail you move away from the center at times. And at other times you are moving closer. It is not a spiral that sucks you toward a vortex but it is something far more interesting. It shows you this way, this Camino, where there are ups and downs or ins and out but if you keep going you will get to where you want to go.

Well did we successfully make lemonade out of lemons there? Ah, five minutes 'til my walk. Wiley and Henna got a new dog and I thought I would get her to join me today for the trail walk. OK, here I go. Thanks for all the comments and emails. Love, Felipé.

SEPTEMBER 1, 2017 / FUTURAMA PART II

The stars are out and the corn is ripe. Well, it is daytime now and that was last night but I'm still gliding along on the energy. Started picking the late corn yesterday which is really the main event. The early corn is, well, early. It is tender and delicate. I know you are early. Yes, yes we love you still. But it's just that the late corn is so much more, well, corny. It's high harvest, it is.

Back to the hospital today. Dana is driving me, the dear. Blue sky out there and it is going to be hot through Tuesday. Perfect corn-ripening weather.

The new addition to our family is fitting right in so far. Wiley and Hanna adopted a rescue dog from Baja, a Belgian Shepherd, female, 35 pounds, 7 months old. I got a feeling we got the perfect farm dog. A Belgian is like a half size German Shepherd. We got like a half-sized ranch here so perfect fit.

So, that's the local news. Was thinking some more about the mazes and the labyrinths. What if they were really the same. Well, what if the journey is the same but it was all in your mind how you looked at it. A reversal may seem a dead end to one person and their walk would suddenly turn into a maze because they couldn't go beyond. Where if you kept going it would be a labyrinth. I might be on to something?

Thanks for showing up today. Alperfect it is really. Love, Felipé.

September 4, 2017 / Caminoism

It is delightful really and I never seem to tire of it, this Caminoism. It is the Way. It is the Way of St. James or a close offshoot of Jesus Christ the Way. Before Christianity had a name, before that word was coined, the movement was called the Way. It's all related, right? And it is real, workable and accessible. That is the beauty of it.

Have to go do some work, Labor Day, no holidays around here apparently.

Miss you, love you, Felipé.

September 8, 2017 / Camino on a treadmill!

I have a Facebook friend Raya who I never met in person. Anyway she posted a pic of the controls on a treadmill that she was using and said that she was starting her new camino. Can a person have a camino on a treadmill? Totally outside the box, right? I love it! She's got us thinking. Buen Camino Raya.

Well, of course her whole school year will be an experience, a walk, a camino so to speak. But I love her thinking. Buen Camino, Felipé.

September 9, 2017 / It's Just You, Me And Saint Francis

That's what I said to a visiting praying mantis. I will have to tell you the story. It all started yesterday when I went in to talk to the bookkeeper at the local hardware store. I had a mistake on my bill and I wanted to get it straightened out. So the bookkeeper is this woman who I have known forever and she is really a people person but she works hidden away in the backroom of the store. So, when you go in to see her be ready for some conversation.

So after we got the work done she asked how I was and I said that I had just been stung by four hornets so the conversation headed off toward insects. I added that there had been a pic on FB of a praying mantis appearing on Vashon recently. She tells me of this praying mantis that she had a conversation with once. Yea, yea, OK. I said that I never had seen one anywhere before much less held a conversation. So, that was that and walking out of the store I was thinking really is it possible to have a conversation with an insect? Sounds crazy but who knows.

So I drive back to the ranch and I am still thinking about this as I go into our wood shop and I am dinking around there for a few minutes straightening up when what do I run into? Yea, a praying mantis. What? I had never seen one before in all my years and all of a sudden there he was bigger than life. He or she was perched on a piece of weathered wood and the same color, a light grayish brown, and I thought they were always green.

So I sit down on the next bench about four feet away. I'm on one bench and he is across the way on the other. So what do you say to an insect really? And I open up with, "Well it is just you and me and Saint Francis." And I go on telling him about my day and he is moving around a little bobbing his head like he is listening. And I'm telling him about getting into the hornets earlier in the day and all of a sudden he takes to the air and flies in my direction and I move over quickly since I already had my bad run-in for the day. He lands on my bench and walks across the bench toward where I am now sitting and climbs up on my hand and just sits there bobbing his head as I continue to talk. Yea, and after maybe ten minutes he evidently got bored with me or had other business to take care of he turned a hundred and eighty degrees and flew away back to the other bench. So, I left it at that and walked away a little wiser and happier.

Alperfect, love, Felipé.

SEPTEMBER 10, 2017 / AND THEN PINK MARTINI!

What an exceptional evening we had! Pink Martini is so much fun. They are so tight and accomplished. China Forbes was singing (she doesn't always apparently). She and Thomas Lauderdale, the leader, have been at this for twenty-three years. And there were nine other members of the band on stage last night.

Some of their songs are in English and some in all sorts of other languages. So last night they invited people up on stage that could sing along with the song. There was a song in French and a bunch of French folks went up to sing. And Turkish there were a lot. And three women who knew Mandarin Chinese. And they did a piece in Arabic and one guy got up there and had his own mike and sang with China Forbes. He was knocked out.

It was at San Michele Winery so we were all drinking wine and it started to rain toward the end but nobody minded. I'm exhausted here right now back at home, we got back just a few minutes before midnight. And just a thank you to Sister Joyce who paid for that whole thing as a gift, what a sweetheart.

So, am jumping up in a moment to pick corn for the day. This is the last day of the stand being open. I almost closed it Friday but decided I could probably stretch it over the weekend. People will want to BBQ and eat corn over the weekend. So we made it 27 days from the beginning of the early variety to the end of Bodacious, the later variety. A good run and it brought a lot of joy to a lot of taste buds.

OK, stop back by tomorrow. Take care 'til then, Felipé. x

September 11, 2017 / What Do We Do With This Day?

Well, Lisa from Hot Springs AK has her mission today. It is her son Caton's birthday. And she and we her far flung friends are celebrating the date for/with him. Caton is no longer with us as he was taken by an aggressive cancer not long ago. Annie and I met Lisa about this time last year in Hot Springs at their film festival.

Lisa drove us from Hot Springs to Little Rock to the airport on our way out. We all had that hour together and it seems we put it to good use. Caton was still alive and in various care facilities at that point. Medical science was doing everything that they could. Lisa was working all day and with him all night. She was impressively strong.

I am clinging to the celebration of Caton's birthday as a sign of hope even in disaster. Yes he suffered. Yes he died too young. Maybe a thousand other yeses. What do we do with all that? Can that be overcome, reconciled? I don't know unless we can grasp onto the idea that there is a bigger picture. This is all a challenge and a lesson, a hurt and a reminder. We really have to stretch ourselves to get anywhere with this, to get beyond the pain.

Somehow this is a little microcosm of the pain that our nation and the civilized world felt on this date in 2001. An unbelievable event had taken place. And what do we do with that? We are still trying to get a grip on it, at least I am. Maybe Lisa is way ahead of us on this account. She is striving to put the sad energy to good use. Bless you Lisa and your family and friends in on this.

What do we do with this day? Love you, Felipé. x

September 12, 2017 / It Feels Like A Monday

We could all prosper by tapping into the flow of the energy of our families and mentors. There is energy out there. We need to figure out how to find it and put it to use. Remember we have spiritual lineage too. The saints all have inspiration and energy to be had, that's what they do.

Love you, Felipé.

September 13, 2017 / 103rd

Numbers, numbers, numbers, they are everywhere here at the hospital. Here all day for my 103rd treatment. And I was down to 171 point something pounds in body weight. Need to eat some more of that corn on the cob. I was 173 after the Camino and I thought that was light, more ice cream for Felipé. Yea, I just don't have it today to write. See you tomorrow. Love, Felipé.

September 14, 2017 / Angela's coming, Angela's Coming!

Yes, yes, did the dishes, swept the floor, took out the trash. Yes, Angela is coming today with her new husband Dave. They are on a round the world honeymoon trip and of course one of their stops is Phil's Camino. Maybe this will be their favorite stop.

Three summers ago when Kelly and I were trudging the Camino we meet Angela and Mary Margaret about the same time somewhere out on the Meseta. Hot, dusty, exposed we clung together. But somehow tapas every night revived us. How does that work anyway? We achieved the rare prize of being "louder than the Italians" on occasion which is our real claim to fame.

Oh, I didn't mention that Ange and Dave are traveling all this way from Australia from Sidney. She and Gracie and Cherry were my introductions to that continent. Thank you ladies you did a good job, felt like I've been there. You were good representatives.

OK, time to walk the Thursday 0900 walk. Sunny, blue sky and cool today. Miss you all. Come see us when you get a chance. Most of you don't have to come all the way from Down Under, no excuses. Plenty of tapas to be had here! Love, Felipé.

SEPTEMBER 15, 2017 / WELL, WE CELEBRATED THE HECK OUT OF IT

You know, once you go through to the training on the Camino it doesn't take much to fire up a tapas party to the maximum. Off to the hospital again later but we are having a special walk this morning for our guests in a moment. Any excuse to tromp around. It is a beautiful late summer morning. It is supposed to rain Sunday/ Monday. We haven't really had any appreciable rain in something like eighty days. So it will be welcome.

Thanks for being here with us at Caminoheads where we try and keep the feeling alive. It's hard or maybe impossible to do it alone.

Miss you, love you, Felipé.

SEPTEMBER 17, 2017 / BLANCHING

Yesterday we had gleaning, today we've got blanching. I had to read up in the *Joy of Cooking* to get the procedure right for some corn freezing. Blanching is boiling or steaming to stop the action of enzymes that are detrimental to freshness. So I am going to blanch, cool, cut off the kernels, bag and freeze. Need to have some of that product for those winter dinners.

There is a little hint of autumn in the air. It is still pretty smoky because of the wildfires but rain is on the way, maybe a week of rain off and on. We tailgated this morning after church, Catherine and I but maybe one of the last. But it is fun, people stop by to chat, people maybe that you don't normally see or talk to. I think they call it outreach.

Oh, more corn to process, be back. OK, that's it for today. Now I am off to deliver some corn to a special person. She is a woman that is a checker at the supermarket. Her father had a sweet corn operation back in the day. He had three acres. I had a chance to use his mechanical seed planter this year back in May. So I try and get her some product now and then although bringing food to the supermarket seems weird.

Walking today at 4 PM. Hope to see you. Love, Felipé.

SEPTEMBER 18, 2017 / "WHETHER WE LIVE OR DIE"

"For none of us lives to himself alone and none of us dies to himself alone. If we live
, we live to the Lord; and if we die, we die to the Lord. So, whether we live or die, we.
belong to the Lord. For this reason, Christ died and returned to life so he might be the
Lord of both the dead and the living." Romans 14: 7-9 from the NIV.

This was one of the scripture readings yesterday at Mass. It resonated with me
and I have been thinking about it since. There is something very comforting about
what it says for me. Having the diagnosis means that dying within months is always a
possibility, always. This never goes away. It is possible to forget about it for short times
but it clings well.

To have this vision of life and death being united in this continuum is important.
Putting things in a perspective that is true and workable is always golden. And this
does it for me. The veil between life and death is getting thinner day by day.

So, as we live our lives we are also assaulted by the diagnoses of those around
us too. It gets to be too much unless we have some way, some healthy perspective to
view it from. How do we deal with it all can be a problem. How do we respond can be
a problem. But this is what makes it easier for me now. This notion that the veil is so
thin and Christ is here for us wherever we find ourselves.

Thanks for being here with Phil. Love you, Felipé.

SEPTEMBER 19, 2017 / LOURDES

Something is developing that is extremely important for me and it really isn't rock
solid but sort of an idea at the moment.

So this is the teaser that I may get a chance to go to Lourdes as in France as in
THE Lourdes. I just can't hold it back, it is way too exciting to think about. I am taking
it as a given but it isn't all figured out yet. It's in the half-baked category. So stay tuned.

As always, love you, miss you, Felipé.

SEPTEMBER 20, 2017 / FELIPÉ MAKES IT THROUGH THE SUMMER

It was tough but he did it! The autumnal equinox is the proper name for the first moment of autumn and the last moment of summer. Pilgrim Farmer John from eastern
Iowa always celebrates by standing out at the end of his driveway with his family and
watching the sunset. On that day the sun sets directly in line with his east/west road. It
is a gravel road, no pavement nearby. Isn't that elegant in a Pilgrim Farmer John way.
It ties so many loose things together.

Speaking of loose things, that was probably some loose talk on my part to talk
about the possibility of a Lourdes trip here at the blog. Everyone has been asking. But
it is an idea, well a little more than an idea. So, I have been chosen to be a candidate for
next year's trip that the Order of Malta puts together from the West Coast to Lourdes.
I am getting the official brochure soon so I will fill you in on the details. But you get
the picture.

This would be such an amazing opportunity for me personally and an opportunity to report on it for all our benefit. I am taking it very seriously in a Felipé sort of way. Right now I feel the need to start thinking about preparing. What does one do?

Well, that is what's new here. Time to pray for the people in the areas affected by new hurricanes and earthquakes. The eye of Maria is going over Puerto Rico at this moment. Man what a bad time for all this.

Off to the wood shop. Building another bench in there. It is slowly getting organized. Time to get stuff done that has been waiting all summer during the nice weather.

Hugs and squeezes and all that. Love, Felipé in a rain jacket.

SEPTEMBER 22, 2017 / MORE GOOD NEWS

Before we get too carried away I still have the washer to fix. But I have a new theory, a new approach to the problem that only seems to develop when one steps away for a time. So that is one corner of my life right now that I am trying to keep contained. That being said, some more good news rolled in yesterday. This was after the deal about the trip to Lourdes, sort of a dessert. I was talking with Cris our Caminohead in Buenos Aires yesterday and she will be up here for a visit in late October. She has a business trip to Chicago and will take a few days afterwards to come to Phil's Camino. That's the plan anyway. Yea, alperfect. I see that my spell check likes that now. OK, but if we can have alperfect it is not too much of a jump to "uberperfect." Ha! I like it! We have to have new words to cover new ideas or visions. Uberperfect love, Felipé.

SEPTEMBER 24, 2017 / LET'S REVIEW

So, let me say because I feel the need to explain that this blog rests on the saying that, "When you get to Santiago your Camino actually begins." just to make things clear. Three years now since Kelly and I got back home the blog has basically been exploring this idea. What does this mean? What does it mean to me, to us? Always remember that you are a completely unique child of God and today was made for you.

Miss you, love you, Felipé.

SEPTEMBER 25, 2017 / EARLY YET

Early morning here before our walk. The sky is gray and uninspiring. Most of the leaves are still green but tints of fall color here and there. The deer are frantically eating trying to put on a little more fat for the winter. They appreciate the cougar being gone I think. What was once a going concern, the corn field sits tired and lonely missing my touch.

We are in transition with summer rapidly disappearing and winter looming on the horizon. Going from salad days to turnip days, going from carefree to careful, going from sun screen to rain jackets. But it is all part of the natural rhythm that ultimately is comforting; you can count on it.

Off to walk. Need my boots this morning. Miss you, love you, Felipé.

September 26, 2017 / My power breakfast

Knock, knock, knock, that is what I woke up to this morning at 0620. It's dark out, who is knocking at our door? "Mike hi." "Hey we got a deer last evening and here is the liver and heart. Didn't know what time you ate breakfast." That's how I woke up this morning. Abundance comes in strange ways sometimes.

This abundant thing started yesterday. My Rebecca and I went out to Gravy for her birthday dinner. OK, just an aside, this is a semi-fancy eatery named Gravy where nothing comes with gravy, only on Vashon. Anyway we had our nice meal, and we were pulling out the card and discovered that an anonymous donor had already paid for our dinner. Well OK then!

We got home after that and Matt, one of my Marine Corps buddies stopped by to hunt the last light and brought fresh caught King Salmon. Some were filets and some was chunks smoked. Well OK then. This is getting hard to handle, right?

So yes, did have fresh liver for breakfast with Catherine y Dana's raspberry jam and will prepare the heart for dinner tonight. Sounds a little primitive perhaps but good eating and super nutritious none the less. I could make some gravy to have with that tonight, yea that would bring things full circle around here.

I don't think you can have all this kind of fun in the city really.

Miss you, love you, Felipé.

September 28, 2017 / Beat Up

Yea, feeling beat up after a hard day at the office yesterday. It was my seventh round of the hard stuff chemo treatment. We were shooting for eight but my body rebelled with an allergic reaction. So, they shut the treatment down and we worked on calming my body down. It is all a challenge. So, it is time to regroup with a scan and a new approach.

Balancing all that is the incredible support that I have in the thoughts and prayers of people that I know and some that I've never met. Ultimately this makes everything right. Ultimately we are in this flow of pilgrims that will take us home. Just like in Spain in the afternoon after a hot day of walking and our group was mostly brain dead someone would be capable of herding the rest of us into shelter. We are all headed to shelter whether we can see it from here or not.

Ok, off to my walk this AM. Looks pretty nice out and according to the weatherman one of our last days of summer. Good, let's get out there and enjoy it, uberperfect, love, Felipé.

October 2, 2017 / The Good, The Bad And the Ugly Once Again

I was all pumped earlier this morning to write about some good news in the neighborhood and we will get back to it shortly. But first we have to cover this tragedy that happened in Las Vegas yesterday and was all over the morning news. It hangs like something heavy on me now. We need to work through at least some of it to clear some room.

It is the killing of the innocents one more time. Two things come up with me at this moment and I need to start somewhere so here we are. One, is the question of how anyone could work themselves into a place where they would think this was a good idea to embrace and implement. Two, I am always struck by how quickly evil can be perpetrated. To do good always seems like life's work and this is the opposite in comparison.

Every week I light candles at church for the projects that I have heard of that are on my mind. People, angels really, get it in their mind to build a dream that would be so good for so many. Maybe it is a medical facility that is long-needed or a program to help a certain segment of the population that needs extra care. And they struggle and struggle to make headway. Everything seems uphill. I light my little candles and pray my little prayers as these certain individuals heroically sacrifice.

Ah, a little room and just enough to say how happy our family is at the moment. Our son Wiley and Henna got officially engaged yesterday. We are so happy for them. It is a moment to celebrate and remember. It is the start of bigger and better things for them and for us. It is a milestone along their journey that will go on to places beyond the horizon. All good, alperfect and even uberperfect, here's to you our children!

OK, a tough day to write a post on. Time to get organized and walk Phil's Camino next. It looks gray but dry out, comfortable walking temp. Maybe someone will show up or maybe I will say the rosary a time or two for our world. Always, love, Felipé.

OCTOBER 4, 2017 / JIM AND GLORIA HAVE ARRIVED

Jim, my oldest friend from Buffalo, is a physician, retired for a few years. His father also was a doctor and was our family doctor back when I was a kid. I remember him making a house call to see me when I was seven years old and suffering with chicken pox. House calls, that's old school.

He and I were up at zero dark thirty this morning and have been talking up a storm trying to catch up on all the news. One thing that we talked about that may interest you is that I want to record a conversation with him about an area of my life that has not been sufficiently explored or documented.

For six years I have been wrestling with cancer and its associated experiences. And for six years the doctors and nurses have been recording millions of facts about my case. Not a misplaced hair goes unrecorded. All this data is available for use. That is a track that is ongoing. So, now on the other hand we have this blog which is another track which has been going on for three and a half years. Every day I have recorded info that relates to the cancer in some way. That is track number two which is very personal in another way.

So these two tracks are moving along parallel with each other, sort of unaware of each other even though they are intimately connected. So I am asking Jim to help me connect them more closely and to possibly explore the area between them to see what we can find. It seems this may be important to someone. So, that is in the works, stay tuned.

The weather is beautiful here but chilly. Hope you are doing well. Love, Felipé.

OCTOBER 7, 2017 / ANOTHER DAY

Hope that you have a bonafide good day. Eat-a-new-apple, drink-some-fresh-cider, smell-some-leaves-burning kind of day.

Love, Felipé.

OCTOBER 9, 2017 / WHAT WE TALKED ABOUT

This is regarding my oldest friend who was here at the ranch for five days. Hope he survived, as I haven't heard from him since. No, I am sure he is fine, just resting up.

One thing that we covered was how diagnosis works. It is not always a one-shot deal that we think that it should be. We are hungry for answers and want them now. But a lot of times there is time involved because the diagnosis needs to be made on the evidence of a pattern that has to develop.

Another thing was the way that things happen and we try so hard to match them up by their cause and effect. This takes time also to sort out because some things that we think are effects would have happened anyway and just look like it was a result of the certain cause that we had in mind.We talked about how God has a way of showing up in bodies that are no longer healthy. Jim had good quotes for a lot of these things but I am repeating just the meat of the ideas. This one is so true in my case as witnessed by this blog. My cancer largely flavors my writings in a lot of ways. And talk of God largely flavors it as well. Without the heightened awareness that the cancer brought, this whole complex dance wouldn't have happened. There is this dance between and among Catholicism, Cancer and Camino that we are always working with here at the blog that influences but is not described in my medical records.

It is sort of like trying to connect art and science perhaps or religion and science. At first there may seem to have little connection or that they are even opposed to each other. But underlying there may be all kinds of similarities. And maybe this knowledge would help both efforts. This is what I am trying to get at.

OK, that is enough for one day. Time to get moving, walk time, love you, Felipé.

OCTOBER 20, 2017 / A LITTLE AFTER TEN

I was awake before dawn and spent a couple hours looking at the sky. The moon is in the final crescent so we see it early. There it was hanging above the horizon. And below it, as if it wasn't pretty enough was another bright body, a planet maybe.

But it was the Big Dipper that stole the show. When looking at this constellation you have to be impressed by its usefulness. The two stars that form the sidewall of the cup away from the handle point to the North Star. This being the most important star in the night sky. This is the same as True North. It saved my butt more than once.

The enslaved people escaping from the South on the Underground Railroad were told to follow the Drinking Gourd, their words for the Big Dipper. But besides its usefulness there is the beauty of the darn thing. There it is setting there like it has for millions of years now. What a treasure.

I was looking at the structure of it, the seven stars. It looks so perfect if not slightly worn. So many have used it, yes it's bound to be a little battered. The cup is in pretty good shape but the once elegant handle has a little bit of a crook in it. Well not anything to worry about really, just reporting. It still all points to the North Star, which is the important part.

And what if that was the really, really important part? What if Christ, the Living Water, is pointing the way for all of us? What if that has been hanging there all this time to show us? Well I am not saying I made some important discovery but it will never be the same for me from now on.

Who knew science could be so fun? And who said the sky is science anyway?

Felipé with reports from the field, x.

OCTOBER 27, 2017 / ONE HECK OF A BEAUTIFUL DAY IN THE NEIGHBORHOOD

Man, the weather is gorgeous. It kind of gives outsiders the wrong impression of Seattle. We don't want to let them know that it isn't always rainy and gloomy. Not a cloud in the sky right now.

Last evening we had a fabulous dinner party over at Catherine and Dana's in honor of Cris being here. We had buffalo pot roast and their own corn bread with a pear dessert. They know how to throw a dinner party believe me, all down home and elegant simultaneously.

Yesterday I put Cris to work on two projects along the trail. We planted some new lavender plants and dressed up some existing ones. Then we planted the cover crop where the corn stood not too long ago. I'm putting visitors to work lately on things that I need done and that are directly related to Phil's Camino. Just a few more things to do to get ready for the winter season. I need to mow the grass on the trail yet so it will be short all winter and that makes for drier shoes. Still trying to get some gravel on the inclines in and out of the streambed to make that less slippery. Not that I want the trail to be too civilized, just Caminoesque.

Well, that's the news from Raven Ranch and Phil's Camino. Hope that it is entertaining for you. Miss you, love you, keep going, love, Felipé.

NOVEMBER 12, 2017 / HEALING AND CURING

One of the most frequently asked questions when we are out on the film circuit is can you tell us more about the difference between healing and curing that you talk about in the documentary.

So curing as I understand it is getting over one's disease. It is all about the human body. It is all about being free from some limitation in our earthly life. This seems very important when put in the context of a certain way of thinking. A lot of effort goes into this endeavor.

Healing to me in the current way that I understand it is about how we relate to not only our particular human body but to everything outside of it. How we relate to God, to our fellow man, to the natural world and I suppose the man-made world becomes important. Are we calm in the storm? Are we at peace with the bigger picture? This is, as I see it, the real challenge in our lives ultimately.

So we see that we can be cured and miss being healed. And conversely we can be healed without being cured. So, it's a little tricky. Yea, well maybe we got a little further down the road on this one today.

One of the lines in the Catholic liturgy that is jumping out at me lately is "say the word and my soul will be healed." Maybe I need to concentrate on asking God for help with things. This is something that we/I seem to forget.

I have a passel of pilgrims showing up today to walk Camino de Felipé. It should be fun. And need to get some work done in the shop beforehand so have to go for now. Thanksgiving loves, Felipé.

NOVEMBER 17, 2017 / THAT'S US

Deep into November now. We have weathered a few storms so we are sharpened up on the drill. Gone but remembered are the lazy days of summer which always appear never ending. Ahh. But we remember we have tough genes handed down to us by our ancestors, people who got through the rough winter on turnips and prayer, living in their stone hut that they were thankful for.

We somehow have to mine our new territory for inspiration or humor or whatever that will keep us afloat. I hear the fire in the woodstove crackling in the next room. Yes, warmth is one of our allies.

Last month Wiley, James and I were sleeping out under the stars in eastern Washington. The experience reconnected me to something very basic. I was reconnected to the fact that nights are cold and a challenge in themselves. We with our insulated dwellings with modern heat lose track of this. A cold night is sort of an abstraction. But sleeping out and waiting for dawn for the sun to finally creep across the landscape to finally warm my bones was not an abstraction. This daily "winter" that we have largely bypassed is a real thing and would be helpful to be reminded of. Somehow there are lessons there that we have forgotten.

Well, I am out of time for now, for this day. There is always tomorrow for the blog, my ever-present companion. Yup, stay warm and stay inspired wherever you find that. Love you from afar, Felipé.

NOVEMBER 23, 2017 / THANKSGIVING DAY

Well, we made it this far to another Thanksgiving and most of the time in good style I might add. Half my brain is working on a prayer for the table today. It's coming along. My Rebecca will be up shortly to get the bird started. What is it 20 minutes per pound?

We are really excited about coming events here starting this coming weekend. Catalina from Berkeley will be here to further our project of the book about Phil's Camino the trail. The film has gotten a max amount of attention the last couple years of its existence but the trail has been in the background. Yet the film grew out of the trail so it will be good to get back to it for an exploration.

I should talk about Catalina for a minute. She came on board to help Annie with the film and she has been in and out of things since way back then. She is a scholar, pilgrim, professor and historian, oh yea, and a wife and mom to two gorgeous children. She has all the bases covered. I see her life as being a balance between the days of Hildegard the Healer and modern-day Northern California.

The idea for the book was hers and rightly so. With her expertise she was able to see things in the mud and the grind and the prayers of our Camino here, something that just wasn't obvious to me anyway. Just as there are shrines to Lourdes in France all over the world which were built so that locals who couldn't get to Lourdes could participate in the healing, she picked up on the parallel phenomenon here. This was all built for/by me thinking that I couldn't go to Spain and do the real Camino. She saw the historic connection. Love her. She calls the project here land art.

So land art it is Catalina. Well, maybe water art too as the season progresses here with the rain and current series of storms. So the book will try and capture this through the eyes and feelings of the pilgrims who have walked here. There have been close to 300 folks from all over the world who have come and participated. I have email addresses for 95 percent of them in the logbooks. So you all will be contacted and asked to write up your impressions of the situation here. Please find the time and energy for that.

OK, time to go. Have and great and meaningful day.

Love your gravy, Felipé.

NOVEMBER 24, 2017 / THE DAY AFTER

Things are cooking here, keeping the Camino energy going for ourselves and everyone around. Isn't it great that we have this calling and have the energy to pursue it? Really I don't know what I would be doing now if I would not have this to concentrate on, to focus on. Probably be worrying myself to death over one thing or another.

See you tomorrow, leftover loves, Felipé.

NOVEMBER 27, 2017 / PART OF IT

You see part of this book is about me, Felipé, part is about you and part is about the new emerging interest in pilgrimage and its importance to us. We are on some sort of threshold to a new way and pilgrimage seems to hold some clues and foreshadowing of what that is. You are a part of that, you see?

Ah, I have a walk in fifteen minutes with folks from out of town. The beat goes on as they say. Well, it's alperfect once again, Saint James is afoot! Love you guys, Felipé.

November 29, 2017 / Something Going On

Back a year and a half ago when Annie had *Phil's Camino* the film in for consideration at the South by Southwest Film Festival something happened to cause me a change of mind. We had been working on the film for nearly two years at that point and we were ready to start showing it in public. And that is where that process all started at that festival in the spring of 2016.

In there somewhere the news got out that the festival team looking at entries watched 800 short documentaries and chose 12 to include that year. Yea, we were one of the twelve, very heady. So, trying to wrap my mind around that lead to a new way for me to think about what we had. We had something amazing in our possession, a pearl.

And now, what I am trying to say to you is that I am having the same realization with Phil's Camino the trail. With Catalina being here recently and us working on our upcoming book about it I saw that pearl thing happening again. And it was magnified by the thoughtful papers that her class had written about our meeting. Here was another wonderful thing with great potential.

I am left humbled and with a feeling of great responsibility with this realization. Holding this pearl in my hand and wondering what our futures will bring, I am amazed as the Camino goes on ahead of me. Recently a realization occurred that the more I do, the more I do. What does that mean Felipé? That means that the more things that I participate in the more opportunities come up to participate. The Camino goes on ahead of me with St. James here in the background somewhere.

In the film I remember saying at the outdoor party at the end that, "This is a great way to wrap up my Camino experience." Very ironic as our dog Sture died a few moments after that happy comment and the dominoes have been falling over ever since and I am foreseeing more in the future.

So that is what is going through Felipé's mind today. Time to go, see you tomorrow. Love, Felipé.

December 4, 2017 / There Was A Question

Friday evening was so extraordinary. That was the showing of *Phil's Camino* on the big screen on Vashon for the first time. It will be talked about for years. After the showing Annie, Dr. Zucker, My Rebecca and myself did the Q and A. We have all participated in these before so we are practiced. But audiences come up with such a wide range of questions that it is always a challenge.

So, there was one man that asked the question, "How do you keep up hope?" Great question and Rebecca jumped on it by telling the joke about the guy who fell off the roof of a six-story building. He goes by the sixth floor and someone yells out, "How's it going?" And he yells back, "So far so good!" And goes by the fifth floor and someone yells out, "How's it going?" And he yells back, "So far so good!" Well, you see where this is going.

And she got a good laugh and it was a good short answer. But I have been thinking about it and I wanted to add more to that. The reason that it was a good short answer was that it pointed to the ability of some people in bad situations to live in the moment no matter how goofy that my seem to the outside observer. Obviously the guy is in big trouble but somehow he finds joy in his place in the situation.

I am going to put a capital on that since if you are in that situation that is the Situation. Somehow I have been able to find peace with my cancer and find myself in the very center of a whirlwind of my three C's. Those are Cancer, Catholicism and Camino. They swirl around me continually and provide a place for me to work from. I am in the eye of that storm.

Christian faith tells me that I have nothing to fear from death. That is the major key for me and helps with how to live this life gracefully no matter the Situation. Those are my thoughts on the question of hope and a longer answer to his question. At least today's longer answer.

Last night I heard that Bill just passed, another man I walked with and who told me that joke.

Ah, time goes on and I am still here saying, "So far so good!"

Yup, thanks for being here. Love you immensely and intensely, Felipé.

DECEMBER 5, 2017 / WE ARE OFF AGAIN

Yesterday I was feeling like something had to be done so I made a management decision. We have been walking at Phil's Camino for months without a plan or destination just wandering in the wilderness, as Catherine says. So, yesterday I left St. Jean Pied de Port for another virtual Camino Francés on Phil's Camino. It seemed like the thing to do.

I missed the structure of "Camino" walks which gave an additional dimension to the trek. So now you can ask me where we are and I can tell you. Right now we are on the outskirts of SJPP, a start!

Our first trek "across Spain" went from December 21, 2013 to May 12, 2014, six months. Then the second one went from August 16, 2015 to March 14, 2017, nineteen months. Now here we are starting again December 4, 2017. Nineteen months from now will put us in September 2019! Wow, will I make it that long, that far? Well, you guys will have to finish it for me if I don't, OK? Anyway, here is to Bill, Harry and Steve.

We have another walk this afternoon. It is pretty cold out these days but sunny. So, come and join us. Love, Felipé.

DECEMBER 18, 2017 / HEART OF THE CAMINO

Jane, one of our Island neighbors is making a tincture of hawthorn from our hawthorn berries along Phil's Camino. It is supposed to be good for the heart. So she is calling it Heart of the Camino. Nice, right?

Just had a nice evening walk with three new people. They all saw the movie the other night and that got them to come. The last lap it was getting pretty darn dark. I'm threatening to make some medieval torches to light the way.

There was a very cool comment from Mary Margaret, our Camino buddy, who bought a property in France and wants to set up a trail, a Camino trail. I think it is highly advisable that she hire a person with experience in such matters to come over and engineer it. Let's see, who do we have on staff here?

Well, have to go and cook breakfast for dinner and watch one more football game. Good for the heart loves, Felipé.

December 18, 2017 / Ah, A Few Moments of Quiet

It is a foggy morning out there when even our limited vistas are further limited. Everything is quiet and close. If you keep moving you will be warm. A good morning for the rosary to be said or just to be with. Yesterday afternoon's walk was very social and gabby, not maybe like this morning's.

Both are good. I trust that the right kind will be there for me exactly when I need it. The Camino provides, again, still, always.

It is apparent that today will be just what I need. It is yet to unfold but it will have a life of its own and it will whisk me along to where I need to be. This is total stream of consciousness, channeling along here.

Yup, time to boot up and get out in the air and the rough. Thinking of you, praying for you, love, Felipé.

December 21, 2017 / Birthday Party And Agricultural Report

Yup, my seventieth birthday today. Yikes! Party preparations for tonight's gathering are slowly starting to happen. But what is really cool about this date today is that it looks like our new granddaughter will be arriving today also. Yea, a double birthday!

We are flying out tomorrow night to be with all those guys in Massachusetts. Hope I survive the red eye flight. Then we will be back on the 30th so no walks in between there.

Maybe for the last time in the blog the I-5 highway is now open and traffic is flowing between Tacoma and Olympia after the big train wreck. That is good news for Christmas.

Lunchtime, and off I go to get ready for the party. Nice to be with you again, freely flowing traffic loves, Felipé.

December 22, 2017 / Donning Our Gay Apparel

Yea, we got the birthday out of the way with great style and now let's don our gay apparel and get with Christmas. The outdoor party was awesome though with lots of lanterns, a bonfire and some torches and lots of friends showing up to celebrate. And I was given the best birthday gift ever with the new granddaughter coming in a half hour before midnight EST. We have the same birthdays, yah.

Her name is Freya or maybe Freyja. A last-minute change from Cheyenne was made. So, Julia my nurse just Googled it and we got the scoop:

The name Freya is a Scandinavian baby name. In Scandinavian the meaning of the name Freya is: Lady. Derived from the name of Freyja, the Norse goddess of love and fertility and mythological wife of Odin.

That's hard to follow with anything I got. Pretty cool, a new member of the family. Well, maybe I will leave it at that today. You don't have time for lots of reading, too much to do, right? OK, I will let you go early, love, Felipé.

December 25, 2017 / A White Christmas Here

That is nothing new for New England, snowing on Christmas but here Vashon has it too. That's news! But snow or no snow it's a very Merry Christmas everywhere.

I hiked out to 8 AM Mass. Somebody tell me how the snow could be blowing in my face both ways. The service was nice with carols and the Padre had a plate of Christmas cookies for us as we exited.

I am waiting to hear the Chipmunks do some singing. Oh, kind of out of vogue I suppose. But I do hope that Martin Luther really did write "Away in the Manger." Well, a really big Merry Christmas to you all where ever you find yourself and whatever you are doing. Big loves, Felipé.

December 26, 2017 / Cold And Clear And In Love With Freya

This New England weather is the perfect Christmas weather like in Norman Rockwell illustrations or Currier and Ives prints. So intense one needs sunglasses to see it.

Anyway, the real news is Freya's arrival. And guess who is totally in love? I finally got to hold her and see her close up.

At Mass on Christmas Eve I got the message that "where I came from is where I am going." It is the notion that me going toward death is the same as going toward my birth or where I came from. All of a sudden that made sense. The only problem is that my birth was seventy years ago, can't quite relate or remember. But holding Freya connects me to a place to touch that mystery. It's really that easy and amazing.

Well, that might not be very Christmasie but it is happening at Christmas. It's a gift for me. Thanks for listening. Love, Felipé.

PART V

Abundance

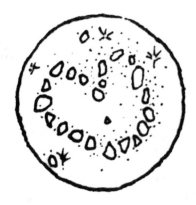

January 1, 2018 / The Spanish Table Goes On Into 2018

Welcome to the very new year, can't get much newer. Here we are on the threshold of a new space, a blank canvas ahead of us. What are we going to do with that?

On the coffee table sitting next to me is the *Spanish Table*, a cook and wine-pairing book, a birthday gift. Our dear friend Michelle from down the road just gave it to me for my seventieth. I like the title and maybe that is close to the mission statement for the new year.

That's a lot of what we do here, re-enacting the Spanish Table. We walk and converse and then we sit around that table to rest and celebrate our time together. It's a communion of souls meeting for a time to re-enact, to remember, to reinforce our memories of a special time, of a special community.

We don't need a lot and we don't ask a lot. It's all a simple thing really. It just requires an uncluttered space to unfold. Maybe that is what we should look for in our upcoming year, an uncluttered space. It will be a place where we can unfold together and share in what we have known and have learned. Thanks for being here, so far so good, love, Felipé.

January 8, 2018 / Checking In With Saint James

We are having a streak of rainy weather here. And that brings balmy temps as compared with other places in the States recently.

The walking is a little soggy though, and companions are few and far between. Standing water is starting to collect in spots and the creek is running. Some trees have gone over giving the trail through the woods more of a random look. The cover crop on the corn field is giving it a greener look as it slowly pushes skyward. The birds and the squirrels are busy harvesting sunflower seeds from the feeders.

So it is all different from the warm glory of summertime. Now it takes a little prep and care to be comfortable on the trail. But the rain always seems less of a problem when you are actually out in it as opposed to looking at it through the window. Once you are out there you get into the swing of it and it's fine.

I have been renewing my conversation with Saint James and perhaps that is what this time of year is good for. Time to review, as Kelly would say, the things that are important. Time to check out priorities and keep them straight. Time to organize, to build strength. Saint James guide me. The best to you there, love, Felipé.

January 9, 2018 / Back Home

My conclusion is that our time spent in Spain on the trail was participation in a training program. We were having such a good time that we didn't maybe realize that. But as we floated across Spain on good vibes and sweat we were learning the way to be.

So when we get to the end of the trail, the trail suddenly begins? Or when we have done the work, there is more work? Or just when we can't take another step there is another journey? Well, apparently so. For my only conclusion to this is that we are supposed to go back to where we came from and find a way to live that life that we have practiced, as best we can.

We are here, in our small place on the planet "still walking." Still ministering to ourselves and those around us, just like we learned. It's no different really. And hopefully our get together here, this blog/book, helps this happen. Welcome, Felipé.

January 20, 2018 / Beauty And Genius Require No Explanation

I just heard that on a hockey show out of Canada just now. What is really taking up my attention right now is that my hair seems to be falling out. I had some loss way back when and lost maybe a third of it and then it held so I really didn't get bald. Not that that would be the end of the world since guys with no hair is in vogue. So, practically, I think I will take a shower and see what happens.

In reality there are numerous side effects from the abuse of chemo and they are all a pain but hair loss seems the most obvious and gets the most attention. People in general don't know this and sort of glom on to hair. Obviously, dealing with this for so long, I have had experience with the many facets but ironically had little trouble with hair.

Well, beauty and genius require no explanation but apparently hair does. I guess we are a vain group of campers as a whole. Well I will let you know what happens with my situation.

If I haven't told you guys recently that I love you I will right now. I love you, you are the best. Bald loves, Felipé.

January 29, 2018 / Striving For Connection

Dr. Brené Brown is a researcher and she has been exploring loneliness. It is her observation that over the last twenty years we have "sorted" ourselves into "ideological bunkers" with the result that as we become more and more sorted, we become more and more lonely. We are "forgetting" our natural state of being connected to others on a grand scale.

Members of a particular bunker are united because they hate certain others and not because they particularly like each other. A recipe for loneliness. So more people are getting more and more lonely as they become more hateful of outsiders. Yuk! And what becomes really scary is that as this gets stronger there is an ability to move the hated group out to a place where they can be dehumanized. And so that means that we are free to do anything to that group.

So, where does Caminoheads come in? I think that our spirit is a breakout from this movement. We strive for togetherness with as many as possible. We strive for understanding of people and things that we are not familiar with. We don't like bunkers, we like universality of the open road. I think Caminoheads is a bright light in this view of the world. We aren't lonely! We welcome people into our lives whom synchronicity places there. We trust what we so painfully learned in the dust and the mud of the Camino about our fellow man, about ourselves and about God.

I am so enthused this morning not by this darkness in the world but about our little light shining. Let's turn up the wattage! Love you all, Felipé.

January 31, 2018 / A Tenth Of A Second

At the hospital today for a treatment after my two weeks off. I don't know if off is really the right word as it is more like work. Fun side effects to sort out and figure out how to minimize and work into a functional life. Anyway, enough of that. But the whole fascinating medical mashup buys me time, time to be with you.

So with all this time let's get on with it. I said the rosary on the ferry this morning, for the trip is about fifteen minutes. It's not an ideal place but it is a place. So, I was praying for two specific people that I was asked to do. Normally or most of the time I am praying for the rock pile at Phil's Camino which holds about three thousand stones, representing three thousand cares, wishes and thank yous, some of them mine. But today I was trying to concentrate on these two specific individuals and to tell you the truth I wasn't doing that great a job at it. But somewhere along the line it occurred to me that maybe if I was just clear and undistracted for one tenth of a second in there somewhere, that was all it really needed.

God is close by and He can pay attention to all of us at once I'm thinking. Everything that I got can be transmitted by me in an instant so I picked one tenth of a second as a working number. Why not? Most of prayer is for me really, to change me. I hear God already knows my thoughts anyway, right? So I am practicing one tenth of a second prayer. Just the shortest instant that a conscious thought can be. Kind of a zap. This is on my mind today.

Looking forward to Super Bowl. Alperfect, love, Felipé.

PS—Tonight is the night that St. Brigid will be afoot. We put out a handkerchief or bandana spread out on a bush outside 'til morning and that dew that is collected is from her, a healing liquid

FEBRUARY 1, 2018 / I HAVE A RANCH TO COME HOME TO

In all its funk and glory, I love Raven Ranch. Please let me express my gratitude for this tiny oasis in the turmoil of it all. We have light bulbs out and dead meal moths on the counter and scotch broom weeds sprouting up in all the odd places outside. But that is it, part Felipé order and part Nature reclaiming. Or is it part Nature and Felipé reclaiming. It's yin and yang swirling before my eyes.

And my lungs and liver are a tiny microcosm of this ten-acre play that is working itself out on the land. I have tumors which we, the royal we, have been able to blast, coax, coerce, zap, pickle and bully into very slow growth. It's party time for Felipé in the short term but obviously this glacial movement will crush him eventually without some sort of balance achieved.

We had a meeting this morning, my tumors and me, and I apologized for my treatment of them but it has been my only option so far. I acknowledged them as being part of me and not some alien entities. They are a rebel faction, a very robust one. But my job as I see it, as guardian of my whole being, including all rebel factions, is to strike balance. My intention is not to eradicate but to strike a workable balance.

They do their jobs these tumors with amazing tenacity in light of all we have been throwing at them and they just show up "Monday morning" with their lunch pails ready to go back at it again. And they are like the light bulbs and the meal moths and the scotch broom in that they have a job to do and I don't hate them for it but I just have to play my part to keep them within what I have visualized as a workable balance.

So, many great blog ideas have crammed into my head lately. I have material for a week ahead. One, just a sneak preview, is that Our Catherine has written a book which I just started on last night. So, now we can say Catherine Johnson, as her name is out in the world. Although lately I have been calling her Dr. Johnson around the ranch and environs. And it is entitled *Finding Mercy In This World: A Memoir*. Way to go Dr. Johnson!

Well, I have to go outside and collect my bandannas with St. Bridget dew on them. I will stack them up on my chest and shiver. Love you, Felipé.

FEBRUARY 8, 2018 / CHICKEN SOUP WITH SALTINES

Weak but hopeful is how I am characterizing my current condition. Had a rough 48 hours. But just finished a bowl of chicken soup with rice and a handful of crackers and that seems pretty normal. I know I missed writing the blog post yesterday and that very rarely happens and will give you some indication about how I felt.

But lovely angels are watching over me. My Rebecca is here at the ranch ever-present. Catherine y Dana swooped in with the chicken soup like they slide down a pole, a couple of firemen. Then, am in phone contact with my trusty nurse Alice at the hospital. They have gotten me through this hard spot.

Walking in a few moments. I will give that a go, one lap at a time. Charlie our neighbor has walked on the last few Thursdays so maybe he will be here.

Ever hopeful, love, Felipé.

FEBRUARY 11, 2018 / A SPECIAL BLESSING

I am here at Providence Hospital to attend a Mass and to receive this special blessing from the Archbishop. It is the Day of the Sick and that is me these days, one of the sick. The folks from the Order of Malta are here also to talk to me about the future trip to Lourdes, France. A future trip that I am trying to finagle my way aboard. Maybe finagle isn't the right word but I just wanted to use it. I have some gaps in my paper-work, and then hopefully I will be an official candidate.

Finally I am feeling better with my body and nearly normal on things of concern. Without whining I have to just say that these new treatments are a major challenge. I think I have expressed that over the last few weeks; maybe I should move on to something more interesting.

The Order of Malta is an interesting topic. This is an ancient organization that goes back to when the first pilgrims started venturing from Europe to the Holy Lands. They were first called the Knights of Saint John, that is John the Baptist, that John. They were tasked with protecting and caring for the travelers on these holy pilgrim-ages. They are credited with setting up the first hospitals anywhere. Sometimes they are referred to as the Knights Hospitalers. They are overall known for their work with basically the sick. And that's where I come in.

They want to include me in their annual trip to that famous healing place, Lourdes. All the chapters of the Order of Malta from around the world are converging on Lourdes during the first week in May. I don't know the population of all that but know that the West Coast outfit is sending 50 of us and each has a helper. So a bunch of us.

OK back at the ranch for a little rest. Then My Rebecca and I are back to Seattle for a dinner. Hmm, I am supposed to be recovering. Love, Felipé.

FEBRUARY 17, 2018 / GET TO WORK FELIPÉ

We are off to a very solid start to Lent with hope for a lot of progress. This reminds me so much of the Lent I spent in the spring of 2014. I was reading chapters of Annie's book as she emailed them to me. It was such a high time getting ready for going to Spain. We were working on the physical stuff and the interior stuff. And this now, this Lent, seems similar at least in its intensity. Our pilgrimage to Lourdes is on the horizon and is flavoring my walk at the moment.

Mass tomorrow with Father David. I am in such a great spot now with all the internal drama of my treatments and the energy that is coming in and the looking forward to France. It is a heady brew. Love to you, Felipé.

FEBRUARY 18, 2018 / FEELING BLESSED ONCE AGAIN

We have a walk in a few minutes. I think that we will be walking the Joseph trail today with all this wind. There are actually two trails here that we got to come out 4 feet in length from each other. One is our standard trail that we walk almost always which I call the Mary trail. Then when it is too windy to be in the wooded area of the property we switch over to the Joseph trail for protection from falling limbs, since he is the Protector.

So that is what it looks like here with the Felipé Family today. People are coming to walk and have tapas. Maybe I will go and start the prep on the food. Thanks for coming by, love, Felipé.

FEBRUARY 19, 2018 / WHAT HAVE YOU FIGURED OUT?

Yesterday we had a nice walk even though we had to cut it short because of the wind and cold. We retreated to the tapas table to talk it over. One couple was new to the walk although I have known the male component, John, for years. So Lin his friend was in from California to brave the locals and the local conditions. I was giving my usual sort of tour guide talk early on in the walk and at some point when Lin and I were together I said, "We have sort of a salon going on here in the French sense of the word. We walk and talk and figure things out." And she said, "Oh yea, and what have you figured out?" I was gathering my thoughts at that moment and then somehow we got distracted and the thread got lost. But I have been haunted by that simple question since. Yes, what if anything have we figured out in all this effort, expense of shoe leather and empty bottles of wine?

I know for one thing that we have figured out enough to perpetuate our togetherness. That could be enough although I am certainly trying for more. It would be nice to have a long list of accomplishments but perhaps we don't. I will ask around.

Here we are on the closing end of the first week of Lent. Are you making progress? Only the best, love, Felipé.

FEBRUARY 20, 2018 / REFRIGERATION NOT REQUIRED

Yea, saw that on my Mrs. Butterworth's Thick and Rich Pancake Syrup this morning. I thought, that's a pretty good idea on a personal level. I think I would just be fine getting through the winter without freezing my behind, thank you.

Yup, that's our big emphasis these days, keeping warm, and of course looking for signs of spring. And there are some of those. Crocus, Snowdrops, Indian Plum blooming now, that's a good start. Starting to snow now, tiny flakes.

Also, on a personal level it feels like Passover for Filipe. I have entered the time of my chemo cycle when I have had such a hard time in the past and it seems pretty smooth sailing so far. Some changes were made in my cocktail and in my diet and that could be the difference. This is very welcome.

Catherine called early this morning to see how I was doing. What a good buddy to have, checking in on my "walk." I am really leaning on her lately but that is what pilgrims do sometimes. We are supposed to learn how to ask for help and be humble enough to accept it gracefully.

Rho, a pilgrim from San Diego, is coming on Thursday. She is very much an archer and will get me out to do some shooting which has been on the back burner for me. Also she has a connection with Italian pilgrimage which will be good to learn about.

Well, little bits of news for you today. Thanks for stopping by to the ranch and keeping us company. Alperfect, love, Felipé.

February 21, 2018 / Ah, What a Morning!

I can't tell you how happy I am for getting through the night so easily. Last chemo cycle I had a very hard time, the worst that I ever had, but this time I was passed over. So the morning looks more beautiful. We are getting a grip on the side effects of the new chemical treatment and that is very heartening. I want to talk about that soon since I want to thank some folks for helping me.

Well, time for me to go. My Rebecca is making her world-famous mac and cheese tonight for the family. Have to finish up my tax prep. A February day here. Love, Felipé.

February 24, 2018 / Villatuerta To Ayegui

Here I am inside on the blog couch and Rho is out doing some laps before breakfast. Seems so odd to change positions. I am always the guy going past the window on the outdoor side. Oh look, I think she is doing another lap.

Yesterday we reached Villatuerta, Spain on Phil's Camino. It is approximately 40km west of Pamplona. The pic above has the beautiful bridge over the Río Ega. All the old bridges were so impressive. How many pilgrims have funneled over them since their building in what year?

Oh, there goes Rho and she has Henna with her. Wow, some kind of movement going on out there. I'm just going to hang tough on the couch.

There has been some bad news in the neighborhood. I don't often talk about the neighborhood here on the South end of Vashon. There is a very talented woodworker down the road here who has just gotten injured in his shop. He and his family belong to St. John Vianney Parish. Please pray for Marcus.

OK, that's what it looks like today. Rho is back making her breakfast. Thankful loves, Felipé.

February 26, 2018 / Gains And Losses

Monday morning and have a precious hour to be with you. I am going to walk at 0900. Blue sky out there right now overhead.

Well, we lost Rho. Well, we didn't really but she isn't physically present this morning. Ah, she will be missed. Like all our guests she left certain jewels and hopefully she took some with her from here. By jewels I mean inspirations or methods that we can now employ. One lovely practice that she played with was picking up three things from the environment and making little collages. Then rearranging and maybe rearranging once again. The pics of my rosary with various other items were her works.

I walked only one lap on Phil's Camino with her and then I had bad symptoms and couldn't continue. But when I said that she could walk alone and it would count in the logbook she just took off and did seventeen more laps in the next few days. Yea, enthusiastic!

We had some time to talk about archery and we got one archery session in. We will have to continue later as we just hardly made a start on it. I did get a chance to give her a beginning lesson on praying the rosary. Hopefully that is a jewel that will stay with her.

Well, that is sort of the bad news that Rho has had to go. And the good news that I have been waiting to announce is that I have been chosen to go with the Order of Malta on their annual pilgrimage to Lourdes, France. Just got the official phone call yesterday afternoon. This is happening in early May.

And the bonus to that is that Padre Tomas, the official unofficial padre of Caminoheads, will be going with me as my caregiver. This is an unbelievable occurrence really. There is some sort of chemistry that will certainly take place. Fasten your seatbelt Felipé!

Now in this time before the pilgrimage I will be preparing. Lent will help immensely just as it did for me before Spain in 2014. All good loves, Felipé.

February 27, 2018 / Scan Day

Off to the big city with Catherine in a while to get a scan to see how my lungs are doing. Two months of treatments accomplished, and now to see what is happening. Thanks for all your thoughts and prayers.

Wiley and I were out pruning our plum tree yesterday. I worked for half an hour before I ran out of steam but it was a gorgeous day and I couldn't resist trying. It is right along where we walk the trail and Wiley found this brand-new pair of reading glasses in the grass. They are 2.50 strength with brown frames. Who knows how long they have been out there. Are they yours?

Hope everything is well with you. Love, Felipé.

FEBRUARY 28, 2018 / JUST COMING UP FOR AIR

I went in today for news of the scan and for treatment. It was sort of a good news/bad news deal. The scan was good, showing a 10 percent shrinkage in the tumors. But the two-month effort has left me too beat-up to get treatment. So Nugget sent me home to recoup for one cycle. Try to gain a few pounds back.

I am home at the ranch. Please pray for me. Love, Felipé.

MARCH 1, 2018 / BACON MILKSHAKES

Yea, whatever appeals to me, I'm consuming. It's open season. I need to turn this weight loss around pronto. But it looks like a beautiful day happening here also. Maybe I will get outside a few times. We are working on pruning the few fruit trees that we have, I could maybe finish that up.

As a boomer born shortly after the Second World War we boys often related to the history of all that. I was always fascinated by the guys who would go in to disarm unexploded ordinance. Sometimes it would be sort of a routine operation where a known piece would be worked on and things would go smoothly 'til a safe outcome would be achieved. Other times, maybe a new never-seen-before device would show up. So, our guy would be out there on his own with a radio, reporting each move as he made them, to try and find the way to a safe resolution. Everyone else is back two hundred yards listening and learning. So, maybe that guy dies in the process but eventually with enough guys and enough radios a way will be discovered.

So, that is how I see my mission as I approach my tumors. At this level one doesn't know what is important or not. Everything is reported and a body of knowledge hopefully begins to form. I will probably die in the process but something valuable may be learned and that is the point. So, that is the basis of what I do. I am not sure that I individually am able to figure anything out. But when people get together and we talk our salon talk, ideas do come together and interesting notions start to form as a result. So, going long today, sorry. Recovering loves, Felipé.

MARCH 5, 2018 / A FILM

Last evening I watched *The Song of Bernadette*, the 1943 version, the story of Lourdes, France. Over two hours long in black and white. At some point I had read a book about her so I knew the basic story. But this filled in some of the blanks for me. Check it out when you have some time. But be prepared for suffering. Somehow these apparitions are never easy affairs.

Lin's question of what have we figured out is still ringing in our ears. It's all good and alperfect, our quest.

I think I will go and get my day started. Steve-O, our good friend from Ashland, OR, is showing up this afternoon and I have work to do before then. Thanks, love, Felipé.

March 7, 2018 / Getting Spoiled

Man, another nice day in the making. Sherie is coming to be here for the day. We are going to shoot some arrows and do some clean up on the trail. It is spring cleanup time after all the wind storms that we have had. There might be some wind coming in tomorrow yet, so not quite "out like a lamb."

I guess I got all philosophied out with all the figuring out we have been doing lately. That was all great, right? I have to balance all that with some physical activity. That was another aspect of the Camino that was so great: the balance of the physical with all the other stuff that was going on. Of course we had better ask our feet that maybe. They might have a little different story.

Kelly my good old Camino walking partner is to have a hip replacement this month. Please say a prayer for the guy. I should give him a call.

OK, I'm good, you're good, the sky is blue. Work hard, play hard loves, Island Felipé.

March 8, 2018 / So Far So Good, Hey?

Sherie, the dear, when she came yesterday brought me a very special gift. It was a quantity of holy water from Lourdes that she had brought back with her eighteen years ago. Yea! I am starting to put it on myself whenever I think about it throughout the day. My pilgrimage has started!

I talked with my group leader yesterday who called in from Utah. Getting details hammered out. Padre Tomas is working on securing my travel arrangements between here and LAX, where the international flight is originating from. I can feel the energy building. We are coming, Bernadette!

What a great week it has been, very restorative. Charlie will maybe be here in a few minutes for the Thursday morning walk and will add to that. Just had a thought that the restoration to myself not only included my own body and spirit but also the visible work that we were able to accomplish on the trail this week. It just makes me personally feel better to have the trail improved. It was in pretty rough shape after that winter, like me too.

Well, time to find my boots and logbook. We are approaching Viana on our third "walk across Spain." Maybe come and join us one of these spring days. Love, Pilgrim Felipé.

March 10, 2018 / We Are Continuing

No big thoughts. But realizing that we have inertia. We have momentum. At this point it is easier to walk on than it is to stop. We have gathered so much energy over the years that movement is what we do. We have to think of ourselves that way.

I continue to treat my skin with holy water from Lourdes. I continue to get stronger day by day. Yesterday I planted an Oregon Grape plant that neighbor Charlie brought by. And am continuing to make progress on my church cabinet job that has to be done before I can leave for France. That's a little over six weeks away. Keep going sort of loves, Felipé.

MARCH 12, 2018 / MY HOLDING CROSS

Yesterday we had a lovely group of pilgrims come from the mainland. Sui, who is an oncology nurse, listened to a talk that My Dr. Zucker gave recently. He showed some *Phil's Camino* trailers with his talk. So, Sui came here yesterday with a whole gaggle of family to meet us. What a treat for us! We walked our three laps and had tapas outside, first of the year!

It was special yesterday. And Chris, a neighbor, joined us. It must be spring with all these people showing up and crowding the trail. Some of the folks had been to Lourdes, the Camino, Fatima, and Medjugorje amongst others. And now they have walked Phil's Camino. We are on the circuit.

But Sui brought me a holding cross which has been blessed and it is a prayer just to hold it. Like on the Camino when we were too breathless to pray with words, we learned to pray with thought. This cross is for me to hold and there will come a day when I am too weak for words and all I have to do is hold on to the holding cross. Thank you Sui.

So many nice folks have come and gone out from Phil's Camino over the years. They spread the healing that we have been able to gather to other people and places. And they come and the dust on their boots comes from other amazing and holy places to enrich our trail here. These folks have even been to a place in Taiwan where Mother Mary appeared to a group of Buddhist monks, we have that dust too! Such a richness.

Well, off I go again. Our Monday morning walk. Time to find my boots and the logbook. See you tomorrow. Dusty loves, Felipé.

MARCH 13, 2018 / THE FLOW OF PILGRIMS 2018

Our dear neighbor Michelle sent in an email reminding me that I am a part of the "great cloud of witnesses." Yes, remind me, remind me, constantly remind me! This should be a constant hum in our consciousness!

Here in the past we have talked of it as the "cloud of believers" and the "flow of pilgrims." Same, right? But what a powerful notion to be caught up in. To be swept along by the magical inertia of those around you. We do that for each other, or it is what we do when we are at our best. For this I am joyful!

Thank you, Michelle. Thinking of you in your greenhouses planting all those seeds for the plants that you will sell later in a few months. It is the start of a busy time for you. Maybe I can break away for an hour here or there to help.

I am still high on the flow of pilgrims that we had here on Sunday afternoon. Sui and her magical mystery tour came to Phil's Camino. Am I lucky or what? They come and talked of the mighty pilgrimages that they have taken. I listen, I learn, I am inspired. Just tell me, how can we go wrong?

Time to go. Shopping day for Felipé. Have to buy the corned beef and cabbage for Saturday's dinner. Oh, I start treatment again tomorrow, pray for me please, it will take courage. Thanks, flow-on-loves, Felipé.

March 16, 2018 / OK, I'll Have A Coffee, Sunrise Eggs and Some Holy Water Please.

Here I am having one of my favorite hunting camp breakfasts: eggs cooked with corned beef hash fresh out of the can. Then there is good strong coffee. And then there are three dashes of Lourdes holy water, one behind each ear and one on my chest. I am a happy guy.

Sometimes the components of sanity seem pretty simple. I am walking through my fifth new treatment with the chemical that I need to know how to love. It is helping me, it is helping me, it is helping me but it is a hard relationship. It takes all my powers to deal with it and to try to come up with a way to live with it. Yea, but I am confident that this will happen with your prayers and coaching and hovering over me.

Speaking of hovering, Catherine and Dana are back from their two-week junket in Hawaii. I have missed them immensely. They are the best at hovering over me. It is reassuring to feel the pulse of that soft breeze their wings create. I'm a happy guy.

What else is new? My Rebecca made the bestest spaghetti sauce ever. I am always trying to make the bestest but I was humbled by her entry. She built it around a pound of ground venison gifted by Brad and Amy, other great neighbors. I am eating well when I can and have turned my weight loss around. Once again, happy, happy.

My Rebecca dragged me off for some culture a couple evenings ago here to the Vashon Theatre. *Big Sonia* was playing. It is a feature length documentary about a very active, kickass little, as in physical stature, woman who survived the death camps of World War II Europe. Very moving film, you'll laugh, you'll cry, you will receive an education.

OK, time to get ready for my trek to the big city and the treatment center. Happy loves, Felipé.

March 17, 2018 / A Saturday Morning

Well, we can get hung up over things we don't understand or we can travel on with the knowledge that we know enough for today. Tomorrow is another day with its own revelations, that today is enough for today.

Somewhere along the line I have picked up the idea the God has the three attributes: Truth, Goodness and Beauty. Which means to me that I can move toward God or God can move toward me along any of those three different pathways. To understand beauty is a whole different ballgame than understanding goodness or truth. Each has its own logic and method and rhythm for instance.

This is a tremendously freeing notion to have these three ways to progress. This is what is coming out of me today. Hope this makes a little sense. Morning loves, Felipé.

March 19, 2018 / Looking Forward, Looking Back

I don't think that there is a day that goes by without me thinking of my stay on the Camino in Spain. Kelly says that too. Fascinating that such a short time could have such an impact on us. Cathy and Tim were here yesterday to walk in the afternoon. They are such a joy. Easily I can see myself walking with them on the Camino or most anywhere. Thanks to you both for your energy.

Looking back in the way that it occurs to me is not something nostalgic. I don't seem to dwell on it in that way. It just pops up matter-of-factly and says hi in a tidy little memory package.

But I am looking forward also. My corn seed came in for this spring's planting. That will occur in May shortly after the Lourdes pilgrimage. The whole corn ritual seems more important to me as the years pass, planting being only one part of it. I look forward to the different stages and the anticipation of the harvest. So much of farming is planning ahead, a little gambling and faith in the way the future unfolds. Well, it is to some extent looking backward in the sense of keeping track of all the mistakes made and lessons learned, but it is basically forward looking in my book.

So, yes, we can't forget about leaving enough energy for the cultivation of the present, that most fertile area. Are we leaving enough of ourselves available for that? We can't get too wrapped up in the past or the future to its detriment. Of course, that happens sometimes but aren't we getting smart enough to recognize it? I hope so.

Off to walk my Monday morning walk. It is dry and overcast out, the fog has broken up. See you tomorrow, present loves, Felipé.

March 20, 2018 / Keeping Afloat

The cloud overcast has got to be very thin and fragile. It is half blue and I expect a gorgeous morning when that breaks up.

We have a walk this afternoon. It is so springy on the trail. All the puddles are dried up and leaves are pushing out. And we have it cleaned up after all the winter wind storms. It almost looks like a different place. Come by when you get a chance. Yea, keeping afloat. That is what we do for ourselves and for each other. I think at this point we are getting pretty good at that. At least I feel the beneficiary of that kind of love and I hope that you do also as we continue to buoy each other up.

Well, here we go, meeting a buddy for breakfast in town. Thanks for stopping by. I'm getting to feel like Mr. Rogers. Thawing out loves, Felipé.

March 22, 2018 / Amenities

Jim has been staying in too many hotels lately. This morning before breakfast I was scurrying around getting things organized in the kitchen and he was working on his first coffee and he was seeing the things around him. He said, "You have some nice amenities here." I wasn't even sure I knew what that word meant. He started listing things that he saw that maybe a hotel would list as plusses.

One was that he could hear the rain on the house giving us a connection to the outside, the outdoors. I forget most of them maybe because I live with them on such an immediate basis that I take them for granted. His best one was that the fire in the woodstove that he could see through the glass in the door was there for a reason, to warm us up and not just for looks.

I know we have lots of visitors and they all see different things that may be memorable to them because they are out of their ordinary. When I am here working around I may have thoughts about paying the bills or how do I beat back the jungle this week, a different view, and miss those essentials.

When Edmund and Irene were here from China and who live on the 23rd floor of an apartment building, what do they see? When I have a group of my Black friends out from the city what do they see? When I have the Taiwanese family here, what do they see and take with them?

This is good for me to think about as it forces me into the present. It puts me in a better place to view my surroundings. And in this new light I may have things that I notice anew. One that I have been thinking of lately is when I get up at six-thirty in the morning and look out the window to the north toward our son's house his lights are on as he gets ready to go to work. It is a reassuring thing for both of us I hope.

Well, Jim and I are off to walk in the rain here shortly. It is a light rain watering the beet and green onion seeds that My Rebecca and Jim planted yesterday. It is a spring rain. So, as always, looking around loves, Felipé.

MARCH 26, 2018 / OVER THE HUMP

Seems like I am out of the tall grass, out of the bad side effects, with this particular chemo cycle that I am in. So happy! Man, this last three months has been hard but it looks like we are making progress to find a way to coexist with this particular chemical treatment. This last cycle was way easier on me. Thank you, thank you, thank you!

God continues to keep me alive for his own reasons. We are all participating in this project obviously. And we continue to blow on our little flame, the Camino spirit. It is such a deserving entity. We are obviously in love with it and we continue to be. That is the story here early on a Monday morning in the Holy Week of 2018. Easter awaits at the end of the trail.

Walking in a moment. Where are my boots? Where is the logbook? Gray skies with lots of rain and snow in the territory surrounding Puget Sound but dry here so far. Thank you loves, Felipé.

MARCH 27, 2018 / UNTANGLING

Of course when I was mentioning components to my wellbeing yesterday I left out whole bunches, whole segments, whole quadrants. It is impossible to untangle and to state truthfully that "X" was the reason something happened or that "Y" was the main component to my success. I am seeing so much love and support from so many places and people that every time I mention one I forget three. We are accustomed to do the old cause and effect thing, or I am. But with complex situations is it possible or recommended?

Thank you Sherie for the holy water from Lourdes. I have my little mustard jar that is half full and I administer it every morning to my body. This is so powerful in my mind.

People like Sui coming into our lives like unchained energy. She would make a good Marauder. The Marauders being the Catholic group from Southern California. I named them that for their endless energy and enthusiasm. They all sparkle.

Sui sent a signed copy of *The Dance of Christian Life* by Scott Connolly. He is a Catholic priest and the last time I heard he was up in Bellingham, WA. Anyway lovely gift, lovely man. I am very familiar with this beautiful book. Way back when in the spring of 2014 Sister Joyce lent me her signed copy. Kelly and I read it and we actually got a lot of our thinking out of it on how to walk the Camino. For sure we copied his pace of 12 1/2 miles per day. We were able to put together an itinerary, well a rough one, so the film crew would know approximately where we were going to be. Anyway it is a lovely big-format book. Thank you Sui. Looking forward to rereading it and savoring memories of the places along the Way.

So yea, springtime along Phil's Camino here at Raven Ranch. We have an afternoon walk today at 4. I think that we may have picked up some new walkers from our shindig at the Eagles Club. I handed out a bunch of my business cards with the walking schedule on the back. Nothing like new people, new ideas, new ways, new walks.

Tomorrow back at the hospital in Seattle. Back to start a new cycle. This will be number six of the new chemical treatment. I am so much more confident now than ever before. I can handle this! Thanks for all your thoughts, prayers, support. I know that I was asking for it and receiving it by the truckload. Gracias amigos.

Time to go, have a big day. Glad that you are here to share some of it with me. Big tangled loves, Felipé.

MARCH 28, 2018 / BLOGTIME AT THE TREATMENT CENTER

OK, here we are, all cozied in with my chemicals in the comfy chair. Time to say hi. Just had a great visit with Dr. Gold where we agreed that we are on top of the situation. Finally we have a workable configuration of agents that agree with me. And my weight was back up to 170 pounds. So royally happy that we turned that weight loss around, was scary. So, all good news coming at you from here at the moment.

I can feel my energies being freed up from all that. It has been three months now when most of my attention has been on treatment and its side effects. What a relief to have a smoother trail for a while. Time to find ways to build my strength again.

Just a bit of Springtime news, Seattle Mariners Baseball opens tomorrow here at Safeco Field. What do they call baseball players sometimes, "The boys of summer"? Yea, I like that. And the temperatures here have gone from 40s during the day and 30's at night to a balmy 50s during the day and then 40s at night. This looks like spring to me and it is going to bring on the blooms that will fill the air with fragrance here soon. So you had better come and help me walk the trail here one of these days soon. Springtime loves, Felipé

MARCH 29, 2018 / CONFESSION TODAY

Yup, Catherine and I got an appointment with Father David to do the sacrament of Reconciliation which is the new word for Confession. I'm not totally switched over yet and maybe that is part of my problem. I struggle with this, and the longer time I wait in between, the harder that becomes.

The heavy-duty portion of Lent has arrived. We are hopefully in our introverted mode and are thinking how to make our connections to God and our fellow man better. That's Reconciliation there. Oh, I am so glad that I am writing about this as it is getting it in better focus for me.

If God wanted robots He would have created them but he didn't, He created us so we could wrestle with it all. He wants us to choose Him and His Way every day. We screw up, we get distracted, we . . .

It is the challenge for us, this choosing. Lent is the time to get that process back in shape, back in good working order, oiled up.

Yea, so a walk here at Raven Ranch at 9:00 this morning. The trail is looking pretty darn dry these days and we are getting it cleaned up after the winter storms.

Reconciling love, Felipé.

MARCH 30, 2018 / A FULL TANK OF GAS AND HALF A PACK OF CIGARETTES

Yup, we are all ready to blast into Good Friday. Sunny here in Seattle. It doesn't have to be dark and gloomy, does it? At the hospital 'til early afternoon and planning on meeting Catherine for afternoon Mass on Vashon.

Just trying to keep it simple as possible today. No tricky moves, no power tools. Just cruise along and take care of the important stuff. I don't think I can go much further with this blog right now with the mood that I am in. So, talk with you tomorrow, yes? Love, Felipé.

MARCH 31, 2018 / NOT JUST ANY SATURDAY

Here we are balanced between Good Friday and Easter Sunday, two polar opposites. This Saturday that is in between looks like something empty sometimes, like a blank spot. Does it have a purpose? It never did really for me until I stumbled on a notion. I'm calling it a notion because as far as I know it isn't exactly spelled out anywhere officially. It is an idea. And that starts with as it says in the Apostles' Creed, Jesus "descended to the dead."

Yes, and what did he do there? The notion that I love is that He preached to the multitudes of past eras and offered them His Covenant. I like to think that is what happened so that no one is left behind for not hearing about it. It seems a perfect fit in my mind and a sort of puzzle piece that I enjoy putting in place even if I don't have proof of its existence.

And how about Notre Dame's win yesterday in women basketball? Catherine and Dana were over yesterday to watch as Catherine is a huge fan of ND. So they are in the finals tomorrow against Mississippi State. The finals! So we have more basketball thrills and chills tomorrow. Easter and Catholic basketball, that seems a fit.

OK, on my way to do some tilling with the tractor. Beautiful day here. Love abounds, Felipé.

APRIL 2, 2018 / EASTER AND A LINE FROM A HYMN

Yup, Easter 2018! There was a line in one of the hymns that grabbed my attention, "manna of the ages." I don't know, I wish I had more today but maybe that is enough. A special day today, may we always feel that and understand that. Love, Felipé.

APRIL 2, 2018 / A BIG THANK YOU

There is a fourth-grade class at St. Joseph's School in Upland, CA. They are lovingly being taught by a friend of ours, Loretta Bowen. My Rebecca and I met Loretta last summer and got a chance to meet her class last fall. What remarkable meetings they were.

This crew is very intent on connecting me with God's healing power. They want to see a win for Mr. Phil at Phil's Camino. Every school morning as a group they pray for me and my situation at 0815 at the start of the school day. Like right now as I look at the clock thirty some intent school kids are sending out their energy. You gotta love this!

So on this last Saturday, the between day that we were just blogging about, I received a big envelope from guess who? Yes, Mrs. Bowen's fourth grade class. And inside were thirty some handmade Easter cards. There were bunnies and eggs and crosses and rosaries and chicks and rainbows and one lone space alien. Yea, for Mr. Phil and Mrs. Rebecca. What a blessing these youngsters are!

I am going to think of something to brighten up their school year. What if I put a donation can out on Phil's Camino for the "St. Joseph's Fourth Grade Class Party"? What if we collected a little cash for their fun. And I would get to tell their story about how they pray for us because people would ask. OK!

OK, I am glad that you know about that. Off we go now for the morning walk. The sky is blue and the trail is dry. One lone space alien loves, Felipé.

APRIL 3, 2018 / THANK YOU

Here I am at the very beginning of April and I am feeling the pull of the Lourdes trip which is four weeks away. In terms of treatments, I have one more to go. In terms of projects, I need to finish and install the cabinets for St. John Vianney's. Getting close.

It was a wonderful Easter. I was much inspired by the whole thing. But one thing that really got me was the new converts that joined at the Easter Vigil just like I did five years ago. I am trying to find them all and welcome them personally. Love you guys, Felipé.

April 5, 2018 / Reporting On A Fun Day Yesterday

Exciting things were happening yesterday, some kind of confluence of the old planets I suppose. Catherine had her book reading and it was standing room only, ridiculous. Us old deaf guys had to retreat across the street and drink wine. We were all so happy for Catherine on the birth of her memoir, a milestone.

In the morning Karen from Chico rolled in with her sis Robin from Seattle. Karen had seen *Phil's Camino: So Far So Good* (the long version) down there in California with Annie recently. Karen did the Camino Francés last summer so she was full of that good energy. Robin is being talked into going which didn't sound that hard to me.

We talked of hospitality, Camino-style. That still is the one word that I can boil down my Camino experience into, well at least at the present. I suppose it could be twenty or fifty other words also.

We also talked about how we wish that we could give certain people the experience, if that was in our power. Probably have to win the Lotto for that one though. But is it possible to win over or pass on "Camino dust" to folks like that without the direct experience of the walk itself. Isn't it our inner glow that is that? Isn't it Dana so warmly welcoming people to the reading last night while Catherine prepared? Isn't it our own personal hospitality that we show to everyone that is that? We have to think on this.

Off to walk here in a moment, my trail awaits. Get that glow going loves, Felipé.

April 6, 2018 / Now What?

The best thing that has come out of this week is the idea of "Camino dust." And there must be "Easter dust" as well. It is a notion in my head that occurred after talking with Karen and Robin. One was freshly back from Spain and the other was contemplating going soon. So there was this differential happening there between them.

So back to Camino dust. If I derived benefit from pretending I am on the Camino, and if we as veterans of walking in Spain can influence someone to go and do that walk, then isn't there something that is being passed around between us that is this inspirational dust that just happens? There is this buzz, this energy that is palpable.

Can we transport this dust and will it be potent when removed from any props that we have used in the past? Am I making sense here? Is it a commodity that just is? Is it a glow or a glint? Do we have to go back to the Camino to get more? Is there some along Phil's Camino? Or can we get it from each other?

Well, obviously more to sort out. Thank you Karen and Robin for your influence. Off again here in a moment. Am going to try and visit Kelly today. He has had a new hip put in recently and is receiving visitors. OK, the best to you all, love, Felipé.

April 11, 2018 / Last Treatment, Next Stop France

Am getting things checked off of my to do list. This is my last treatment day, then back on Friday to the hospital to get disconnected and I am done with this for a while. Dr. Gold gave me my next treatment off and wished me a good trip, so I feel blessed.

Cloudy out now looking out the window. It was so beautiful out yesterday at the ranch along the trail. It was that day that everything looks so beautiful that you finally call it spring! A little regression in the weather today but we'll bounce back.

I am trying not to think too much about the pilgrimage to Lourdes at the moment. I have this cabinet job to get installed before I go so that has my attention. When that gets completed I can relax and change modes. Not that I wouldn't like to get "prepared."

So fortunate to have this chance at another pilgrimage. This is so timely for me. Will be reporting from there daily. Padre Tomas will be by my side to help me interpret the happenings.

One thing that I haven't given enough time to lately is the new flock of ducks happening next door at Wiley and Henna's. They got four baby ducks that are pretty dang cute.

Yup, that's the way it is today. Time for lunch. Ducky loves, Felipé.

April 20, 2018 / Things Bursting And Ricocheting Around The Venue

OK, I really don't know where to go from here. There is so much energy here right now that I am barely holding on. Spring energy and end-of-project energy which we have talked about. Visitor energy with Annie and Esther coming tonight. I'm not even getting to Lourdes energy which I am trying to keep the cork in for the moment.

Esther had an awesome comment combining the robust fecundity of our descriptions of springtime with the blossoming of Caminohead energy. Camino dust abounds, it is thick in the air like the tree pollen right now. The air seems visible right now. Yes, certainly, this could all be.

It is wild and wacky but deep and wide. It is slick and slippery but something you can always count on. It is visible and then disappears. It seems to travel well but can be found everywhere. It is timeless but then always here at the very moment. It is friend and foe. It helps you move forward and then trips you up. You can always give it away but you will never tire of it. Just have to surf on it all right now, the only thing to do. Blue sky, rising barometer loves, Felipé.

April 23, 2018 / Thinking Of The Weekend

Just got back from an action-packed weekend with Annie and the gang in Olympia, WA showing *Phil's Camino: So Far So Good*. It all went pretty wonderfully. So, part of the audience there at the church hall was made up of a cancer support group that was meeting there at the same time and came over. And while the questions that Annie and I fielded were, as memory serves me right, all about pilgrimage and the Camino, nothing much came up about cancer and that whole world.

I don't know if I have anything particularly new to say on that front but there are some basic ideas that I could review. This is all beyond and/or in conjunction with your treatment. One, from Dr. Zucker's teaching, exercise can be used as a form of medicine. Movement strengthens the body and that gives the ability to do more. It builds on itself. Movement actually cuts down on fatigue which seems counterintuitive. I have found that exercise outside in a peaceful environment brings added benefit.

The ability to cut back and limit fearfulness is something to be pursued. Fear and worry are huge wastes of energy. Any amount of that that one can save can be plowed back into health and that grows on itself and pays off.

Beware of isolation. Be open as possible about your condition. Meet with others who have similar problems and are positive about it. Stay away from all forms of negativity. You have little time to waste on that.

Dwell in the bigger picture. Dwell in the Spirit. There is peace, energy, hope, nimbleness and joy there. You deserve all that, every bit. You can learn to live in this musical.

Be with family and friends who know how to support you. Community is a form of medicine, thank you Erica de America. Practice buoying each other up. Everyone is playing injured, they need you, you need them.

Have a purpose. That could take many forms I suppose and would be as unique as you are unique. You are the only you that ever was or ever will be, give it to people and expect it from them.

Learn to spend as much time in the moment as possible. Trust and don't worry too much about the next step. Concentrate and celebrate the step you are on. You are the beautiful flower that is growing up out of the crack in the concrete, be there! Love, Felipé.

APRIL 24, 2018 / A TUESDAY AT 8:05

Was thinking about yesterday's entry and wanted to add to it. We were talking of facets of wellness during the cancer journey.

I think that was all a description of a zone. It was a place to be that gives meaning and a sense of possibility. I like to be there as much as possible but can't always. It is a way to think about a goal or a way, a camino I suppose. It is a place away from the doctor's numbers and the hospital's rules and regulations. It is a different sort of healing. I am grateful for my doctors and nurses and the hospital, don't get me wrong, but it is not the complete answer to the situation. To be able to operate and think in such a way that one has less fear, worry and general wear and tear must be a positive in placing the cancer in its proper place. It is, in the big picture, only so important, remember.

My cancer in my body appears persistent but lazy. It likes me and doesn't seem anxious to leave, but at the same time it seems to be like a plant growing on a bad patch of soil. It is sort of maintaining or existing and stunted. I am not giving it the proper conditions to thrive. Well, yes. Thinking of my father-in-law who taught me an important lesson, if you can't stop something bad from happening then learn to control it. OK, yes exactly.

Sometimes, I say to people that God is keeping me alive for His own reasons. That would be another way to say all this but maybe a short answer. All these aspects of the situation that we have talked about are maybe the long answer to the same question.

OK, off we go to the wood shop. Making progress loves, Felipé.

April 26, 2018 / Taking Folks With Me

My emails this morning told of two people who I am taking to Lourdes with me in prayer. They need some TLC. One is short on the Spirit and good on health. And the other is short on health and long on Spirit. They are both going.

Months ago I decided to take in prayer all the people that wanted to go but were too sick to go. There has to be a bunch of those. I was once in that group that couldn't go to Spain to walk the Camino. I guess that is what empathy is.

Somehow this all feels like I am going to blast off to another planet, or time or dimension. It has a sort of other worldliness about it. Must be because it is such a holy place, holy meaning set aside, or not ordinary. Yes, that it is.

Have to go for now, duty calls. Another beautiful day here. Beautiful loves, Felipé.

April 28, 2018 / Genesis Chapter 32, I Was There

Here I am Saturday and I am trying to make myself pack for the Lourdes trip. Had Bible Guys this morning and we are working our way through the very first book, Genesis. We very seldom study Old Testament but I try and suggest it, love the stories. One of the chapters we read today was 32, which includes the story of Jacob wrestling with God.

This is how we learn about God, how He chooses to reveal Himself, these encounters with real people. There never is a list that says God is this and this and this. That would be real tidy. But tidy isn't big on His priority list apparently. But we have these stories.

Every once in a while there is a story that I can relate to. I so related to this one today where Jacob spends a night wrestling with God and lives to tell the tale. He is injured in the process and always walks with a limp afterward as a reminder I guess, a badge or medal so to speak.

This is what I have done for an extended period now I am seeing, wrestling with God. I live to tell the tale but carry this cancer with me always as a reminder. The important part is done for me. Carrying the cancer afterward I have to remind myself is the reminder of this event, it's my medal.

Working to prepare for this new adventure: pack, find passport, pray, wonder. Will take you with me, dusty love, Felipé.

APRIL 29, 2018 / GETTING READY

Have to give you a report on our first supermarket parking lot tailgate theology party of the season. It was nice and warm in the sunshine for Catherine and I to eat our bagels, donuts and coffee and talk theology. People pass by and say hi or they linger for a few minutes to talk and we sprinkle Camino dust on them.

It is quiet and peaceful here right now. Time to take a few deep breaths and be grateful. Ah, that is very good. My Rebecca's homily today was on gratitude so I am in the groove. She brought up some great points and possibilities. One thing I need to look up as it deserves more study, and that is Jesus and curing the ten lepers. One came back to thank Him and Jesus told him something like go you are healed. Healing only comes after thankfulness? In the feeding of the five thousand also before the food was passed out Jesus prayed and gave thanks. Thanksgiving precedes abundance. Thank you Rebecca.

If you have anyone that I can pray for in Lourdes let me know. I will try and make that happen for you and them. Later, love, Felipé.

MAY 2, 2018 / ON THE BIG BIRD

This is an Airbus A 340. We are learning how to put on our life vests in French. Hope I really don't have to do it for real. It feels like we are all off to camp, that's a good thing. Synchronistic events are happening that are very interesting. Yes, I am on a pilgrimage. Yes, something important is occurring. Pay attention and let it happen Felipé.

I can feel it—that old pilgrim thing of living close with others that you have just barely met. Sort of letting your space be infringed on continually. Just relax and keep smiling. They are all good people and they will be your companions for an extended period so get into it. We are all in the same litter of puppies and we are all in a pile.

Padre has been fabulous. He is my caregiver, handler and shepherd for the trip. So glad that he wanted to go and take on this challenge. And it's all so far so good.

Oh, what a fabulous airline dinner. Had chicken with mixed veggies and rice. There was a hard roll and butter. Cheese from Tillamook! All the cheese in France and we got cheese from Oregon, yea I like it. There was a corn salad with shrimp on top. There was cheesecake. And best of all, free wine.

Well, our team leader was suggesting that we get some sleep but I'm just getting wound up. Half the people in the plane are up in the aisles talking to the other half so I don't see hardly anyone following that advice.

Well, eight hours to go loves, Felipé.

PS—We're here! Safe flight and bus ride completed.

MAY 3, 2018 / WITH THE KNIGHTS AND DAMES

First full day of activities here at Lourdes. Raining outside but nice and warm in here in the bar. Just having a café con leche with the Padre

There are numerous knights, dames, priests and nuns that I am traveling with. They are all very competent and accomplished. It all makes me feel like an artist. Yes, Father, I have a trail where I paint with mud. Catalina is right, I am a land artist.

Having fun with the Padre. He seems an artist too. He paints with rough and tumble fellows like myself. Padre—a man of the soldiers and sailors. He knows about mud.

Be back later, clean feet loves, Felipé.

May 3, 2018 / Today's Report 5/3/18

We were in the Immaculate Conception Basilica this morning for foot washing. Padre washed and kissed my feet. I don't know what to say but it was very moving. We got a rosary there and did Confession. I just did Confession at home but figured I needed the practice. Father Jordan, a Dominican priest was helpful with a fumbling Felipé. Then we returned to the hotel for lunch and to warm up.

In the afternoon we did the famous dunk. That was breathtakingly cold water. I prayed for all the malades that were too sick to make the trip as I went under. Coming out there are no towels, just get dressed and get marching. But it feels good to have that water all over you and be moving.

After that we entered the Rosary Basilica with maybe two thousand other pilgrims. It was all the people that had come from the US. It was a Mass with seven bishops and dozens of priests celebrating.

It is raining and will be for a while. They are expecting the river to start flooding the lowlands. That doesn't look like the little stream that Bernadette crossed in the film *Song of Bernadette*. There is a lot of water right now looking for the fastest way downhill.

Tomorrow more big stuff and it is topped off with the nighttime candlelight procession. Will be back to give you the exciting details. Well-washed loves, Felipé.

May 4, 2018 / Hour of Sleeplessness

Last night in an hour of sleeplessness I had a meeting with my tumors. I did the night before but forgot to report on it. It seems like an odd thing to bring up now but we have talked of it before. And now here in Lourdes I am striving to connect my inner with the inner of Mary. Well, last night I did invite Mary to go with me to this meeting. These meetings always have essentially a nonverbal quality. More later, we are off to do the Stations of the Cross. Love, Felipé.

May 5, 2018 / Knights and Drones

Doesn't happen too often that one gets a medal but today was our day. They handed out medals to all the malades and caregivers. So I am wearing mine now, proudly.

I am way behind on describing all the goings on. The Order is putting us through a lot of experiences, as much as they can providing the time and the weather. Last night's Candlelight Procession was exceptional. There were malades and caregivers and Knights and Dames from all over. Every country in Europe and many others were represented. There is even the country of Malta, which I am trying to connect with.

Anyway, I feel like I am finally over my jetlag, which is helpful. And despite all the hoopla and goings on I am trying to figure out what is really important here and what is the take away. What is the basic idea that is being presented to me. I am slowly realizing that it is roughly the words that Mary said at Cana, "do whatever He tells you." Mary always points to Jesus.

I was out by the river in one of the more secluded areas of the Domain (the acreage that is officially the grounds) and was very happy to watch the water go by. Right now I crave some communing with nature and some quiet.

Also, some of the hotshot young knights have been doing drone shots of the place, daytime and nighttime.

Have to tell you that last night I had dinner with the Bishop (of Sacramento) and the head Medical Officer for this trip. We spent most of that time talking about what? Why the Camino of course! Who are you talking to but Felipé?

Today I had a great time talking with a Marine Corps vet who was in at the same time as I was. We had lunch and gabbed for another hour in the bar. He has a sailboat and I may have a trip in my future.

OK, have to wake Padre up from his nap. He is sawing logs here and we need to be assembling for the next activity. Thanks for checking in, love, Felipé.

MAY 7, 2018 / LIFE OF A PILGRIM

We are off to a fourth-century monastery, St. Savin. I see that we are saying the rosary on the bus ride up there, the life of a pilgrim. So, off to the assembly point. Later, love, Felipé.

MAY 9, 2018 / FRANCE TO LA

Never been on a charter flight before. I know, I have to get out more often. An interesting thing has happened onboard. On the way a week ago we were mostly strangers and it looked like a normal airline flight. But now we are traveling home after being together at camp and we are joking and hitting each other in the arm like old buddies in the barracks.

The Padre is on one side of me here watching the Smurfs and snickering. And Jan is on the other side. Jan and I have a mutual friend that lives in her neighborhood and who reads Caminoheads. So, we both came into this being on the watch for each other and guess what —the organizers put us exactly next to each other on the plane. Huh, coincidence?

Yea, Jan got up last night and spoke as a representative of her team giving everyone a glimpse of her and their experience. She said something that neatly encapsulated it. And that is, many seeds were planted in us here and it would take some time for them to sprout and grow. It is an elegant way of saying that we will need time to process the busy experience that we have had. Everything is not so obvious at the moment.

Yea, I am not ready to say in a definitive way what has happened either. A lot of moving parts have moved for all of us. Well, how about a couple of observations then Felipé?

I heard a pilgrim say that they were describing Lourdes to someone back home as a place where a lot of sick people come. And that someone said, "Oh, it must be a depressing place"? But far from that, it is quite a joyful place. A place where we are learning to celebrate our predicaments, our disease, our problems.

APPROACHING GREENLAND

The common perception is that there are cures here. And there are some, a few. And there are miracles here and they happen. But generally it is a place of healing in a deeper broader sense where pilgrims discover the role of their suffering in the big scheme of things for one. We go home with a new attitude, a new way of looking at ourselves and our place in the world. And we see that we are not alone. We never were alone really but it takes getting together in the same place to get a sense of that. Again, a time and place to celebrate. As always, Felipé.

MAY 23, 2018 / EASE

One of the things that I noticed on our trip to Camp Lourdes was that the malades (sick people) seemed to be having more smiles on their faces as the week went on. Well, I can't say that was everyone but it was in general true. Is this a sign that we were more at home with Lourdes, with Our Lady, with ourselves? I am thinking that these are the kind of miracles that were occurring. They were subtle but apparent.

People were feeling more at ease in many ways. And maybe ultimately the biggest challenge would be if we are to feel at ease with our problems, our maladies. If we can find a way to use our situation to some positive ends. What are we going to do with what we got?

Well, in other news, I found out an interesting thing about Father Tom my care-taker on the trip. I often call him Padre or Padre Tomas. It was so great that he agreed to go along with me. We had fun being who we are and letting the rest take care of itself. Not too many demerits were accumulated. But what has come to light recently is that he is actually the long lost third Blues Brother. Yea, how about that, right in our midst.

OK, that's about it for the moment. I am off here in a few moments to get an appointment to put in a replacement for my worn-out chemo port. More fun to come. Tomorrow, love, Felipé.

MAY 24, 2018 / GO TELL IT ON THE MOUNTAIN!

The unpacking from Camp Lourdes continues. A major puzzle piece appeared to me yesterday at the hospital that I tripped over on my daily camino. It appeared so obvious because of the newfound abilities on my part to see it.

I learned at Lourdes. I learned about myself at Lourdes. I am a new Felipé who sees his own situation in new light. We live with ourselves so closely we rarely have a chance at a perspective that is telling.

Someone asked My Rebecca in the last few days whether I saw any miracles there at Camp Lourdes. Well, no it didn't happen quite like that. I didn't see anyone with a "throw down their crutches" moment. And that can be disconcerting if that is our only definition of a miracle, our only measure, but consider: that doesn't mean that our inner lives weren't changed. And maybe those changes are not apparent 'til we return to our homes and communities and use these as a place to find measure. We can only see our new selves when comparing to the space our old self left behind.

That is what happened to me at the hospital yesterday when I stumbled over something that had been there for a while but I didn't see it for what it was. Let me explain. Chemotherapy patients have a port where the liquid treatments can enter our bodies in a clean easy manner. It is basically a small titanium gizmo that lies under the skin and it has access to the blood stream. So at each treatment a small needle is inserted through the skin and into the gizmo so the treatment can be administered that day. It is really an amazing innovation. So this is sort of a permanent situation where on a different day the same port is there for access of more treatment through a new needle. It stays in place covered by the protective human skin with its natural healing ability.

So my port was put in just shy of five years ago and I am so much at home with it that I don't give it much of a second thought anymore. But here is what is happening, the situation is worn out. My skin in that particular place is not able to keep up with the demands over time. OK, but why? Because that is longer than the vast majority of people get chemo except for iron men like Felipé. I see that the doctors and nurses are not used to this situation of having to give me a replacement in a new spot and therefore I am seeing my situation in a new light. THE MIRACLE IS ALREADY HAPPENING! I have had the blessing to be still here time after time to be treated by my medical team over this extraordinary time period. Felipé the Ironman is still here on his feet to be the gosh darn amazing positive influence that he is. THAT IS ALREADY A GOSH DARN MIRACLE!

Gratitude in buckets that I am here and have great things to do with that time. That fits together nicely in the cosmic equation. You are a part of that too. Thanks, love, Felipé.

JUNE 1, 2018 / GOTTA GET THE COFFEE GOING

Please stay tuned to upcoming days as we will be "reentering" our common world with new eyes. If the Camino was a teaching place, then Lourdes must be a teaching place also. If the Camino was life changing then Lourdes must be also. What is it that we have learned and how do we put that to use? How have we changed and what are the implications?

Well yes, and it is the first day of June. The corn is five inches tall. I am making a valiant attempt to keep the weeds down around it. The sunflowers are up also. They need more water right now. Yup, I'm coming! Love as always, Felipé.

June 6, 2018 / Switching Over

I was so conditioned to thinking in a Camino way that it was a stretch for me to encompass the new ideas coming in from Lourdes. I had to make room for them and more are coming in daily. The best way that I have to explain the situation is to say that I have been reporting on roller derby so long now that switching over to consider opera has been a challenge!

Camino pilgrimage is maybe something very horizontal. It stretches on for 500 miles or more and it is continuously in motion. I see that and feel that in my bones. There are regular times of rest but only for the purpose of recharging for the next stage. It is immensely restless. I remember thinking of it as a river when I was walking especially the last 100 km where it was so crowded and the river seemed to be overflowing its banks.

But by contrast, the stay at Lourdes revolves around the Domain. The Domain is the grounds or sacred territory of the city of Lourdes. There is no commercial enterprise inside its gates. All the hotels, restaurants and gift shops are outside. The very center of the Domain is the Grotto where Mother Mary appeared to Bernadette. So everything there is centered around activities inside those gates which is maybe a quarter square mile, that's it. So it is not horizontal by any measure.

So then is it vertical? It sort of must be. The river that runs through the Domain and right by the Grotto is a great foil to this. It is the epitome of restlessness in its springtime rush to the sea. I found myself greatly attracted to it while we were there. Maybe I subconsciously related to it like that while I was puzzling over the rest of what was going on around me.

But I am worn out for now. Let me see what comes forth overnight. Ideas always seem to appear when we need them so we will have faith. Thanks for stopping by today, your presence is always appreciated. Lourdes loves, Felipé.

June 8, 2018 / Peace

Mother Mary's appearance there in 1858 is still sending out ripples. Bernadette's simple reception was a marvelous thing. I search for Mary and have been serious about it since my diagnosis in 2011. It is mostly comfort that I am after.

Is comfort another way of saying being at peace? This idea of being at peace becomes more important every day to me. And personally it seems to have largely replaced the idea of being cured. That's pretty earth shaking when I think about it. Earth shaking loves, Felipé.

June 10, 2018 / It's Sunday

It's Sunday and I am going to take a break from the Camino/ Lourdes Intersection for something completely different. I was just out trying to make some progress on the weeds in the corn. The corn could almost be a full-time job if I let it. But in the corn news is something else. Our son Wiley unveiled his latest tattoo to me minutes ago.

And he said that it was in my honor. So what could that be but a nice big ear of corn on his bicep! It's the Cornmino! Well how about that?

I have the Sunday afternoon walk in moments. The weather has been totally goofy the last few days. Sun, wind, clouds, hail in different combinations. Well, we will see who shows up.

I just received a new rosary crafted by my friends in the fourth-grade class at St. Joseph School in Upland, CA. We had a fund raiser here at Phil's Camino and raised a few dollars for a class party for them. I hear that they voted to do a three-way split with the funds. Some went to a charity, some went to materials for the rosaries and some went toward their festivities. So a good time was had by all. Full house loves, Felipé.

June 11, 2018 / Something That I Have Been Meaning To Say

Ah, the sun is breaking through our clouds, the so-called marine layer. Nice, let's dry this place out a little. I am looking at a full and fun day with some work and some play. Camino visitors coming from out of town which is always exciting.

So, Lourdes, it sits in my mind like a door that I am still trying to get through. Or a possibility still not connected to. Or perhaps I am baffled by God and God's goodness. I know that we are all struggling in our own ways and in our own times. I don't mean to add to your confusion. What I have to say will be helpful to you hopefully, if I can just get it out plainly.

After mulling this situation over and over actually over the last month one thing becomes apparent. That one thing is the importance of peace. Our own very deep inner peace is the sort that I am talking about. Of course that fits into peace at other levels but this is the basic first step so to speak. This is peace of mind or peace of being or peace with God or some such foundational situation that is the first step.

That sort of healing, this connection, is available at Lourdes. It is a thing way deeper and broader and more complex than the simple idea that a malade throws down his crutches and walks away. If anyone goes to Lourdes and is disappointed because they didn't have this throw-down-the-crutches experience I am sorry. If one felt that they were somehow lacking because they didn't have enough faith to make that happen I am sorry. And maybe their problem became greater because of carrying this new burden. See that?

We need to be good to ourselves, we are beat up enough. We have faith and we should feel good about that. We don't need more of a burden. We need something positive. What is there at Lourdes that is available to everyone? I think that this peace is there and waiting for us. It may be something way more valuable than simply being cured. Just the world according to Felipé. Sunny morning loves, Felipé.

June 16, 2018 / New Kid On the Block

Maybe there is a parallel to my relationship with two pilgrimages, one to Santiago and one to Lourdes, and with the two versions of *Phil's Camino*. I become so sort of loyal to the former in each case and then there is a new kid on the block and I have to make room for that. Not only make room but try and encompass it, see it for what it is by itself and then integrate it. Love, Felipé

June 19, 2018 / The Day I Dream Of

We have a plan for this afternoon and evening. Our walk is at 4 and some folks from the mainland will be here plus Catherine and Dana. Then tapas and off to see the Pope's new film at the Vashon Theatre!

Right now Steve and I are going to put in some time in the corn which is teetering on the brink of weed-dom. And a deer got in and thought the sunflowers were tasty. It's all a constant battle. I need some minions, maybe a dozen please.

Well, you see the picture here. Will be blogging from the hospital tomorrow. The two sides of the same coin. But it is all do-able and with the right attitude, enjoyable.

Oh, the horses are here from next door. Yup, well time to go and battle the weeds. Have a great day where you are. Summer loves, Felipé.

June 20, 2018 / What A Beauty!

We went after the walk and tapas to the Pope Francis movie last evening. That was My Rebecca, Catherine and Dana. It was a beauty, very moving for us all. If you get a chance take it in. And it is not really a Catholic thing but a humanity thing. He cuts across traditional boundaries to bring people together is what I see. He is very humble throughout, a breath of fresh air these days.

The way I look at Pope Francis is that he is not your typical Pope. He seems bigger than the position. He is someone that seems to transcend the current situation. And even transcend Catholicism. How does that happen?

I don't think that there is a person alive that he doesn't challenge with his message. We all could do better, maybe way better. But Papa is a compassionate man and he ends the film speaking about the importance of the smile and of humor in our daily travel as to lighten his message to each one of us. It was a nice touch.

The turnout at the theater could have been better. I don't know the exact reason for that but I think it seemed light for such a good film. Maybe there is the feeling that it is a "Catholic" movie but I think that would be a mistake.

My Rebecca is off to Boulder, CO for the national gathering of the Threshold Choirs. She has participated in it for years and it's great that she has a chance to go to the big powwow. These are small groups of women that sing for people that are dying to ease their transition. What a bunch of angels, right?

Good to see you again. Walk and tapas love, Felipé.

June 21, 2018 / Short On Time

Steve-O has been here with his current flat coat retriever who is a giant puppy. So that says a lot, he's big and powerful, playful and goofy, learning and making mistakes. That's the dog, Rasmus, not Steve-O. Just wanted to clarify.

Anyway, we were all out and around the property and Ras picked up one of my handmade-by-Phil garden stakes and was carrying it around because that what retrievers do. So he got bored at one point and started gnawing on it which is what puppies do. And I in my old self or past self would have been mad about that thinking that that was destructive but the first thought out of my mind was, "Oh look, he is celebrating his teeth!" See the difference?

The property is a giant growth and decay laboratory. Or it's creation and destruction together. Or it's celebrating and/or madness. We have to at some point start to embrace those two sides of the coin. Ah, up, up and away, celebrating loves, Felipé.

June 22, 2018 / A Cloudy Friday

Overall summer is getting a rocky start this year. Must be some bad switch somewhere in the works. Looking out the big window at the treatment center Downtown Seattle is in the distance. And there is St. James Cathedral.

Yesterday I was telling you that I was realizing our land, our little ten acres is a creation/destruction machine. That is so much like my body these days. My body is that same mixture or has the same dynamic. I am having a hard time finding the words for this right now but seeing this is one of those overarching realizations that seems healthy. One does what he can to keep everything in some sort of balance.

Yea, and back to thinking about the land, I will be back there this afternoon with time to get some things done. I know you are probably bored hearing about this but it is the time of year when there is incredible green growth and most of my energy goes into weeding and mowing. Need a couple of clones to keep up.

So that's what it looks like from here, it's alperfect, love Felipé.

June 24, 2018 / Pilgrims Coming

Just as the Camino in Spain attracts an interesting set of people so does the Camino here. And what we do here I have likened to a salon in the French sense. I see the mix of all these folks to be a rich brew and I get inspired and new ideas flow. I get something important out of all this and pilgrims leave with little treasures I know.

Cris has been calling this a neighborhood. I am liking that a lot, the Camino-heads Neighborhood. I think actually she was referring to this blog but it works for the walk also. Maybe the walk is part of the blog or vice-versa. Anyway sort of a Mr. Rogers thing going on here now apparently. Where's my cardigan?

The sun is out and the sky is blue and we have a walk at 4 PM. And tapas afterward of course. My Rebecca might be home by then from her convention in Boulder. That would be perfect. But it is always alperfect anyway.

Well, I am going to mosey on, dishes to wash and weeds to pull. Always good to see you here at the Neighborhood! Be at peace. Loves, Felipé.

JUNE 28, 2018 / A CASCADE OF ROSES

Right now sooo busy, a summertime frenzy of activity around here. And as I eat my meals from my chair at the dinner table I am looking out at a rose bush that My Rebecca planted decades ago. It so totally loves it in that spot that it outgrows the ability of the deer to eat it. It outgrows my ability to civilize it as it climbs all over anything around. I do my best to keep it from coming in the door and occupying our living room. It is the very definition of happy plant!

And there it is now in the midst of its summer flowering right out the window from my chair at the dinner table. Actually it is a little over its prime, which was probably a week ago. But that is making my point. Am I, are we appreciating the many blessings around us? Here is this crazy wonderful rose that is basically shouting at me to take a minute and appreciate before it goes into its fall and eventual winter. Right now sooo busy yes but, take a minute, some of the best things are sooo fleeting. Catch 'em while you can loves, Felipé.

JULY 4, 2018 / THE FOURTH

Here we are once again at the birthday party for our nation. It is still early in the day before the noise and hoopla. Our usual round the Island boat race got canceled because of rough water conditions. But our amazing Island fireworks show will go on this evening at dusk like always.

Rebecca was just telling me that one of her teaching associates is leaving on a two-year stint in the Peace Corps to rural South Africa. She is a two-time cancer survivor and now seventy years old. So, apparently they do make them like they used too! Way to go Georgia! Think about that Camino for a minute.

We had a whole family here yesterday to walk and they stayed for a tapas get together afterward. Plenty of time for great conversation and sharing. In this group there were three generations, two nurses and a cancer patient all happily traveling together. Obviously a lot of good dynamic going on there. They were here April 12th of this year, we looked it up in the logbook. I am pretty sure that we will see them again down the trail.

Those of us that are the intrepid little flowers that are growing out of our particular cracks in the concrete need to cheer each other on. As for Felipé, this pulls his 3C's together nicely. Let's review now, remember the 3C's are Cancer, Catholicism and Camino, not sure of the order. In other words those might be thought about as the Crack, the Seed and the Bloom.

It is a place that we find ourselves that we as yet don't totally accept but we are learning to make the most of it no matter what. That is the name of the game so to speak.

OK, the corn calls me. Glad you stopped by loves, Felipé.

July 10, 2018 / Shoveling Manure

We have a walk this afternoon at four. The daughter of my oldest friend is coming. I haven't seen her in many ages. And maybe Father David will show up, he's been threatening lately. We could talk about his last homily. One line of it has stuck with me bigtime, "healing is a form of reconciliation." Let's talk more about that Father.

What is that line from *Phil's Camino*, "healing is being reconciled with the bigger picture"? I think that we are on the same page there. Perhaps there is more that we can uncover if we work at it. Some of this stuff is akin to, "you can have your cake and eat it too." In other words, they are way better than they even first appear.

Sometimes words fail us and that is a sign. If we are talking about a topic that is hard for us to articulate then perhaps we are on uncharted ground, it is an area that we are unfamiliar with, we don't have the words. I think that is an interesting place to be, a place of discovery where we are not just shoveling our usual manure.

I think that Wiley and Henna are back from their short California trip. They got in at midnight so they are probably sleeping in. Maybe they need some milk from town? Miss you, love you, Felipé

July 11, 2018 / Time Was Getting Short

Just like on the Camino, it is better to think about the miles that you have accomplished than to dwell on how many more you have to go and how that will happen. I really don't know where all this is going, this effort of ours. Well, other than ultimately, "This train is bound for glory!" We know that. But I think that Caminoheads, instead of a movement toward a goal or an effort designed to accomplish something, is more of a zone to be in. A place to be, a sanctuary as our friend Terry Hershey calls it. Lately we have been using the word neighborhood, thank you Mr. Rogers.

A place to be. A place to be at the tapas table again. Ah, that brings a tear. No big explanation needed there. We are grateful that somehow we were called to be a part of this.

And at the same time it is not some sort of exclusive club. We don't say that we are somehow special. This Camino dust that we have been inoculated with is free for anyone everywhere, at any time.

And then the trail here at Raven Ranch is another part of this neighborhood. It lives on because it seems to fulfill what we need, what we have been waiting for. Always ready for us to tread on its back.

I guess that I needed this today, to look back at where we have come, the miles already walked. Always remembering though, that it is this present moment that is most important, that is the address of the neighborhood where we want to be.

A long way dusty loves, Felipé.

July 14, 2018 / My Quest

I don't know how many darn times that I've tried to answer the "why me" question as it relates to my cancer. Wish I had a nickel for each one. But it is a maturing process to try and come to grips with that. My quest goes on. And that journey reveals so much, as a pilgrimage is more about the doing than the destination. That is something to consider as we sit in the shade in between chores. Love, Felipé

July 16, 2018 / A Bright New Morning, A Bright New Week

The wedding of our son Wiley here at the ranch approaches. The frenzy intensifies. I know it is all for a good cause but please everyone—keep it to a dull roar. I guarantee that we are going to have a good time no matter if all the details get worked out or not. That's my call.

Gorgeous morning here at the ranch. This is the July that we all wait for. I am working hard getting firewood split and stacked for the dark days of winter. It always looks so good freshly stacked like so much money in the bank. We had two little city boys here yesterday who were full of questions about everything at the ranch. They were especially intrigued by the firewood. "What is that?" "What do you use it for?" They have such fresh eyes.

The Sunday walk yesterday was with a family from California on a road trip in the Northwest. The man I met on one of my film trips. He is a medical doctor working in cancer rehabilitation, my favorite topic, well next to the Camino of course. So we gabbed and gabbed. I think that this is the genesis of some more trips down south.

The corn is tasseling out in the field. It is a run-away scene out there with the weeds gone crazy and the deer eating the weeds. We are getting to that time of year, due mostly to the dry conditions of late summer, when the deer suffer for lack of suitable eats. I have cut down whole trees in the past to feed them during these times.

Those little boys asking questions left a big impression on me. It gave me a sense of how maybe out of the ordinary we are here on our little island with our little island life style. Things that I take for granted are out of the ordinary for others. Well, I guess that is what travel is for, mixing it up. Mixing it up loves, Felipé.

July 19, 2018 / 0131 And Awake

The three C's are important to us here right? I don't really tend to talk of Catholicism as much as I should but I lean on it in a big way. It supplies me with inspiration and connection that I frankly have not been about to find elsewhere. People from its ranks have been immensely helpful to me. I thank them sincerely. I may not have written that before but there it is on post 1641. This "C" could also have been Christianity but I, in the world of Felipé, don't think that is as accurate and descriptive given the situation. This is all very personal.

Cancer in an individual creates a situation that is life changing and that calls for new and more powerful medicine. Meeting this challenge also takes more than singularity.

And last but not least comes the Camino. The Camino is the big limb of St. James on the tree of God and the 1200 years of pilgrims that went before us late comers form the branches on that limb. And we are hopeful little twigs on those branches. And the leaves, flowers and fruit that are displayed on us the twigs in this time are our expressions. Caminoheads blog is there along with millions of other expressions, wonderful expressions. Besides being numerous they are varied and all beautifully crafted and well-tended. Can you see it all moving in the breeze? The breeze is something important too. Twiggy loves, Felipé.

July 20, 2018 / Little Signs That Work

I was driving on the Island the other day and saw a walker by the side of the road that was walking the same way as I was going, so I couldn't see her face, but I knew who she was. Something was different today though. For years now seeing her movement was always like a soldier on a forced march. Today she looked so peaceful and relaxed as she ambled along, as in, "I am enjoying myself." It made my whole day and no words were spoken.

Today driving to the hospital I saw a garden springing up on an unused little corner on First Hill in Seattle. It won't be unused for long but for just right now there are rows and rows of green things reaching for the sun. Not landscape but agriculture. What a pleasant vision. It is sticking with me.

Living here in the Northwest blue sky comes and goes. I don't know if you are going to get the full significance of this if you don't live here. It can be very rare at times of the year but when you see a small patch of blue sky it is beautiful. It is beautiful in the sense of yes, it still exists, not that it is over my very head but that could be possible. The possibility of it is important, maybe tomorrow you say.

Or maybe it is the little flower in the crack in the sidewalk as you walk along that just randomly cheers you up. It is nothing really in one sense and a miracle in another.

I remember climbing all those hills on the Camino and coming to the end of my ability at various places and I would rest there. And I don't know how many times my eyes would light on a heart rock there in the dirt as I wondered whether I could go on. OK, OK, I can do this!

Just little stuff really, all these things. They will never be in history books. They will never win awards. But boy when they happen at the right moment, they are priceless. Just little thoughts here today. Little loves, Felipé.

July 24, 2018 / Spritz

My Rebecca is a writer who can relax into the scene and produce something nice. She did this on our "daycation" yesterday. Just give her paper and a pen and a lake full of laughing kids and off she goes.

I, on the other hand, seem to need some obstacle or bother to spur me on. While she was outside on the deck happily writing away I was a few feet away inside trying to write my daily post. I was having a hard time. Guess it was too nice there, right? Nothing to push back against. Give me a good problem and I am all over it, but too nice and I'm lost. It's kind of being like a spritz cookie. I get under pressure in that little tube and out I squirt in a beautiful star shape, no problem. Yup loves, Felipé.

JULY 25, 2018 / ST. JAMES DAY 2018

It's the feast day of St. James the Greater, our mentor, today. He was one of the of the twelve apostles. Yea, so this is his day of the year, a day to celebrate St. Jamesness.

Four years ago Kelly and I were in Madrid on our way to the start of the Camino Frances. We didn't run into any celebration but then we were busy and focused on figuring out the Spanish trains and buses. But St. James is the patron saint of the whole of Spain, so it must have been going on all around us.

Here at Caminoheads blog we have a saying that maybe needs reviving since it is good and we haven't used it in a while. And that is SJA. That stands for Saint James Again or Saint James Afoot. This is what we used to say when some unexplained good thing happened on our daily camino. It is an acknowledgment that St. James is alive and well in our lives. Yes, it is time for that.

Well, Happy St. James Day to you all the world over! Loves, Felipé.

JULY 27, 2018 / AH, THE FRENZY

I am getting a chemo vacation next week to celebrate the wedding. So, I will have a month free just like I had in Spain. Dr. Gold suggested it, the guy. I am just getting half-way normal from treatment last Wednesday, over a week ago now.

Well, I need to get a move on it. Got fuel and sharp blades for the mower so look out world! Catch you guys tomorrow. Summer loves, Felipé.

JULY 28, 2018 / READING A NEW BOOK

Not long ago I started reading *Radical Remission: Surviving Cancer Against All Odds* by Kelly A. Turner, Ph.D. It was given to me by a couple that were here walking Phil's Camino.

A brief summary of the book would start with the author, who is "a researcher and psychotherapist who specializes in integrative oncology." She spent ten years interviewing and studying people that had reversals in their cancer situations. In other words these people somehow figured out or lucked upon cures to their maladies, improbable as that seems. It is pretty phenomenal news when this happens and she was intrigued by it. So, in the end she discovered nine traits that this group had in common. Not that each had all of these but that these items kept showing up time and again.

Well, now that I have gotten this far I see that I will have to type up the list from the table of contents because I have piqued your interest:

> Radically Changing Your Diet
> Taking Control of Your Health
> Following Your Intuition
> Using Herbs and Supplements
> Releasing Suppressed Emotions
> Increasing Positive Emotions
> Embracing Social Support
> Deepening Your Spiritual Connection

Having Strong Reasons for Living

Yea, nine, a good round number like 909 laps on Phil's Camino equals one Camino Frances. That is all sufficiently untidy to be real. Anyway, I am so relating to most of these topics and it is the kind of stuff that we talk about here frequently on the blog. As I read down this list right now I would say that six of those are very important to me already. And maybe three I don't understand or that I haven't dealt with sufficiently. And perhaps those three hold the biggest potential for me.

This is so highly personal and at the same time universal. The book talks about the idea that the tumors are messengers. I had thought this also although I had never cracked their code. It is suggested that they bring the message that my life as I have been living it is out of balance. Ahh. Yes, I see that now although that may always be hard for the individual to grasp at first. Like isn't my life perfect? Isn't it just exactly what it is supposed to be? Doesn't it fit exactly the set of situations that it occurred in?

Well, the tumors at the door of your conscience is somewhat like Genghis Khan being at your door. He doesn't really have to say, "Yes, I am here to rape and kill you and yours." But that isn't the end of the story, there is more to it. Yup, as always, love you, Felipé.

JULY 31, 2018 / AT THE RANCH

It's all happening here right now, family and friends gravitating in for Wiley and Henna's wedding. I don't know if I will be able to write much of a post today as I am needed for this and that here starting at this early hour. Maybe I will make it out to the tapas table with my coffee cup. Ah, quieter out here and amazingly chilly.

I am just trying to "sing" along over the increasing frenzy. Sing seems like an apt word. I suppose I am not used to this many moving parts in my life. Maybe it would seem simple to juggle all this stuff to others. But one's own challenges always seem harder somehow. Anyway, I am a half hour away from making noise. I always try and keep things quiet after nine at night and before nine in the morning, stuff like mowing and running woodworking equipment. I have to go in a few minutes and mow the pasture that we are using for parking first thing.

Pilgrims are coming and going too. I am doing my best to keep Phil's Camino running during this period. So if you were thinking about coming still come, we are working around all the preparation commotion.

So, we will continue tomorrow. Please pray for me and my family during this period. The best to you. Joyful preparation loves, Felipé.

AUGUST 6, 2018 / RECOVERING FROM THE SHINDIG

We had a heck of a wedding here at Raven Ranch. It was all outdoors in a big pasture that we have been grooming for months. The weather was warm and dry, not hot, just perfect. The ceremony was short but not too short and full of love. Wiley and Henna's vows were so thoughtful and sweet. We were all bawling.

Our good friend smoked a lot of meat for the feed. There were three kegs of different brew, one a local Vashon one. There was no wedding cake but a wedding cobbler. All very down home.

I really did enjoy myself at the event. I have been involved with so many deals in the past where it was all I could do but to be glad they were over. But I did have a good time although I only made it to 11 o'clock and the party went on all night. But the cops never came so I guess we are still loved by our neighbors.

We had a nice walk and tapas yesterday afternoon. I wanted to keep the trail open even with the wedding going on and we were able to do that. Three pilgrims showed up yesterday that were really fun and energetic. One had taken a class with our buddy Catalina down at Santa Clara so we got some news from down there.

Off walking again here in a few minutes. The morning is bright and cool and the blackberries are ripe for the picking along the trail. So come by when you get a chance and see for yourself.

Blackberry loves, Felipé.

AUGUST 7, 2018 / THE PIPELINE-O-LOVE

Still doing dishes from the wedding amongst other things. What a disaster area, but we are working our way through it.

Yesterday I wanted to announce the opening of a pipeline to deliver tens of thousands of gallons of love to my chest cavity. It will be focusing on the area of the disturbance that I also call my cancer. I have gone through all sorts of ways of viewing and thinking about my tumors and lately seeing the area where they occur as a site of disturbance has been a good way. I am flooding the area with every sort of love that I can come up and in major volume.

A walk and tapas this afternoon, don't forget. Cardigan loves, Felipé.

AUGUST 8, 2018 / FIRST CORN!

We picked a dozen ears of the early corn, Sugar Buns, last evening and enjoyed the heck out of it. Freya our latest grandchild was keen on it too, I'm glad to report. Oh, this is a beautiful thing and the start of my favorite season. Time to fatten up for winter.

And it is time to start picking blackberries. For all you locals that aren't lucky enough to have your own patch going, swing by. What a crop! These brambles are so productive and after all I abuse them. I guess I will have to explain that. There are at least three species of what we refer to as blackberries growing here. And not merely growing but wanting to take over the place. They will grow anywhere that has been cleared of forest and they need absolutely nothing from us. In a few years they will form these patches that nothing can penetrate. Old-timers would wire the throttle open on their tractor, put it in low gear and point it toward the blackberries and then catch it as it came out, hoping to divide and conquer.

But the blackberries are just one example of the terrific life force that is really all around us here. The trees they say we can grow by accident around here. It is a jungle.

I realized years ago that ninety-five percent of my relationship with plants was hacking and burning trying to beat back this jungle. And that mode is needed. But lately I have been studying this life force that surrounds me and marveling at it hoping to learn something. What if I had that kind of energy and persistence in the face of all sorts of abuse and obstacles? What if . . .

Yup, that's it for today, the jungle is calling me. Wednesday loves, Felipé.

AUGUST 14, 2018 / PLOWING BACK THE ENERGY

For the next few diary entries I want to talk about the nine factors that Dr. Kelly Turner distilled from the thousand cancer survivors that she interviewed for the book *Radical Remissions*. The garden of our health needs numerous components to thrive and we have to pay attention to a broad field of notions.

I, being Felipé, have to tackle this in my own Felipé way. I can only speak for myself on this really. Please read the book if you are hot on this topic but know that the book speaks of these notions in a general way and they may have slightly different meanings to the individual.

When I am really in the groove with my spirituality, things happen to place me outside my former self and outside the norm. Having my feet on a good foundation gives me the position to shed large quantities of fear for one thing. Fear is rampant in normal life but for a person with a diagnosis it can quickly go out of control with the fear of the unknown and of death. Deepening my spiritual connection was a way to get this under control and even to be able to use the energy that I would have wasted for positive purposes.

Energy that is saved can be "plowed back" into our health instead of having it wasted. This is a must. Having a strong spiritual connection means having a trust that whatever happens I will be upheld. This is a must for me and I can't see anyway for me to continue without it. So, this is where I choose to start and as we move through my reorganized list of the factors we will get to ones that I am weaker and weaker on. And that far end of the list is where I have to concentrate my energy as there is so much room for improvement. Strong Connection Loves, Felipé.

AUGUST 15, 2018 / COMMUNITY AS MEDICINE

I have heard of cancer patients trying to keep their disease a secret. This is the worst form of isolation that I can think of. Isolation is what one doesn't want, it is the opposite of support. And even at the hospital all the privacy rules and regs. serve to keep patients isolated from one another and leaves them to largely navigate alone.

My four hours of walking every week here at the ranch are an opportunity to connect with others. I never know who will show up and, sometimes no one does, but great getting together does take place here in this venue. I learn a lot in the give and take of it all and so do others hopefully.

So, there are a lot of facets to this factor for me and you can see that it is very strong. It is one of my biggest assets. It is community as medicine as Erica De America would say.

OK, I think that you get the picture on that one. The best to you ever and always, love, Felipé.

August 19, 2018 / Increasing Positive Emotions

Somehow my encounter with cancer brought about something that put me working on not taking life too seriously. I don't know how or why, but it happened. Also included in there is the resilience that resides in Catholicism. And also included is the belonging and the trust fostered by the Way of St. James, or the Camino de Santiago. I have no idea of how this dynamic worked but it did.

If one is to reside in the place of positive emotions one has to come to grips with negativity. Worry and fear have to be put in their place, not boiling away on the front burners of our life. It takes a certain amount of trust to unlock this, to move in this direction.

I think we are talking about finding joy and being able to dwell there as the ultimate connection to the positive. To find peace in our lives is a major component in this process. I saw peace in thousands of malades (people with a malady) who had come to Lourdes when I was there in May. That was my major takeaway—that peace is possible in the middle of sickness and suffering.

I have time to get some projects worked on before our walk at 4 PM. Stop by when you can. Peaceful loves, Felipé.

August 20, 2018 / Diet

My parents and ancestors never had that much trouble with diet. They ate what was in season and largely what they or their neighbors grew themselves. This makes the most sense to me at the moment.

We had a wonderful walk yesterday with old friends and new friends. The Camino continues to provide. We are fortunate. Summer loves, Felipé.

August 21, 2018 / Worry and Anxiety

Worry to me seems distraction in another word. Three times during my cancer journey I was in near car crashes. Maybe they were my fault or maybe I wasn't paying attention like I should have been, doesn't matter really. The safest way for me to be is to live in the moment and actually see what is going on around me. If I am worried I become distracted and miss important clues in my environment. I finally realized that, what good is it to worry about my cancer and then die in a car accident because I was distracted.

And on to anxiety. I am thinking about this as an unsettled feeling in the gut, a nervousness maybe. I put it in a line of things: fear leads to anxiety leads to nausea leads to not eating right. I was able to avoid 99 percent of the dreaded nausea that is associated with chemotherapy somehow. And I am attributing that to the taming of fear in my being and its taming of anxiety.

Smoke-filled morning here in Puget Sound. Love you, Felipé.

AUGUST 23, 2018 / AT LAST—TAKING CONTROL OF YOUR HEALTH

Through this entire journey with my cancer I have always disliked the word or designation "patient." It sort of gives you the image of a passive being that just takes in. Like a stump could be a patient. We are more than that right? Maybe that is what this factor is getting at.

Well, as for me so far, I have been closely relying on my conventional treatment which has done so much for me. Having stage four cancer and prolonging that for five years now is proof that my treatment is effective although I am not "cured." I do credit my conventional treatment with a lot of that but I feel not all, for I have been able to do this for so long and beyond the normal range of things. Some of it comes from me and what I have been able to add.

I used to say that my cancer is very lazy but now I say, well, maybe I am just not giving it fertile ground to grow in. There is a slight difference or a big difference maybe in the sense of me being more involved in the process. So I think that is where we are going with this factor, that the patient has to be more than the patient. That it takes effort and imagination to navigate a successful journey through this maze.

Well OK, I am walking in a moment. It is such a cool morning, a change from the hot smoky days of the last few weeks. Thanks, Love, Felipé.

AUGUST 28, 2018 / A BODACIOUS VIEW OF THE LABYRINTH

It's here! The Bodacious sweet corn is ripe. This is high summer right here. The time that we dream about all the rest of the year. Or in other words it just doesn't get any better than this.

A minute ago I was reading an article about labyrinths. It stated that there were 3,800 in the US. That is amazing.

But what are you getting at here Felipé? Well, I was just remembering my impressions of labyrinth walking and I am a newcomer at this, so no expert. For years I shied away from them thinking they were maze-like. Which they are not! There are no dead ends nor any decisions to be made. Well, there is one basic foundational decision and that is a pledge to keep the faith throughout.

To walk this means ultimately to arrive at the center or to arrive at your destination or to arrive at God. But the going, the doing of it, is not a regular progression. Sometimes it seems so easy as you progress nicely and then sometimes you are as far away from the goal as when you started. It can be disheartening at times. What is needed is a faith in the whole process, that if I just keep going, I will arrive no matter what.

So, part of the year we are eating Bodacious and warming our relaxed bodies in the sun. It is easy and fun and we are generous and smiling. And then there are times when it has been raining for a month. Times when the ability to pick fresh vegetable seems a dream. Times when our bodies are all crunched up from fighting the cold. Times when it all seems to be working against "our plan." Times when life seems so dormant. But the year goes around and we move forward through the thick and the thin of it, our own personal labyrinth. That's what I am getting at.

Ah, time to go. I have a favor to do for a neighbor. See you later. Bodacious loves, what else, Felipé.

August 29, 2018 / Maybe There Is More

That was kind of a fun entry yesterday working on walking a labyrinth. It looks so simple, a labyrinth, but it is really ingenious. It is stripped down, like a good poem, to its essence.

Annie was here in the spring and we went down to Olympia, WA to St. Michael's for a showing of *Phil's Camino* and to do our usual fantastic Q&A. There at the St. Michael's campus is an outdoor labyrinth that is very neat and tidy. I had some time in between things so I did the walk. I had a vision where the flat labyrinth changed into a mountain and I was walking around the mountain on the trail and working my way upward to the center at the mountaintop. The tight 180 degree turns of the flat labyrinth changed into switchbacks on the mountainside. That makes total sense, right? Can you see it?

I wonder if there is such a thing as one that is big enough to say a rosary while walking. That would be good to figure out. I like the idea of that where the walker has something to do, to concentrate on, rather than just plain checking his progress continually which can drive one crazy.

Maybe I will find some paper here and work on a different design while I am tethered to my chemo. Lunchtime now though. I think I will investigate the cantina here on this floor. OK, all good once again, alperfect really. Walking along loves, Felipé.

August 30, 2018 / The Four Campañeras

Here we are blogging while under the influence of chemotherapy. Well, under the influence of steroids more specifically, and it's 2 in the morning and I am wide awake. I have an hour or two now to write and be with you. Having apple cinnamon tea with blackberry honey to help while away the time. This is what Jerome K. Jerome wrote on my teabag, "It is impossible to enjoy idling thoroughly unless one has plenty of work to do."

I don't know what category we are in on that account but I am here to talk about four very inspiring women who I light a candle for every Sunday. That is such a nice little practice and to say a prayer too of course. It is a visual prayer mostly with the little flame shining. To back up a little bit we have been blogging about labyrinths the last two sessions and we could segue nicely into today's if we would view these four women's efforts walks on the crooked course of a labyrinth, their personal labyrinth. They would be four different but similar labyrinths each as unique as the Four Campañeras are.

My goal here is to encourage them to continue on one day at a time. What they are doing is so important and so under-appreciated that I am here to help. They are bigger than life stories from four bigger-than-life women, but we all need buoying up.

I am going to attempt to write a paragraph about each. I am sure that you know people with similar energy and goals where you are but these are mine to cherish. Let me start with a story of early Seattle. Way back when, during the Yukon gold rush, there was a nun that traveled around with a burro and begged money from the miners. Her goal was to build a hospital for them, for all of us. I just drove by it yesterday and that is Providence Hospital in West Seattle, still there and running.

So, my first compañera is Suzanne, who we joke together about the idea that all she needs is a burro to accompany her on her fundraising tours to really "strike paydirt." She is a nurse by day tending to characters such as myself and by night she is doing her other work of building a facility the likes of which is rare in these parts these days. She has been nursing many dying children and there is no place for them to make this passage comfortably. Now it happens at home which many times is woefully bad because the family is usually drained of energy and resources by then and it lacks the technology and care that a hospital could give. And then there is the hospital that lacks the whole important warmth and familiarity of home and all that brings. What is needed is something halfway between that can bring the best of both worlds simultaneously. Read about her idea at their website: www.ladybughouse.org .

Allison I have never met, although her brother is one of my best friends and I get snippets of news from him about her in Pittsburgh. She has a studio where she works as a sculptor. Mostly this is welding and grinding to create. Remember Pittsburgh is a steel town. The twist is that she brings in vets with problems to help them work on their own projects. Her personal labyrinth is to build a facility worthy of that. We don't have her contact info but we know where to ask.

Third is the latest that I have added to this list and she is Kim from Marin County, CA. Kim knows a lot about gardening and combines that with new technology and new ways of thinking about it and new ways to get people together. One of her projects which I just heard of lately is putting together gardens where prison inmates can work in the soil. I know that this sounds like it has been done before but she is bringing it back as a therapy rather than forced hardship.

And last is Annie the Producer/Director of *Phil's Camino* the documentary film. It is about me but it is about all of us. It is about us as Camino people and cancer people and people who view life in a Christian manner. It has been such a success in the sense of all the countless folks that it has inspired in its three years of existence. And now Annie has created the hour-long version. And it has been a labyrinth for her to be sure. There have been fat times and lean times on all sorts of levels and categories. But Annie has tremendous energy, smarts and drive and through plain hard work, smiles and perseverance this train is going down the tracks. She can be found at: www.philscamino.com. Kudos Annie.

So, life goes on but quality of life really hinges on efforts such as these coming to fruition, making life better for all of us. Thanks, my campañeras. Your inspiration is my inspiration. Your effort is our effort. Making it better loves, middle of the night Felipé.

SEPTEMBER 2, 2018 / FEELING WARM AND COMFORTABLE

Seems like Labor Day Weekend, oh but it is. Gone is the heat and now it is just right. Gone is the smoke from the wildfires. Boy, perfect day today.

Sunday, so Catherine and I went to Mass and then had our theological tailgate party at the supermarket parking lot. People stopped by to give us bits of news or they hung out for a while enjoying the sun. It is the time to savor the rest of the summer. The tomatoes are ripe, the corn is ripe. All is well.

Please stop by to walk if you have been putting it off and haven't made it yet this season. Conditions are perfect for conversation and low blood pressure. You may have to put a few dollars in the bird seed fund, time to put the donation can out for the upcoming season. We usually feed our feathered friends October through March, so that is on the horizon.

Oh, I spy the moon, how pretty. There it is in a cloudless sky. What part of perfect don't I understand here? See what I mean?

My only thought outside my little bubble here today is for John McCain and his family. I will pray for them today as I walk the Camino. It seems to have brought us this moment of peace to our national conversation when that is exactly what was needed. Hopefully we can continue on remembering this when the weekend is over. Thank you John.

Bless you there where you are. Pray for me when you get a moment. Off to my day, sunny loves, Felipé.

SEPTEMBER 3, 2018 / YAY US!

Well, there are times when we need a pat on the back, a little encouragement. We had our Sunday afternoon walk yesterday and tapas after, as usual. And Catherine and Dana were here for that just like old times. Our summers were so busy that they were barely here at all and this is the first time since Spring that we got to slow down and just walk, tapa and laugh together. At some point in this Catherine said, "Yay us!" That is where I'll start from today.

Just nice to do a simple celebration like that. Nothing major or complicated, just a pause and an acknowledgement that we are here together intact along the trail. Yes, we are weary, yes, we are dinged up, yes there still is a long way to go but "Yay us!"

We are walking in half an hour, part of our Labor Day celebration. Stop by when you get a chance, today or one of these days soon. Bring a dollar for the bird seed donation.

Yay us loves, Felipé.

SEPTEMBER 4, 2018 / SIXTY-SOME THOUSAND

There was a report that just came in from Santiago that 60,000 pilgrims came off of the Camino in the month of August. August is supposed to be the busiest month there but really? In August 2014 when Rick, Maryka, and I crossed the finish line there were 30,000. Talking growth here, wow! I'm stunned.

I don't have the facts at hand but I know this isn't an anomaly. There has been steady growth over the years but I have lost track of it the last few years. It is more popular than ever, yea than ever.

This seems something to be happy about. People are hungry for what the Camino offers and I am happy about that. It is grabbing them today as it grabbed me four years ago and look, we are still talking about it. There is concern about the overcrowding, but I think that for better or worse that will work itself out with a little time. The Camino will provide in a bigger sense for us all.

I know that Phil's Camino is working hard to do its part. We have at least eight pilgrims coming for this afternoon's walk. It has been a busy summer here for us and things are going to be hopping 'til the rains come. And look, it is that same energy, that same hunger that brings people together here so far from Spain and the "real" Camino.

Come by when you can and walk with us. We all profit when you come. We aren't in danger of overcrowding yet here. Camino loves, Felipé.

September 6, 2018 / Talking Hospitality

I know this is hard and it takes a long time to distill but if you were to put your Camino experience into one word what would it be? Mine is hospitality and has been that for a long while now. It is in the great big definition of the word. It is in, "The Camino Provides." It is one of my things that I say to people wanting to go, "don't over plan, just fall into its arms." I have heard that the King of Spain pays some of the pilgrim doctor bills along the Way. It's in that!

The word goes back to Old French and back farther to Latin. The Knights Hospitaler are credited with opening the first hospitals to care for beat-up pilgrims on the original Jerusalem pilgrimage. These knights remain today in the Order of Malta who took me to Lourdes this past May. They sort of invented the word and are still living by it.

I can't help but think that it is the Golden Rule in practice, in practical application. It is a practice, a discipline. It is giving in a world that mostly takes. This is one of the big lessons that the Camino has left me with. There are others but this to me is my key to loving my fellow man, an important part of the big picture.

Time to go. Ten minutes to the Thursday morning walk, just enough time to get organized. Treating each other right loves, Felipé.

September 9, 2018 / Blue Sky, Light Winds

I know that this blog is supposed to be about the 3 C's: Cancer, Catholicism and Camino but somehow Catholicism gets pushed to the back burner often. Well maybe that will change. I really never know day-to-day the direction of this ship of a blog. Sometimes it goes this way and sometime that.

But people ask me why I converted most often. That is the main question I get on this topic of religion. And I usually play the cancer card at that point saying that I really needed spiritual help from a church that has depth and resources. I needed to lean on something. And I did lean on it and continue to.

That is a very practical reason and true, but there is more to the story. Just for now I might mention the quest for comfort. I sensed that I would find comfort in the Catholic Church and I have. Mother Mary is the font of comfort and I am learning how to open myself up to that, to her. And there is more but I want to think about it a little. Time to go for now. Hopefully will find time to work on my truck and get some air and sun today.

Yours through thick and thin, love, Felipé.

September 10, 2018 / Getting Some Rain

The process of Fall is happening here. Rain is starting to show up to green up our situation. Summer was fun while it lasted, as always. The corn is about played out. The apple and pears are coming on. BLTs on the menu with the fresh tomatoes. We lead a garden-centric life here apparently.

We had a bunch of pilgrims yesterday for the walk and tapas who were really fun. It was Jeannie and her flight attendant friends who fly in once a year for a reunion. So Phil's Camino was on their agenda this year. And they left with two dozen ears of Golden Jubilee corn to remember us by.

And Phil's Camino the trail goes on into the Fall with a few rainy days here and there. But that is easily compensated for by the colors. The fog starts coming in too which adds a certain spookiness and sense of mystery. Gone is the strict clarity and surety of the summer months. Ah and mushrooms sprouting up hither and yon.

Well, time to find the right footwear for the walk this morning, wet grass situation out there, been a while. All good all the time, wet grass loves, Felipé.

September 13, 2018 / The Storm Is Blowing In, We Left

The forecast of this monster storm headed for the Carolina Coast is bringing back all sorts of memories for me. I was there in 1968 when a massive system came through. About thirty of us Marines and all our fancy radio gear were being loaded aboard ship to leave Morehead City, NC with a destination of San Juan, PR. We left in a hurry to get out of the port and out to sea.

Ships are safer at sea in bad weather than in harbors where the wind and surge can raise havoc in the confined space, literally stacking things the way that was never intended. So, we left quickly, and cleared land safely but lost a lot of government property off the deck because it wasn't chained down to meet the conditions.

We were aboard an LST or LSD which are similar flat-bottomed ships made to get up to a beach so they don't need a dock to unload. The major disadvantage is that this shallow draft makes them very unstable and squirrelly in the blue water, which we the Marines on board found out, not being experienced sailors. We were scared to death and we wound up after three days 300 miles north of where we started; and we were headed south remember.

But we made it to Puerto Rico after that and we spent the winter there in the warm, a good trade-off to the harrowing opening experience. I never put this together but in 1975 I was sailing out of Hilo, HI with a destination of San Francisco, CA. And something very similar happened but in a warm and sunny way. We left the harbor a couple of days before a tsunami came in to land and devastated the harbor. We were out to sea and sailing northeast toward the Horse Latitudes and the massive when surge passed right under us and we never felt it one bit. We were wrapped in our protective blanket of good karma, is maybe how we expressed our luck.

But maybe there is a lesson here somewhere about facing our personal "storms." We are not always safest in the safe places. Sometimes we have to get clear of things that trap or confine us and just wing it to the best of our ability. Yes, let me mull this over.

Well, walking in a moment and then archery lessons. I hope I haven't been too off topic with that but it just "blew" in on me so to speak, a memory storm. 40 knot loves, Felipé.

September 16, 2018 / Sunday With Some Rain

Just thinking of our pilgrim friends on their journeys. Catherine y Dana are walking the Dales Way in England. And also right now Sybil and Mary are somewhere around Burgos I would guess. I hope they are all carrying on like quality pilgrims being brave, helpful, resourceful, cheerful, somewhat cheeky and hopefully reverent at the right times. Can't wait to see them all again and get the report. Their enthusiasm will fuel us. I just know that. That is how it works. It is all so contagious.

It is such a good antidote to those times of isolation that we are all susceptible to. Standing next to someone fresh off the trail or just hearing about it can give me the goosebumps. You know that feeling. It's alperfect in all its glory and imperfection. Take care on this Sunday, love Felipé.

September 19, 2018 / New Places

Catherine and Dana reported from the trail in England yesterday. That route is called the Dales Way. Because of our enthusiasm for pilgrimage we are overburdening the Camino Francés. Is it time to branch out? Time to discover or rediscover new and old places?

Way back in 2014 when I was walking the last 100 kilometers on the Camino de Santiago and the flow of pilgrims seemed like a river overflowing it banks, I was happy. Happy in a sense that wasn't it wonderful that all these people are here to participate just as I was. And yes, it is good to see the increase in pilgrims, but there is a limit to that. The old too-much-of-a-good-thing comes into play. So, it is fitting that we think about branching out to other trails in Spain. How about the trails in Italy and Ireland and Japan? How about trails that are not so famous? Trails where there are no trails?

Well OK, thank you Catherine for your inspiration on this. Off I go to the day. More thoughts tomorrow. Walking loves, Felipé.

September 20, 2018 / What If . . . .

We have been talking about other Caminos, about the idea of us branching out to see what we can discover. And the old tried and true definition of a pilgrimage may need to be stretched and grown to accommodate this. It has been the thinking that the most important thing about a pilgrimage is the destination. That we go through hardship to get next to something in the end. That the value is in the completion of the process, to getting to the goal.

What if. . . . What if it is almost the other way around? And not that we don't need you Saint James, but what if we could redefine pilgrimage just for now? What if we take into account what we bring as individuals and groups to this? What if we are really talking about a gathering of "teachers" as Catherine calls us? This is what we have stumbled across on Phil's Camino. We don't really go anywhere physically here, just in circles, thousands of circles, but we do it together, willingly and enthusiastically, which is the key.

But the goal does seem to set the theme for the journey. There needs to be a theme to give it a "something." Then there needs to be a shout out to gather a critical mass of "teachers" or the "someones." Maybe the "somewhere" doesn't matter all that much really. Oh yes, it needs to have a certain quietude so the group can make its own music so to speak. And it needs some level of facilities to accommodate the needs of the "teachers." These are all things that occurred to us here at Phil's Camino, a little tiny miniature situation, but a situation.

Not long ago here at Phil's Camino the idea came up that what we are running here is akin to the French salon. That is what we are talking about, right? We walk but we also talk and then we "figure things out." Things, ideas and solutions start to occur, don't they?

Time to walk. A little wet out this morning here at Phil's Camino as I look out the window. Salon loves, Felipé.

September 21, 2018 / A Friday In September

Back again to say hello. All the talk about Caminoing in the last few days was exciting. We covered a certain view of it that we hadn't done before in our four years, which is hard to imagine. And if we stretched our definition of pilgrimage a little more maybe this diary would be a Camino for me, for us.

So, we walk on into the future. We cherish the whole situation. We plan on making the most of the day. It could rain, it could shine. We have faith that it will all work out. The Camino provides. Having faith loves, Felipé.

September 22, 2018 / Check This Out

Yes, here we are September 22, 2018 and we have the first random sighting of a Phil's Camino patch on the Camino de Santiago. Annie had these made for the movie and Mary spotted it on a pilgrim's backpack on the Meseta.

Steve-O is enthused about the expanded versions of the Camino that we have been talking about. He calls it Camino-X. And we in our conversation realized how close we are to having the Camino be talked about as a state of mind.

We who are fortunate enough to realize that it is possible to keep the flame burning are growing in numbers. This I think is the real lesson of the notion, "That once you get to Santiago your Camino begins." It's happening!

Have to go and get things started for the day. Happening loves, Felipé.

September 25, 2018 / Heartship!

Hey, a great new thing has happened! My spell check came through and invented a great new word, HEARTSHIP. What do you think? I think we can work with it. It must be defined something like the state of having heart, right? Yea, I was trying to write the word hardship and heartship was substituted. A thousand times this is frustrating and then once it coughs up a gem!

Speaking of that, I myself need to cough up a gem later this afternoon. Have a scan this afternoon to check out my insides and could use some good news from way in there. Pray for me just a tenth of a second.

We have been talking for years about the Camino, pilgrimage, walking and related issues. It happens quite a bit here at the blog that just when I think I am dry for inspiration, something new comes appears to work on. Somehow this image came to mind of us walking, of moving forward, of accumulating experience, of being together as "walking into the bigger picture." I like it so much. That is really what we are doing. Yes, I think we can work with it.

Well, time to shower and get the tractor dust off me for my hospital visit. See you soon. Maybe send a note to My Rebecca wishing her a Happy Birthday. OK, heartship loves, Felipé.

September 26, 2018 / The Old No Coincidences Department

Apparently it is International Book Week and you are supposed to grab the nearest book and go to page 52, the fifth sentence, and post that sentence with the instructions for the next person. Some interesting sentences have come up amongst friends.

And you know how recently we have been kicking around ideas about expanding the definition of pilgrimage. We talked about including Phil's Camino in the realm of pilgrimage even though it has no "real" destination. We had so stretched the definition of Camino to the point of being on the verge of it becoming a state of mind. That's a good thing to me.

So, the no coincidences part is my quote:

"But along with the monastic peregrinatio ascetia, another form of peregrination, the peregrinatio ad loca sancta, developed starting in the 4th century under Constantine."

So with my mighty Latin skills I am interpreting that to mean that the pilgrimage to holy places started in the fourth century and before that was something different. And that was the ascetic pilgrimage, whatever that was. That sounds challenging, if not sorta grim. But the important thing is that there was something different and it looks like it was happening locally inside or around the monastery, sans destination.

So, that is what I ran into recently. Had to work around all the partying that has been going on. Oh, and my scan report came back "stable" meaning no growth of my tumors. That is good news. God has me where He wants me these days. No "Get Out of Jail Free Card" but nonetheless I am left with something challenging but doable.

Thanks for all your thoughts and prayers. No one has support like I have. It is unbelievably powerful. Thank you one and all.

No coincidences love, Felipé.

September 28, 2018 / We Recognize and Respond

I feel like I am turning from the Tom Sawyer to the Henry David Thoreau of the Camino. I spent years now cheerleading and hopefully getting people excited about walking the main Camino in Spain and then now to moving to alternatives to alleviate the crowding. The Camino is suffering from its own success. It is all wonderful really, so many attracted.

But we are starting to see alternatives appearing where the same lessons may be available or other valuable lessons may be had. And maybe some of these walks are close by and don't require jet fuel. Maybe we don't have the time, money or health to pull off a far-away extended trip but can prosper from something close by just the same.

Close by loves, Felipé.

September 29, 2018 / Good Stuff To Come

What is on the schedule for today? We got Autumn coming here and trying to get all the chores done that relate to that change. Visitors are still coming to walk on the trail. BLTs are prominent on the menu with ripe tomatoes in abundance.

There is talk of having a get-together next summer for as many Caminoheads as can make it. Just starting to put together timing and logistics. Stay tuned for details on that. This is exciting stuff. Good stuff to come loves, Felipé.

September 30, 2018 / Crockpot News

One of the great joys of Autumn is the dusting off of the old trusty crockpot. I picked up the makings for a beef stew and I think that today is the day for that. A real Sunday dinner is happening. Catherine said they have plenty of cucumbers so will run over there and grab a few for slicing.

Yes, Catherine and Dana are back to the Island after their Pilgrimage to Dales Way, England. They will be here for the Tuesday afternoon walk and tapas so we will get the report in full for you.

Oh, there is the waning moon in the blue sky just for me. Well, it is not just for me but maybe . . . Little puff clouds are marching across the sky and the sun is coming and going. All very exciting. There is moisture at higher elevations but I think that it will be dry here today. We had a little rain overnight though, perfect for my little itty-bitty clover seeds that I planted.

Hmm, plenty happening here at the moment in my natural world. Time for me to move around in it. Thinking of you, joyful thoughts. Life is a poem loves, Felipé.

OCTOBER 1, 2018 / OUR ALMA MATER?

That's what I'm answering from now on, "Santiago Class of 2014!" How can I not? It was my finishing school this Camino. It didn't take four or six years but just a month or two. It didn't cost major money but 30 euros a day. What is this thing?

I can't believe that I have been writing this blog for over four years (1700+ posts) and I am not sure that I am any closer to answering that question. What is this thing? We have sliced and diced it a hundred ways. We have put it back together in different forms just to learn. We have studied its long history. We have slept on it and dreamt about it. We have day dreamed about it. We have remembered it every day since.

We continually long for people to come along who are willing to hear us prattle on about it, the poor folks. Every little detail seems important and relevant and worth repeating. Little things seem to become big and big things somehow get put in place. It seems a perfect balance after all.

We finally understand the statement, "When you get to Santiago your Camino begins." That took a long while to accomplish and was a Camino in itself. People around you were patient, bless them.

And over time you have influenced others to go and walk their own Caminos. You are sort of proud of that. It seems part of your new configuration that has come about. You are now the evangelist, who would have thought?

And mysteries have appeared but they no longer bother you. They seem a natural part of the landscape and have come to be cherished. You seem touched by that, the mystery. It lingers like a smoke or a mist but doesn't hinder you. And maybe that is the final thought, that the Camino is part of that mystery to be cherished rather than to be figured out. Yes, "Santiago, Class of 2014!" Plan on meeting me there. Love in the mist, Felipé.

OCTOBER 5, 2018 / OUR PARTICULAR COUGAR

Well, in case you haven't heard, Vashon Island has a new cougar, a puma, a mountain lion. And this one is way new and improved. The last one we had (and the first one in a long time) was cool and did a fantastic groundbreaking job but the new one has panache. Well, he or she is on Facebook with his or her own page for one. Pretty funny and probably only on Vashon.

Having a cougar around takes a little getting used to. They are a class A predator and very capable. We say as locals, "Yes, he will take care of some of these darn deer." Yup, we will put up with so much as long as he is helping out. But the other side of the coin is that we all have big cats in our DNA memory and this adds interesting spice to being outside with this guy.

And personally, these guys have meaning for me. A while back we had a small group of us known as the Cancer Commandos, that was Jennifer, Bill and myself. We would have some fun with our situation and try to do some good. They both have passed away now leaving me the sole survivor. But I remember one of the things that Jennifer said to me in her last days hooked up to all the tubes and medicines was, "You won't have to do this, the cougar will get you." I think about that a lot.

So, you can join this fun by being FB friends with Vashon Cougar. There is some pretty fun and creative stuff on there. Tell him Phil sent you. Yea, love, Felipé.

OCTOBER 10, 2018 / A LABYRINTH FOR A DEAR FRIEND, MAYBE

Well, I don't even know if she needs help but if she ever did, we would be ready. Right now we don't have much to work with but we have enthusiasm and we know how to work a shovel.

And of course, someone else may need help also. Labyrinths may be the next big deal springing up hither and yon. Wouldn't that be great to see. Of course, they are not as exciting as devices with screens. Maybe they would be a good alternative. Or time spent in that form of contemplation would be a good alternative to the time spent on our gadgets.

As I understand it the labyrinth was an invention to give a person an idea of what a pilgrimage would be like. I really have to stretch my imagination to come up with that but yes, there is something there. I will work on expanding that for myself and for us.

And who knows—maybe we could come up with some innovations in what a labyrinth looks like. Maybe there are other forms or ways to do it. We could maybe reinvent the wheel on this one. It has been known to happen. Thanks for stopping by loves, Felipé.

OCTOBER 29, 2018 / ATTAINING HEARTSHIP

Sometimes it seems a long way to anywhere from where we stand. And sometimes we have a certain clarity because we seem to be near the center of things. Ah, that seems so like being on a labyrinth, yes? There we sometimes get very near the center as we travel and it benefits us even though there is more trail and we are not at the end yet.

We must operate here on this earth from a position of occasionally glimpsing the truth, the goodness and the beauty. We charge our batteries while we can because the glimpse is a glimpse and never permanent. It slips away for one reason or another just as the trail snakes away from the center of the labyrinth to send us exploring some misty byway.

It seems to take a lot of energy to maintain when we don't feel at our best out there at the edge of things. Our solid feeling that we grasped so well yesterday is just a memory. What sustains us to have the faith that we need to continue when things are ragged in the outer reaches? I think now this is the purpose of this new word, heartship, that has come along. It appeared a few weeks ago as a mutation of the word hardship in my auto correct.

Having heart or fortitude or toughness or resilience is what we need. Not that we are inventing a new thing here; we are reviewing something long-known. But that's fine and as it should be as many have walked on this trail before us. Heartship, we are seeing where it fits in all this.

The Monday morning walk is coming up in a few moments. It is a little foggy and very still out there. The rains of the last few days have soaked in the ground. Getting close to starting to fill the feeders for our birds.

Monday morning loves, Felipé.

October 30, 2018 / The Ebb and the Flow

Most of all have faith. Remember, joy is our main job. Let us bridge the gaps for ourselves and those around us. Let us work with the ebb and flow.

Geographically we are all separated. And we may be separated by a certain amount of political hoopla. But we have knowledge and power that keeps us floating individually and keeps us united as a group. Let's build on that and see what happens.

Having touched the face of St. James loves, Felipé.

November 1, 2018 / We Have A Neighbor

We have a neighbor that is actively dying. Got that term from My Rebecca's Threshold Choir. They sing soft songs for people that are actively dying. Anyway, as this goes on next door I pray. Sometimes praying seems a feeble gesture and sometimes it seems a mighty mustard seed capable of who knows what.

Interesting that we are here with this situation on November 1st, the Day of the Dead this year. This holy day isn't something that I grew up with so it all seems a little weird to my sensibilities but maybe this convergence is going to educate me. "No coincidences" strikes once again.

I told My Rebecca that I wanted to die in the Elk Hotel, our expedition tent. I don't know how practical that is really but hey, it's my occasion right? Going out like a Civil War General seems appropriate, conversing with my Captains about battles won and lost, passing on the grit.

Ah, walking in a moment. Good morning to say rosaries. Alperfect once again loves, Felipé.

November 5, 2018 / An Inspiration From St. Paul

St. Paul wasn't always a saint. At his early worst he helped out in the stoning of Stephen, considered the Church's first martyr. Stephen after his death was seen as St. Stephen. But back to Paul, or actually Saul, who met the risen Christ while on the road to Damascus. Life-changing that was, and Saul's name was changed to Paul to commemorate the event. Anyway the upshot is that Paul turned out to be the chief carrier of the Christian banner to the Greek world and thus to us.

But this was not easy on him personally. One, he had a physical ailment that plagued him. And he was continuously running from, and hiding from, the critics. He suffered beatings and imprisonment, and was finally beheaded in Rome for causing so many waves in the empire.

All this hardship makes a bright point all the brighter though. And what has been inspiring me is the tale of him being in prison somewhere and being chained to a series of guards, his time there being closely supervised. And Paul, never missing an opportunity, even in there was converting these guards left and right. He could probably do it in his sleep, but still. They definitely had "a tiger by the tail, it is plain to see," as the old Buck Owens song goes. Who has who?

We are so used to hearing, "He or she has cancer," "I have cancer," "What if I get cancer?" "Living with cancer," "Dealing with cancer," or "My cancer." Those are all the same in that they start with we are the ones that HAVE cancer. What if all of a sudden we said screw that, what if cancer HAS us. It obviously doesn't know who it is dealing with here anymore. Who has who? That is where we should head toward and get to!

Can you see it? Monday loves, Felipé.

November 7, 2018 / Voting Days Past

At the hospital today to get my share of chemicals. I was talking to one of my nurses about voting days past and it was kind of fun trying to remember the details.

It would be November in Buffalo, New York and you went with your parents to vote, a kind of a Ralphie pilgrimage (as in the *Christmas Story*). You walked because each neighborhood had a place. It was cold and dark but not quite snowy yet. But maybe you didn't have your new Sears and Roebuck winter coat yet so staying warm was a little dicey in the coat that you had outgrown.

The city had these little wooden structures all painted green that they would deliver to all the neighborhoods maybe a week before the big day. I could guess and say they were something like 10 by 16 feet in plan. Not a lot of room in there for more than one family at a time.

So there must have been a table for check-in although I don't remember that, as there were other things more important. The white-painted interior of the building was lit with a couple of light bulbs which was such a contrast to the darkness outside. In the corner was a potbelly stove burning coal which was pretty exciting. But the main event was actually going into the voting machine. Yea you sort of entered it and there was this lever that swung and caused the heavy curtain to close behind you for the privacy required. Of course, only the adults voted and we would just peek in as they entered and exited. All very mysterious for us short people.

My parents never ever talked politics at home and people in general out and around did a good job avoiding it too. Our neighborhood was probably 90 percent Democrats I would guess, blue-collar guys for the most part. My mother probably voted on the Democratic side most often, reflecting the neighborhood, while my dad was more involved with the Republican side of the ballot, having more country influence. But again, they never talked about it and it didn't seem like it ever caused a problem between them. You just voted and then walked home and set the table and ate meat and potatoes like always.

I remember registering to vote when I was eighteen and choosing Independent to describe myself, seemed like a balanced thing to do. Yup, and those were the days of 15-cent hamburgers but that is another story for another day.

Thanks, love, Felipé.

November 15, 2018 / One More Digression

I just happened randomly to watch a Public Broadcasting program last evening about the big cave rescue in Thailand. Remember that? It wasn't too long ago.

There were 12 boys who went exploring a cave with their soccer coach. Unfortunately the first monsoon rains blocked their exit as the cave started to flood. It was an amazing joint effort of different experts and rescuers that was put together in a rapid manner.

I am always drawn to these dramas where people get together and perform at their very best to pull off a rescue or solve a problem. The Chilean mine rescue back maybe five years ago was exactly the same. Remember that one? There was one funny incident from that one that just popped into my head. One of the miners, as he hit the surface, was welcomed simultaneously by his wife and his mistress! Oops, slight problem.

Well, have a walk in a moment. Love you immensely, Felipé.

November 16, 2018 / Exploring Our Digression

As we walked yesterday Dana and I were asking the question, why do we need a crisis to perform at our best? What is that temporary state that happens to us only once in a while? Can we tap into that and be there more often?

I don't know, big questions that probably need big answers. Could it have to do with decluttering? Both situations have a "deck clearing" aspect. We don't have the burden of all the trivia that normally inhabits our lives. There is one thing that may be bigger than we think.

Then there has to be a need and not only a need but one that has to be addressed immediately or quickly. We were pretty needy the whole time on the Camino from what I remember. We had to help each other when our self-help ran out, which it seemed to do daily. Desperation is present.

Being in this groove with others offers a high, a high state, where we seem to feed on each other's energy. There is that! It is rare but we know it when we see it and jump on it if we can. Am I right?

Just a few thoughts to pass the time. A gray morning here with a little wind out of the north and the leaves are falling one by one. Thanks for stopping by loves, Felipé.

November 20, 2018 / It's Quiet Here, in the Morning

My Rebecca is going to bake corn bread today with the new cornmeal that just came out. Two big batches will go into the making of cornbread stuffing for turkey day. She makes that in big flat pans so the bread gets crunchy around the edges, oh boy! I am a convert to this, having grown up north of the Mason-Dixon Line but I'm a believer now!

So are you working on your thanksgivings for Thursday? Our whole largesse is one big blessing of course but we need to be more specific. This is important because children will be listening to our expression.

All good, alperfect on the Camino. We travel on wishing each other the best. The morning sun warms our backs and our shadows stretch out before us. Wait, I think I smell coffee.

OK, good on ya loves, Felipé.

NOVEMBER 22, 2018 / HEARTSHIP–THANKSGIVING DAY 0553 WITH COFFEE

At the hospital that was the topic of the day, who is cooking what for whom amongst the nurses. And a lot of the younger nurses will be tasked with being on duty today so they may get the meal in take-out form this year.

We are off to a potluck meal at a rented hall with old friends here locally, no big travel. My Rebecca is bringing her signature cornbread dressing to share. We have been processing our dried corn into cornmeal for this. And we have lots more meal that will be vacuum packed and stored in the freezer for later. It is part of the largesse that we are thankful for today.

I'm trying to get my brain around my crowded life and all the wonderful things that have come my way over the last decade in the guise of serious illness, its genesis. But if I could pick one thing that points to our gift of largesse it would be for me the phenomenon of corn.

I am going to make up a little demo for our guests at the meal today. I will shuck two ears of our dried corn and put that in a Ziploc bag for them to handle and view to see what one seed will produce. This will be an excellent show and tell. Yes. And an excellent prayer.

Remember to bring calm and peace to the meeting today. People will be there with new hurts and old hurts and new hearts and old hearts. Quite a minefield to navigate through, but that is our job. Bless you loves Felipé.

NOVEMBER 23, 2018 / THE LAND OF NO COINCIDENCES

Somehow it is not Kansas anymore. All that is in our rear-view mirror now. But where are we? What are we doing here? Can we be comfortable here in this new land? Comfortable is not the right word, but what is the right word? Can we flourish here once we figure it out, like our ancestors who came to the geographic America threadbare and hungry with nothing but a desperation/hope double-combo, full-meal-deal within them?

We have fallen through a looking glass. That is it, isn't it? We were equally threadbare, hungry, desperate/ hopeful. We have discovered Heartship so far though. Our Caminoheads are changing to Caminohearts before our eyes. We are in the process of internalizing the situation, the Camino experience. After the Camino things are never the same. Yes, something massively significant occurred AND continues to unfold for us.

There is something that has overtaken us. Something strong but stealthy like fog, and subtle like a mist. We can't quite put our finger on it but it seems to have stalked us. We are the hunted. And maybe there is a time of trying to figure it out being over soon and we can surrender to a time of enjoying it. Maybe it has been all figured out for us all along and now we are just catching on to that fact here in the Land of No Coincidences.

Right now I am so happy with the blessings that this holiday of Thanksgiving has brought to us. It all seemed more poignant this year. A drop of gratitude in the mix of our lives can go a long way to healing our many rifts. Enjoying you loves, Felipé.

NOVEMBER 24, 2018 / BURNT SIENNA SATURDAY

Yea, maybe every day needs a color designation. Well, personally I didn't go shopping yesterday. OK, I ducked into the supermarket briefly to grab a half a basket of items. But gosh, I don't know whether to laugh or cry about the Black Friday activities.

I hope to take this day at an easy pace after my time in the city this last week. I am off to LA in the middle of the coming week to do some work there, patients and doctors to meet. That is all very exciting and intriguing but still in its formative stage and I will tell you more as things gel.

This evening Catherine and Dana are coming over to "gobble" up Thanksgiving leftovers. I am making mashed potatoes and gravy which somehow I missed on Thursday. Notre Dame Football is on tonight and Catherine is a big fan, so that is the central focus.

Burnt Sienna in my mind is a good color for a horse or a saddle. Seems like the perfect color for the day ahead. Thanks for stopping by. Here we go loves, Felipé.

NOVEMBER 26, 2018 / RAIN, COFFEE, WOODSMOKE

Here we are, Monday morning. Yesterday was the last Sunday in Ordinary Time on the Church calendar. Advent approaches! Or *we* approach Advent . . . that seems maybe more pilgrim-like.

After the tension of the elections Thanksgiving was something to grab on to and a place to rest at. In less than a month the solstice will be here and the good news of more light, more heat and the promise of easy living will be upon us. The longer I live in the Pacific Northwest the more important this shift seems to become.

Walking in a few moments here and then an archery lesson. Oh, Catherine just called to say she is coming to walk also. OK, the warmth of friendship to accompany the last few leaves falling, Buen Camino! Good day loves, Felipé.

November 29, 2018 / Beverly Boulevard

Just had a good safe flight in to LAX. Up in my hotel room taking a few moments to enjoy the quiet.

I have a bunch of meetings with doctors and patients tomorrow which is the reason for my trip. I hesitate to say too much beforehand. This is all about meeting folks and learning how things work in the cancer rehab area basically. I have things to contribute and they have things to contribute and we are trying to see how that will interface.

Well, I brought my jar full of corn with me to keep me company. It was something that I put together for Thanksgiving as a demonstration of abundance. Two seeds that I planted in May made this much corn is what it says. And am so glad that it made it through TSA at the airport security, where it got a lot of attention. More to come loves, Felipé.

December 1, 2018 / Back Home

Back here just in time to watch Washington Husky Football. Big game tonight. Playing Utah and the winner gets to go to the Rose Bowl, so pretty darn exciting.

I want to let you in on what I have been doing these last few days. Went down to LA to work with the staff at the Cedars Sinai Cancer Rehab Department. They have developed this wonderful program called GRACE to teach resiliency to cancer patients.

They have been using *Phil's Camino*, the documentary, as part of this class. So Annie and I showed up down there to do a showing for a reunion of the students and then a Q&A. We were told that maybe eight would show up and there were thirty-five. It went really well.

We did a luncheon showing for hospital professionals and following a Q&A. One hundred and forty crowded in for that. Another success.

I really don't know what all this means for the future but we got a start on something. This is cutting edge in the world of cancer treatment, that's important to say. We are in the process of putting together some amazing new stuff.

OK, back to football for now. See you tomorrow. Amazing new love, Felipé.

December 1, 2018 / Abundance Some More

I miss my corn buddy. I gave him to Dr. Asher in LA. He will have a good home there. Maybe I will make another next year at harvest time.

My Rebecca and I did try and take a stab at figuring out how many kernels were in the corn buddy jar and came up with the number 800, give or take. If you need a number, there it is. Or we passed it around with the folks at the patients' meeting and the weight of it was impressive. One way or another we need to be impressed with this abundance thing.

I wish Pilgrim Farmer John were here at the moment to talk to us about this phenomenon. Maybe he will contribute when he reads this. Farmer Michelle said that dandelions have 1000 seeds. Farmer gallows humor there.

I challenged the patients' group to pay attention and see whether they couldn't discover abundance in other areas of their lives. Surely there are productive avenues in our minds that are waiting to be discovered that will yield answers to some of our problems. Surely our spiritual roots are connected to riches galore ready for the taking.

That's what is on my mind today. Thanksgiving really took a hold of me this year and won't let go! And Advent starts tomorrow. What a season loves, Felipé.

DECEMBER 2, 2018 / ADVENT!

The opening of Advent today. Officially the Christmas season according to the Church. And our Padre was right there with a great homily, To Live the Usual Unusually Well. OK, we can do that.

Yea, there is a broken sky here with the sun coming and going. It's chilly and we are going through firewood at a pretty good clip. Comes with the season. So we will hunker down as usual.

Catherine and I did our weekly tailgate session after Mass. We were talking poetry and that attracted attention. Like people listening for stock-market tips. Maybe that is a sign of changing times. Or maybe that is just usual for unusual Vashon Island.

Just have another minute to be with you. But I had an image just there of hanging Christmas lights around in my mind. Let me see if I can color my doings with the addition of that cheerful ambience. Mind ambience, decorating the mind.

Alperfect today loves, Felipé.

DECEMBER 6, 2018 / THERE WERE ABOUT FIFTY OF US ATTENDING

I am so fortunate to have witnessed a very special event. I can't stop smiling. It was incongruous to the max. Here I am with time to "kill" between chemo treatments and what should happen? Outrageous!

Let me calm down. There was a wedding performed here at the Swedish Cancer Institute Treatment Center, right before my eyes. I am so amazed and delighted. I am here watching happy young people eating cake and sipping what appears to be sparkling cider. Well, you can't have everything.

We are finding joy in a new way here in the very heart of the beast. Just who said that there couldn't be a full-blown real wedding here where you would least expect it? Oh, maybe that wasn't sparkling cider after all; they are all laughing and giggling so. We are all higher than kites.

But alas I must go and address business. What a day. Thank you newly-weds. Off we go down the Camino. Congratulations to all loves, Felipé.

December 10, 2018 / A Table for Catherine and Dana

Here on the red leather couch covered by my Camino sleeping bag I drive my universe.

The cloud layer seems thin and sunshine could appear maybe in time for the walk. I confess that I only made one lap yesterday instead of my normal three. It was pouring and I talked my way out of it. This happens occasionally but not often. Raven Creek is not running yet. The still-dry ground is still absorbing.

I am lucky enough to be working on a table for Catherine and Dana. It is a seven-foot-long dining table made from solid oak. It was crafted by someone they knew and has lived with various folks and now has come to them. They asked me to clean it up and put a finish on it.

When approaching a project such as this I have to get to a place where I am in awe of the piece's history: all the meals, all the Christmas presents wrapped, all the science projects completed, all the tears and the joys are all there in the burns and the scars and the glitter.

How to clean it up and not disrupt this rich history? How to make way for the next act and still honor all those that came before?

Hey, time to find my boots. Time to get outside and air out my brain. See you soon. Love and stuff, Felipé

December 11, 2018 / One Flower

My Rebecca keeps a Christmas Cactus in our living room which sits in the winter light of the southern facing windows. It has always been off-schedule preferring to bloom at Halloween or sometimes Thanksgiving than the standard Christmastime. You could say quirky and that would cover it and a lot of what goes on here on our beloved Vashon Island.

So this year, back to the beloved cactus, it decided to not bloom at all in the Fall and what should appear now but a single blossom. Sometimes a Halloween Cactus or a Thanksgiving Cactus but now an Advent Cactus. OK, so an Advent Cactus, yes we can work with that, no problem.

And the blossom looks out in the direction of My Rebecca's chair like a messenger with a little pink message. But it is more active than pink really, more energetic. Pink would be an understatement.

In contrast, it is extremely gray outside and the rain pitter-patters on the skylights, the Big Dark has arrived in all its dampness. We, like the Native Americans before us, hunker down in our shelters and wait it out. Our focus comes close, gone are the views of the mountains and the stars shining. Our world is small where things like a thought, or a smile, or yes that single flower, grow in significance.

We adapt to survive in this desert in reverse. We dwell on that thought/smile/flower longer that we would have in the expansive summertime. Now we milk every single droplet of essence to nourish ourselves and each other. And the thought/smile/flower is happy to give and it doesn't seem diminished in any way for the giving. Maybe that's the miracle if we need one at the moment. Waiting smiley loves, Felipé.

December 12, 2018 / Simple and Singular

As thoughts do, my mind went to the square miles of sunflowers blooming on the plains along the Camino in August. What would our one flower be in that show, one among millions? But really in December here in the Northern Hemisphere, here at Raven Ranch, it seems totally sufficient and apropos.

It stands out just being itself. Maybe so much like the Christ child in the manger. All very simple and singular. It is what it is or He is who He is. We should be that pure, that straight forward.

Off I go to build a fire in the shop and put another coat of finish on the table. Maybe I just saw a snowflake? Hmm, could be. All that I can gather loves, Felipé.

December 17, 2018 / The Crazy Positive Attitude

The robins are here by the tens and hundreds. They think that this general area is a good place to winter. They seem glad to be here, a break from the frozen ground to the north.

There was a lone fawn out in the pasture yesterday when I walked in the afternoon. No one showed up to accompany me so it was the deer and me. It was moving from apple tree to apple tree looking for some fruit that had fallen over night. I could see that there wasn't much there so I shook branches as I went and got some feed for it.

I'll pick up some more sunflower seeds on my next trip to town. The seed-eater birds need help this time of year. It's always a challenge to keep those feeders supplied. And my favorite scene in *Phil's Camino* is the juncos at one of the feeders hanging in the hawthorn hedge. There is no talking, just the birds busy.

The other day a hummingbird zoomed into the area by our kitchen windows. And it hovered where we had a feeder hung two years ago. That was the last time, as we didn't get it together this year nor last to hang it. So we are led to believe what? This tiniest of critters has been checking on us all this time. I'm amazed.

Ah, I feel better, can you tell? Time to find my boots and the logbook for the walk at 9. A lull in the rain this morning but it is back this afternoon and continues all night.

Oh, and I am back to the city tomorrow. Time for my every two-month scan. OK, later, love, Felipé.

December 18, 2018 / A Glimpse

I caught a glimpse of Mt Rainier yesterday. Gone were the icy glaciers that reflect the sun's rays, gone the rocky ridges. The whole thing was a-white from head to toe. While we get the endless rain done here, it is snowing like crazy up at elevation. Skier's delight.

One more week before the big day. As of the moment I have done a big zero. Well, My Rebecca did corral me into helping with the tree so that counts. I just have a hard time traditionally getting cranked up.

Off for my scan this morning. I should be scared out of my shoes but I've had so many that it is kind of easy for me to think my way around them now, sort of.

I will go now. Need time to panic on a number of fronts. The best to you. Time for a rosary loves, Felipé.

DECEMBER 19, 2018 / LET ME TELL YOU ABOUT MY DAY YESTERDAY

I was on my way here to the hospital yesterday when I got involved in a traffic accident. No one was hurt fortunately and we were all very cordial throughout. But I just wanted to relate the aftermath as it has some comic aspects.

This is all sort of in a day's work for trying to get to my appointment yesterday on time and in one piece. And I did make it and with my blood pressure in pretty good shape to boot.

First I had to get out of the street and into an adjacent parking lot so we didn't have to worry about getting hit again. That maneuver was successful with my truck but some horrendous noise was coming from the damaged area. On further inspection it appeared that my bumper was bent inward and was up against my front tire meaning that I couldn't possibly turn to the right.

About that time the owner of the business was out telling us that we couldn't be there and we would have to move. He was having work done and we were smack dab in the middle of things. There was a crew unloading tools and I borrowed a crowbar to try and straighten the offending part but no go. The bend was too strong.

Just then the boss of the crew shows up with a dump truck that needs to be there. So I am looking at the name on the side of the truck and it is a demolition outfit. So, a light goes on in my brain. The boss is looking at me and I'm looking at him and we are both looking at my truck and I say, "I need a Sawzall." That is one of the main demo tools ever and I know they have one there somewhere.

So, even better, he not I, after a little conference, saws off the end of my offending bumper, no muss no fuss. And then and there I was able to drive away and be out of his way and on my way. Wow, everyone needs a demo guy!

That was the salient part of my morning. And everything went more normally after that. Even all the way to being back home again and having our son and daughter-in-law for spaghetti and meatballs. Then we decorated the tree. All's well that ends well right there.

And beyond all that good stuff I think maybe the incident shook something loose in my writing department. You know how they say in hushed tones, "Yea, he was never quite the same after the accident." I'm feeling a bit more poetic these daze. Movin' on loves, Felipé.

DECEMBER 24, 2018 / HALF-DECENT

Oh, feeling that feeling of half-decent this morning. It's been two days of nasty side effects for this guy. But here I am sipping on a cup of the world's strongest coffee and there appears to be some light at the end of the tunnel. Kind of like our vision of Spring right now. Only the smallest of hints that the darkest day has past but nevertheless . . .

Christmas Eve today, yes it is, no matter my/our troubles. It is exactly as it should be here in the year of our Lord 2018, that is for sure. That is one thing we can all bank on.

Maybe the best thing that happened to me in 2018 was witnessing the wedding that was held at my/our cancer treatment center. It was just quirky. The idea was quirky. It was just quirky that I got to witness it. It was just quirky that joy can cling to a small chunk of real estate like a hallway in a hospital so us participants and witnesses will forever be smiling when we pass through it.

There is a need for joy. And most of all there is a need for joy in places where we least expect it, where it is most needed, where we can't possibly miss it when it happens, rare but potent.

Morning walk here in half an hour. Looks gray and dry out. We are beginning to encounter some standing water on the trail and Raven Creek is starting to run. Time for steadfast hearts and hearty conversation in this wintertime. Steadfast loves, Felipé.

DECEMBER 25, 2018 / MERRY CHRISTMAS, 2018!

Merry Christmas to all in the Caminoheads world worldwide! It seemed hard fought this year but here we are once again, maybe not exactly bright-eyed and bushy-tailed but here nonetheless. Thinking of you wherever you are in our far-flung neighborhood.

Know that you are loved and appreciated. Potent loves, Felipé.

DECEMBER 26, 2018 / THE DAY AFTER

Well, we did it, Christmas 2018. My Rebecca is such a champ and the rest of the family rallied to make it all happen with little help from me. I have been hit pretty hard with the side effects of treatment over the last four days and am not much good for anything. But maybe, just maybe, I am on the back-end of all that.

We had a walk yesterday afternoon and the weather cooperated for us. And tapas afterward was orchestrated by Our Catherine y Dana. Having tapas is such a joy and a benefit, but you already know that.

It appears to me at the moment to be a very worthy topic of reflection and thanksgiving. To take a break from our labors at the end of the day is good. To be with those whom you labored with that day. To know that we are all safe for the night. To know that we have what we need to rest and recuperate for tomorrow. To be proud of our accomplishments but to acknowledge that we couldn't have done it without help from each other, from those that came before us and from our God. To be joyful. To toast what is important so as not to forget. To share in the bounty that is provided by Providence. We take the time and energy to internalize this experience not only physically but spiritually. We know that the time and place is special and we treat it so.

Time to rally for Felipé. Work needs doing here today, some, not a lot. Off we go loves, Felipé.

DECEMBER 28, 2018 / HOSPITALITY STILL THE KEY WORD

As we chart the course for the new year the sound of the word "hospitality" still rings true. That is really the main theme on all our levels. "How could it be otherwise?" just sprang up in my head and I am scrambling to surround that with my mind. Yes, it is that central to the whole understanding or to understanding the whole.

After almost five years of writing about things Camino, that is the word that I have come up with when I ask myself to boil the Camino pilgrimage experience. down to one word. That is the essence, the spirit, the Grade A, Maple Syrup of it all. And just like that ultra-sticky substance, that is what is supposed to stick to us as we return to our little corner of the world along with our still raw feet and our sunbaked brains. Those things heal eventually but our vision of hospitality should be permanent like the pilgrim tattoo, a sign that we have tasted it.

I'm inspired loves, Felipé.

DECEMBER 31, 2018 / COUNTING DOWN

So a new year coming up. Maybe a chance for a new start or a different angle on the whole thing. Maybe a different intensity.

These daily writings are still and will be about the "bigger sense camino." It will be more focused on leaving behind a "map" (thank you Catherine) for those cancer patients that are new or struggling. It will be a way of showing "God as a verb" (thank you Janet). It will be more joyful hopefully.

Yup, a few more minutes left before the frosty walk this AM. Oh, I finally have seed for the birds. That will be a project to get all the feeders going again. Hang on birdies I'm coming!

New loves, Felipé.

Part VI

The Veranda

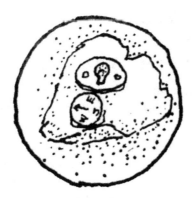

January 7, 2019 / A New Week, A New Year

The barometer is rising and some blue sky is around. Walking in a few minutes.

The Christmas tree is being dismantled. Time to lurch into the next phase of winter. Time to cut firewood. Time to order seeds. Time to contend with taxes. And at the end of that will be the Spring payoff of warmth and light.

Off to walk loves, Felipé.

January 23, 2019 / Dwelling in Mary

Janet and I have been doing some energy work over the phone. I am not totally sure what that means but it seems to be agreeing with me. During our last session over she said that she had a vision of me inside what I figured out was the Lady of Guadalupe. Really?

As the days move on I am so happy to think about that and contemplate on what is going on there. First of all, visions can be staggering to normal sensibilities, no joke Felipé. They can at first seem strange and weird. This one has a certain amount of that. Could be confusing until you can settle on an interpretation that agrees with you.

A literal interpretation could mean that I was the baby Jesus. Yes, OK. But that is not it for sure to me. We can all do our best to mirror Jesus, yes for sure, that's a life's work. But currently I am seeing the image as me dwelling in Mary. Or dwelling

WALKING IN THE MUD

in "Maryness" the epicenter of peace. That seems the closest that I can get to at the moment which is incredible, phenomenally great!

Yes, I am so happy to contemplate this amazing vision. Maybe for the word "happy" substitute the word "enlarged" or maybe a dozen others words. It is a focal point. A place easy to go back to when I wander off. It remains steadfast and visible in the chaos.

Just going back to my visit to Lourdes, France in May of last year, where Mary is known as the Lady of Lourdes; peace was what I took away from that meeting. Peace in the sense of being part of a cosmic equilibrium. Peace in the sense of being part of something larger, something that makes ultimate sense. Peace in the sense of a substance that is at the same time useful in the everyday.

Thank you, Janet, for supplying me with another piece in the puzzle. The vision is a wonderful visual of this Way, Mary's Way. I will be able to see it come rain or shine.

Well, off we go. Thanks for being here today for our meeting. Love you, Felipé.

January 24, 2019 / My Friend, The Padre

We all know him as the Padre. Actually, to be totally correct he is the Desert Padre. He now hails from the desert country of California although he has been on the road or at sea most of his adult life.

The Padre served as a US Navy Chaplain for many years, that's the at sea part. We got to know him through Annie and the *Phil's Camino* documentary where he served as our spiritual advisor. We already had a lot of spirit but what we needed was occasional guidance, which the Padre provided.

The Padre came to Raven Ranch for several days a few winters ago. I felt so honored. Where 1200 Marines have to share him, this Marine had him all for himself. It was very rainy as I remember and we talked and talked.

Our last adventure took us to Lourdes, France with the Order of Malta. I went as the malade (a person with a malady) and Padre went as my helper. Us malades all needed helpers or care persons. The Malta folks said, "You have a priest as your helper?" I said, "Yea, I need a lot of help!" Well, who was helping who, I'm not sure but we had a great time. We might have been a bit much for them, as I wasn't your garden variety malade and Padre is a stand out as always.

Padre is a Paulist Father which is a fairly new order. Paulists specialize in media to get the word out. So it is fitting that I got to know him through our documentary. And below is a link that he just sent me about himself.

You can tell I love this guy. Hope that you get to meet him at some point.

Walking on loves, Felipé.

January 25, 2019 / Wind From The North

Our rainy spell is over. Time for the puddles to drain and the mud to harden up around the trail. Little shoots are coming up, snowdrops, crocus and such. I've been working on our firewood for next year, processing the maple that we felled last week. It's that time of year.

This guy is enjoying his chemo vacation, with missing my treatment last time. Yea, could get used to this. I'm back to the hospital this coming Wednesday and Friday. It has gone way too quickly.

I've picked out my corn seed from the catalog. I will stick with the three-variety succession planting that I did last year, Sugar Buns, Bodacious and Golden Jubilee. That gives us 4-5 weeks of solid sweet corn. Have to try my hardest for a good harvest to feed the pilgrims coming for the Caminoheads Rendezvous. That's August 23-26.

Ah, I just got news from My Rebecca that a friend has died. That's Lauren Lane Powell who was active in the Threshold Choir here in the States. She came here for a visit last year. A bright light and strong spirit finally overwhelmed by cancer.

As a teenager I made an observation that too many people died in late winter. Like it is a big hurdle to make it to spring and it is just too much for many. I have no idea if that really is the case or not but it seems true.

Time to get going for Felipé. Have to take advantage of the weather. See you all tomorrow. Hurdling over late winter loves, Felipé.

JANUARY 28, 2019 / WE NEVER CLOSE

It was a gray chilly afternoon walk yesterday here at Phil's Camino. No one was here to walk with. It was one of those wintertime occasions when "we" try not to see it as a chore but that is challenging. But this trail has a sort of energy because, as Steve says, "we never close." In other words, we are always continuing or always present.

I went around my usual three times to equal somewhere around a mile and three quarters total. The first time I put out two pounds of sunflower seeds for the birdies. The second time I prayed the rosary, which on Sundays concentrates on the Glorious Mysteries. That's a good thing. Then the third time I kind of hurried through it.

It's a discipline and sometimes, as with them all, it is harder to accomplish, but one persists. In lean times and fat times the beat goes on. I like to think that folks always visualize Phil's Camino as an active process. It goes on no matter what.

The other day one of the pilgrims that was with me was talking about a friend of his that had some serious malady and was out washing his car "because he can." In other words, whether it needed it or not was irrelevant and any other reason or motivation was secondary to his belief that he wanted to do it because he still could or "because he (still) can."

It maybe is part of my motivation with this, my backyard walk. It certainly colored my pilgrimage to Santiago four years ago. It is a sort of Don Quixote thing. We just keep getting it done no matter how crazy things get.

So back to yesterday, I came in after the walk and had tapas with My Rebecca. Sometimes in winter with no one walking with me tapas get skipped but this time I felt strongly about it. It was, as I thought about it, hospitality toward myself. See that? Maybe I deserve that?

Have to go walk, Monday morning loves, Felipé.

January 29, 2019 / There is News

As our Midwest freezes over the weather here is spring-like. We have to loll around in our luck. The Indian Plum bushes are unfolding leaves. We are walking at 1530 with tapas afterward if you are in the neighborhood to join us.

There was some news on Facebook this morning about some Israeli researchers having some breakthroughs in cancer fighting. As I read their report I am so happy for their expertise and understanding. They are really bearing down on the Achilles Heels of the situation. I cannot really understand what they are saying but as with our spring weather here I just want to loll around in it for now. Love you guys!!

Well, time to go. You Caminoheads now know everything I do. Springtime loves, Felipé.

January 30, 2019 / Chemo Day Again

Boy, back in the chemo saddle after a month off. And as a bonus I gained some weight and came in at 170.8 pounds. I have been fighting for months to get to 170. Yea!

Oh, yes, have to give you a report on yesterday. Shari from San Francisco made it out to Vashon to walk with us and have tapas. She is on our distribution team for the film. The weather was totally cooperating and we had lots of company for the walk and our party. I got the deck cleaned up after sitting fallow for the winter and we had tapas outside for the first time in a long, long time. My Rebecca was thinking that it was on the chilly side but we crowded together for warmth and made it through. Winter might not be over exactly but we are pushing the envelope as much as possible.

Bundled up but grinning! First outdoor tapas of the season.

Well, time to wrap it up here at the treatment center. Back home to the Rock kind of loves, Felipé

February 4, 2019 / Well, Phil's Camino's Not Closed!

Snowy conditions across Washington State. It has been snowing on and off all night and we got maybe 3 inches here at our 300-foot elevation and more to come this AM. Schools all closed, kids happy. But what about Phil's Camino? According to Steve, "We never close!" That's right, Phil himself will be marching around the situation here momentarily.

I would so love to come across cougar tracks or some such rarity out there. Well, you will be the first to know.

Yup, guess winter is still holding court here. I've been longingly looking through seed catalogs myself thinking we were going to slide past this kind of activity, but no, guess not.

OK, well, here I go. I have fifteen minutes to gear up. We never close, right Felipé? If I'm not back in an hour call the Mounties. Love, Felipé.

FEBRUARY 5, 2019 / WEATHERING THE STORM

Right now we have some snow on the ground, icy roads, schools closed and all plumbing working. So, just a sort of winter vacation here at Raven Ranch.

People are starting to check in for visits here this Spring and Summer. Those are the casual times when we can thaw out from all this present reality. Remember the big get together here, the Caminoheads Rendezvous, is August 23nd through the 26th.

That time in August is the time of harvest and God willing, abundance. Sweet corn season here runs roughly from the middle of August to the middle of September. And tomatoes and other wonders are in full stride then also. The pastures are golden colored after two months of no rain. That's our Mediterranean climate. They will green up again quickly in October.

But for now it is the opposite here and I can only dream. All hunkered down now when Mother Nature is at her sparsest. The cupboard is bare in many ways. Time to grin and bear it for a little while longer for all us God's creatures.

Well, time to go. Need to check all the systems. Maybe I will get back at my books and taxes after that.

Hunkered down loves, Felipé.

FEBRUARY 10, 2019 / THE NEXT STORM

The next storm is coming in around 4 PM today. The weatherman is talking about 4-8 inches in this one. We are all patching things together and helping each other out. I'm about ready to make a big pasta sauce to feed people stopping by.

Just phoned in to the hospital to cancel an appointment I have for tomorrow morning. Don't need an extra headache. Still have to make it in Wednesday and Friday so that's enough fun.

Yesterday at some point when the cable came back on I was watching a clip from the Mr. Rogers show. It was the one where he had Itzhak Perlman on playing his violin. That was lovely but the important part was that he was shown also walking with his crutches. He had polio as a child. So, he was shown in two different modes and his quote (roughly) was, "I had to separate my ability from my disability." I can so relate to that with my cancer journey.

The day dawned today with beautiful blue skies and chilly temps, had that Colorado look. Now the clouds have rolled in and it is starting to look ominous. Well, maybe I'll start the pasta sauce so it can simmer. OK, that's the situation here at the ranch.

Fun times love, Felipé.

FEBRUARY 13, 2019 / MADE IT TO THE BIG CITY

Sticking to the main roads I braved it into the hospital for treatment. The city itself is largely empty as most folks are still on forced vacation. And the new Seattle tunnel is open for business which made the traffic a breeze.

Yea, it will be good to have this storm and its cleanup in the history books. It's been hard to have an independent thought as of late, nose to the old grindstone as it were.

So, Pilgrim Farmer John and Farmer Cathy are off today on the beginning of some fun stuff. They are driving to Santa Monica in the motor home to start their cross-country bike ride. PFJ said it's all because he can. More power to him I say.

I saw a pic of the labyrinth in Chartres Cathedral, France today and it has mesmerized me. I often think that in former lifetimes I was involved in helping out with the construction of some of these structures.

Wouldn't that be a gas! Or how about laying out and doing this labyrinth? I missed my era, for sure!

Looks like my chemo is nearing its end for the day. Time to sign off for now. All good loves, Felipé.

FEBRUARY 14, 2019 / ABOUT OUR IMPOSSIBILITIES

Early in the morn here at the ranch. I am up buzzing on my steroids from yesterday's treatment. Sometimes these are some of the best blogposts when I am "the life of the party" high.

The movement of the freezing and thawing here has shaken a memory out of my brain. It is a memory of years ago with My Rebecca, my new love in my life, and my year at the U of Washington studying art metal casting. This was mid-1970s with disco and those crazy flowery shirts. Nobody but nobody dressed in all black and stared into a cellphone all day, but I digress.

The University kept us gnarly sculpture students out at the edge of the campus hidden out behind the baseball fields where no one would find us. I worked in the foundry where we were casting with aluminum, brass, bronze and iron. I am trying to remember, but aluminum melts at 1200 degrees F, to bronze at 1800 to iron at 2200.

It was all very esoteric and at times scary. We had huge furnaces fired by natural gas and coke. We ran around in silver suits and the heat would blow our long hair back as we poured the molten fun.

And the finished pieces after weeks of work were exciting to view. We made those! And our pieces were durable as they were beautiful, good for two thousand years at least. Well, that is the world that we lived in and it brought on a certain mindset or a certain way of thinking about the world around us.

And these last few weeks with all the freezing and melting of the water in our environment with the four storms that we endured, it shook loose memories of those days. We moved then through the freezing and thawing of metals as easily as we commonly move through the freezing and thawing of water. This movement between the physical forms of water we take for granted, and that is with us in our shared knowledge. But we sculptors were privy to this world where all metals were basically "frozen" as most people normally experience them.

We were thawing scrap aluminum screen doors and making art. And brass plumbing faucets and making art. And scrap bronze from ships to make more art.

And busting up old cast iron heating radiators to put in a cupola with coke and forced air to raise it to 2200 degrees and make some more art. We were nuts concentrating on the art but the process made the world liquid for us. Things like cars, silverware and ships were just temporarily frozen and waiting for us to change them into something else and maybe something better. It was a swords-to-plowshares world.

And now after all these years I bang my knee on the step of my tractor, Juliet, and I instantly feel that it is pretty darn solid and immovable but there was a time . . . More tomorrow.

Good one Felipé. Happy St. Valentine's Day! Love of course, Felipé.

FEBRUARY 24, 2019 / A SUNDAY IN FEBRUARY

Well, actually it is the last Sunday in this here snowy month. March has got to be a notch warmer. And Lent coming up. Wow, Felipé, what are you giving up or adding this time? Well, have to give that some thought.

And Easter toward the end of April, the 22nd I think. This will be my sixth anniversary in the Catholic Church. Wow, time is flying. I must be feeling like an old-timer by now. Love my little Island parish, small but mighty.

They want me to build another cabinet for them. Yes, that will be great. The reason they need one is they are expanding a program and they need more secure storage space for the ingredients. A small group of parishioners run this program called Backpack Pantry. Each week come rain or shine they pack forty-eight parcels of food and drop them off at the various schools. The idea is that a student in need will get a backpack full of food to get them over the weekend if things are lean.

Then at the other end of things we have our dear friend Jessika who I talk about often who is studying Canon Law or Church Law. And in addition, she is working to become a member of the Order of Malta, the folks that took me and Padre Tomas to Lourdes last year. All this very scholarly and knightly.

I guess I am trying to say that I feel at home there from one end to the other. Just wish I had my dear Mother to take to Mass with me. She would enjoy that. But she sees me now and that makes me happy.

Well, have the Sunday afternoon walk here in a few minutes. The snow is melting a little bit more each day and we are getting things more cleaned up. Soon it will be pretty normal. Please come when you get a chance.

Only the best to you, late winter loves, Felipé.

FEBRUARY 25, 2019 / WE ARE DOING FANTASTIC!

Just thought that I would let you know that on this Monday morning. Whatever you are up to, you are doing fantastic! I am here staring out the window thinking I might see snowflakes falling. Maybe not. We have all here have been traumatized by the recent storms and you are probably tired of me talking about it but the feelings remain. We all think we might be seeing snowflakes.

Yes, Monday morning—a time when we hopefully are all ready for the week to come at us. I am off here later this morning for a scan. It is that magic time again to take some pix of the situation and see what's happening with my tenacious little guys. "Okay, I know, you are little but you are mighty." Right now I am seeing them as Alvin and the Chipmunks. Hehe, hehe.

Ah, maybe I have been at this too long. Maybe I could take a little break and trade maladies with someone for a month, kind of a busman's holiday. Sorry, just crazy thoughts from Felipé.

On a different note, we had some frozen sweet corn for dinner last night and it brightened me up with thoughts of August and September coming up with endless corn and blackberries. That's 180 degrees from where we are on the calendar but I can imagine it easily.

Well, enough of this for now. Time to boot up for the Monday morning walk. It is pretty out but frosty.

You are really doing fantastic loves, Felipé.

FEBRUARY 28, 2019 / MOVING ROCK

We move rock here on Phil's Camino when folks put ones that they find on the trail on the pile with their intentions on them. It was a good thing that got started a long time ago by My Rebecca back when we started all this walking and praying stuff. It is in the alperfect category.

So, yesterday I caught up to one of my old hunting buddies that I haven't talked to in ages. We were standing in the sun outside the market telling our lies. I had heard that he had a cancer hobby going also and I asked him about it. When you start asking questions you never know what you are going to come up with and in this case I was richly rewarded. It seems that the major part of his treatment was 7 weeks of radiation at five days per week. Now my friend is a very robust fellow and his response to this ordeal was equally robust. Since he had to catch the ferry each time, he came up with the idea of driving his dump truck over and hauling a load of gravel back each day since that commodity is so much cheaper on the mainland. Yea, when most of us would figure out how to catch the bus just to be easy on ourselves. Love it!

Then today I was at the hospital waiting to see my Doc when I struck up a conversation with a well-dressed man sitting near me. He asked how I was doing and I responded with the ever appropriate, "So far so good!" He got a kick out of that and we started conversing about guy stuff. Turns out he had owned a gold mine in Alaska for thirty-five years. We went on for half an hour on that. And hardly a word about our problems, mostly about moving rock. This is what I like to see.

So what are you getting at Felipé? Well, it is that it is really easy sometimes for people to have their conversation all about their problems. Some more than others of course. It is possible for someone to actually channel their cancer. It is delightful when that is not the case. And beyond that I am seeing that it is possible to guide a conversation somewhat and keep it on the upbeat side. That is interesting to discover.

Yes, back to the ranch from the hospital for me now. I got another two-week chemo vacation in preparation for a possible change in treatment. My scan from a few days ago was the last straw for the chemical that I have been on for almost a year. It hasn't done a great job and we are looking for the next good option to pursue. And my weight is up again to 174.4 lbs. and that is extremely heartening. That is ten pounds heavier than a year ago.

Enough for now. Rockin' loves, Felipé.

FEBRUARY 28, 2019 / GIVEN A GOLD MINE

I have been thinking about this meeting in the waiting room yesterday with the owner of the gold mine in Alaska. Maybe there is more to relate to you.

In the first place I saw this man and he was "well dressed." I try to be well-dressed myself. Maybe not highly dressed but having gone through some thought and care. But the point is he was alone and I didn't know if he was the patient or there with someone who was the patient. Sometimes people don't know that I am the patient. This is a good sign. We are not channeling our problem.

During our conversation he revealed how he came to have the mine in the first place. He had an older friend that was in poor health and he would help this friend by driving him to his appointments and such. And it happened that the old man died and he left the mine to his young friend and not his son. I guess his son wasn't interested. So, it was a thank you of sorts.

It didn't sound like it was a grand gift, in the sense that the mine probably was run down and needed renovation and reorganizing to get it modernized. But that happened and this new owner ran it for thirty-five years and sold it.

Well, being the Felipé, this got me thinking. As strange as this may sound, fate handed me a gold mine of sorts with my cancer diagnosis. Of course that is not in physical terms. And it was a ramshackle mess to start with but somehow there was a thread or a flicker of insight that got things started.

I know that might sound strange but there is something there nonetheless. We, you and I, over the years have woven something together here. It has value, maybe even enduring value.

Off I go, walking in minutes. Beautiful morning, although chilly here at Phil's Camino. Catch you later loves, Felipé.

MARCH 1, 2019 / THAT GUY

Tomorrow or at some more distant point in time there will be someone in my exact shoes. I mean that person will be exactly where I am at today, maybe not geographically but in other important ways. Well, maybe geographically also, who knows?

I must clean up the sink and the toilet just like I found it as on the Camino. There were always others right behind you. You don't want to be a burden on them and maybe you want to make the moment easier for them even.

The point being that we are part of a procession always going onward. It is not just our procession, it belongs to all of us. It is the Camino as I see it today.

Then what about that person that was just ahead of us, whose tracks we are filling? Can we thank them for leaving us some fresh batteries or that little piece of soap which was just enough for us? Maybe they kicked the fallen branch off the path.

Maybe they left some inspirational graffiti. We will probably never know the facts but we can guess that others came to the same realizations that we did, that there are others on the same trail that we are on. We may never catch a glimpse of them but there are hints and clues aplenty.

We must thank that person just ahead of us for making the advances that they did. We will perhaps meet them someday but for now they have our gratitude, all of it. Then of course for the one following us, we wish them luck and offer them the best that we can leave. We only have so much energy and know-how but we will do our best to make the way clearer or easier or more welcome.

This is all just a thought and may turn into a poem one of these days, who knows. Traveling on loves, Felipé.

MARCH 5, 2019 / A NEW TACK

My Cancer Camino moves on day by day and recently we, my Doc and I, came to a crossroads. After seeing my scan of last week, we both were not pleased by the performance of my present treatment. It was time for a change. So, we are getting off one road and making a transition to another.

This new road is a clinical trial that I was lucky enough to get into. There are only so many openings for participants and I have secured one of those spots, thanks to my Doc. There are some technicalities to navigate through yet but he seemed confident. This trial is treating patients with my type of cancer with a drug that was developed for another type. Somehow it was found out that it helped a certain percentage of folks in my category. So, maybe it will help me.

This all reminds me of skipping across a river jumping from rock to rock. Sometimes the route seems plain and sometimes it is unclear. You just keep going with a certain amount of faith that things will work out. Getting a little wet along the way is inevitable but we try not to fall in whole hog.

Yea so, that is one part of my life here in the winter of 2019. Pilgrims come and go and keep me buoyed up. And here outside I have the firewood splitting operation going full bore. We are stacking up fuel for next winter. It's life at the ranch.

Take care for now, see you soon loves, Felipé.

MARCH 7, 2019 / SNOW AGAIN

So, it's the second day of Lent and I am reading Annie's book, *Everyday Camino with Annie.*

Remember this book is about how to get a glimpse of the Camino without actually being there, physically that is. Just as I was walking my backyard Camino to get a glimpse of pilgrimage and of the Camino de Santiago, so is this book attempting to get a glimpse of the essence of the thing. It was auspicious that the book came to me during the time of my effort.

This points to the fact that much of the "work" of pilgrimage is the interior journey of the individual pilgrim. And this is what was happening to me here in my "backyard." I was intensely working on this. It is a process that takes commitment and effort mostly. And I am so glad that this all happened to me the way it did at the time that it did. It is largely a mystery to me still though.

Well, there is so much going on this weekend. I have unconnected from most of it so that I can concentrate on a memorial service for a neighbor of ours that passed this winter. Another death due to cancer. I am so immensely glad that he reached out to connect with our Father David in the midst of his struggle.

Time to go boot up. Still walking, still on pilgrimage. Always room for one more. Snowy loves, Felipé.

March 8, 2019 / The Collision

The inner pilgrimage happens simultaneously with the physical pilgrimage. It is as grueling as the other. If this isn't happening it's not a pilgrimage, it is merely walking or hiking or trekking on vacation. There is something challenging about this that is an important part of the process to strengthen our spiritual connections. Then showing this to our fellow man is "It's light as me, as you." It's learning, internalizing and mirroring as I see it.

OK, snowing more now once again. Hmm. Time to go for Felipé.

March 9, 2019 / The Day I Have Lived For

Really I'm not a big goal setter. But I did see today as something to live to or live for. It is official that we have paid off our mortgage on the northern five acres of our ten here at Raven Ranch. Hurrah! It has been a long haul but the day is finally here when we own it outright!

I saw this day as something important to the family. It is a step in permanence, a bit of security. And I have said to my cancer OK I need to live to today to make sure that this happens. And well, good job and here I am.

It occurred to me a few months ago to start looking for the next thing to look forward to and to live to. Well, that is easy really. And that is the Caminoheads Get Together in August. What could be better! We haven't done a lot of planning as of yet but the dates are set.

Day Four of Lent and of the *Everyday Camino with Annie*. Our quote is one from Rumi: "Out beyond the idea of wrongdoing and rightdoing there is a field. I'll meet you there."

The quote points to a place outside of our intellect and outside of the rules and regulations that govern a certain portion of our existence. It wants us to gather there in this space. It wants us to leave our baggage behind and meet where we can look at things in a fresh manner. This is what I am seeing here.

Either way we are getting to a place that is outside of the norm, an extraordinary place. It is a new place to work from and to launch ourselves from. This is where the pilgrim comes from, this place of being outside the norm or outside of the normal way. It is a sabbatical.

Time to go for now. I have a few hours to work on my firewood project. Then this afternoon is a memorial service for our neighbor Chris. Another person that cancer has taken from us.

Off we go loves, Felipé.

MARCH 10, 2019 / ENTER INTO THE MYSTERY

It is the First Sunday of Lent today. Still no flowers at church. It always looks so bare and austere. Part of my personal ritual upon arriving is to get into the flowers, to get into beauty to begin to enter into the mystery that I will be participating in. Without the flowers it is a different process for me. I have to work harder, just an observation.

Time to go and work on my firewood again. The sun is out and begging me to get out there. A little lunch and get to work for Felipé.

Thanks for coming by. Always good to see you loves, Felipé.

MARCH 11, 2019 / OLIVE OYL

According to My Rebecca this is how the beloved girlfriend of Popeye the Sailor Man spells her name. I don't know, it could be. That is the way I am going to put it on the shopping list from now on:

> wine
> baguette
> olive oyl

Well OK. A Monday morning in Lent with our walk in half an hour. We had a lovely walk yesterday afternoon followed by tapas outside. It was borderline warm out. One of the pilgrims brought some delicious local blackberry wine. We had a good old time.

Here we are at the fifth day in Lent and the *Everyday Camino with Annie* has this quote from Chief Seattle: "This we know: All things are connected like the blood that unites us. We did not weave the web of life, we are merely a strand in it. Whatever we do to the web, we do to ourselves." There is a piece of environmental thinking if I ever saw one. And a big piece of Camino thinking also, right? This one is hard to miss on the trail in Spain as we hobble along and wish for a cloud to come and shelter us. There always seems to be a Camino angel around every corner to give us a hand or a band-aid or a kind word of encouragement. We all felt part of the fabric.

Time to find my boots and hit the trail here. The morning is crisp and sunny. The ending of winter is quickly coming. Everything is just around the corner. Oh, the anticipation!

Big anticipation loves, Don Felipé.

MARCH 16, 2019 / GENEROUS PORTIONS

My friend Roy was telling me that he had gone to the Eagles Club last evening for their St. Paddy's Day dinner. He said that there were generous portions of corned beef and cabbage. Yea, generous portions, I haven't heard that phrase in a long time but it is a good one.

I just got back from my Bible class and we were discussing the story about Jesus saying that it was harder for the rich man to get into the Kingdom than to get a camel through the eye of the needle. And I hope that we the trusty pilgrims that we are, realize how lucky we are generally and that generous portions are available to us. We can do quite well in this life without getting obsessed with the accumulation of things and wealth. Going down the trail with our "light backpack" and gratitude in our hearts is still the way that we see to best navigate the world.

We are lucky that we have been exposed to the lessons that we have. Of course we think that the whole world would be better off if we all went on pilgrimage for a bit in our lives. It is fortunate for us that we had the chance when we did.

Time to go. The beautiful sun is out and I still have plenty of cleanup to do outside. Later y'all loves, Felipé.

MARCH 19, 2019 / HERE ARE TWO

Take what you need and leave the rest. Yes, yes. We want to take the cure for any and every problem that might arise. But we have to pare down to the essentials and learn to trust, there is that word again, that we will be taken care of by one angel or another.

Well, and that goes for "affairs" too. To keep things easy and uncomplicated as possible with people too. There is no need for most of the drama that passes for relations these days. We can make things a lot smoother without much effort. Or sometimes effort is required but it will be well spent.

Yes, and with me, I am off and running with my clinical trial that turns up as my next course of treatment. It is pill form this time and I just took my very first one. So we hope and pray for the very best for the Phil/Felipé team. Will keep you posted.

OK, time to head off and get down the road. A short visit to the hospital today.

Enjoy the weather loves, Felipé.

MARCH 20, 2019/ I'M OFFICIAL

Yea, I'm an official lab rat now. I got all the paperwork and counselling done and am officially in a clinical trial. Took my second pill this morning, it's a one-a-day pill. I guess I am doing my part for the greater good on this one and hoping for some "activity" for my own sake in the process. It's all dreadfully scientific mostly. Lots of monitoring and record keeping making sure Test Pilot Phil comes out of the other side in one piece.

So, this changes my schedule greatly. Instead of coming in two days every two weeks I will be coming in once every three weeks. And then there are some scans thrown in occasionally. So, less time on the road in Seattle which is more time at the ranch. And I'm not sure how long this will last. It all depends on the performance as monitored by the scans and my ability to tolerate the agent. So, right now it is a So Far So Good thing.

The way I see it this will not change the walking schedule at all. That should just continue along as usual. On that account more visitors are showing up with the warmth of Spring. Alperfect.

Annie's quote for Day 13 is "My search is over, and I rest in Thee," from Rickie Byers and Michael Beckwith. I think, if I am not mistaken, that these are lyrics from a gospel song that these two wrote. It shows a certain maturity to finally reach a resting place like this. We might not understand everything but we have arrived to a sense of calm and trust. Alperfect.

Well, have to go. I am giving a talk tomorrow at 6:30 in the evening on my pilgrimage to Lourdes with the Order of Malta and need to prepare. That is at St. John Vianney's on Vashon.

Enjoy the day. Something interesting will happen I am sure. Warm sunshine loves, Felipé.

MARCH 22, 2019 / SO HAPPY WITH MYSELF

I delivered a nice talk last evening about my pilgrimage to Lourdes last year. That was spring, the first week in May. I've had some good time to digest it by now.

Remembering how hard it was to blog about when I first got back. It takes time to break down anything that subtle. I had to gnaw on it for many hours. My old friend Jim says to understand some poetry you have rub up against it like those smooth shiny boards in the horse's stall that only get that way over time. Yea, like that.

I had to admit that I didn't see people "throwing down their crutches" or experiencing any exceptional sensations. But life always seems larger, deeper, broader, more brilliant, more exceptional than my expectations. And Lourdes was like that.

Let me list a few of the perceptions that one could come away with. One could get outside oneself. One could get beyond the "why me?" One could see plenty of others that have bigger problems than they have. One could see suffering in others and relate to it, relate to them. One could start to understand suffering as Christlike. One could understand Christ better because of their own personal suffering. One could start to understand the purpose of suffering. One could also become closer to Mary, as I was striving to do.

Could be endless really, what goes on there that to me would be in the category of healing and not curing at all. We understand the situation better and therefore live more joyfully and at peace with our problems. And time will tell. God has a totally different feel for time than we do. We want everything yesterday and when things take time, we may not even recognize their significance.

Peaceful loves, Felipé.

MARCH 23, 2019 / SATURDAY, A DAY OFF?

I don't know what I would do if I had to take a day off. This is Saturday and once I get this written I will be off on some project or other here at the ranch where something is always calling help. Help to finish the firewood, to get the winter damage cleaned up, fix the trail up, all that. The good part of that is that I no longer have great anxiety over it. I just find it rewarding to be busy.

It came up in Bible Guys today, "What would you do if you only had one week to live?" A very telling question, this one. I've been through this more times than I can remember with my cancer hobby always looming. Something to think about.

Annie quotes Thomas Merton on day 16 of her book: "Let me seek, then, the gift of silence, and poverty, and solitude where everything I touch is turned into a prayer, the wind in the trees is my prayer, for God is all in all."

Oh, how totally lovely. This could really be every day but I am thinking how well this fits with the earlier question about how would you spend your final week? This seems like a plan here to me at the moment. We should have that kind of peace to just be and be in touch with God so intimately.

Yea, it is classic gray sky overhead here at Raven Ranch. Time for lunch and then a few precious hours of being outside. Ivette, our old friend is here, and Cathy and Tim and another couple are coming later today. We are all having dinner out and a concert here locally.

Later loves, Felipé.

MARCH 26, 2019 / SOMETIMES I THINK . . .

Sometimes I think that we all live on an island. It's a big island, big enough to give us the feeling that we are all that is. And rushing by this island is a mighty flow of a river. Only thing is we have never seen it.

We think that we know that it is there. But most of the time we are too frightened to even get close. There are stories of those who ventured out in that direction and failed to return or come back babbling. So we just don't go or even think about it.

But there is a certain curiosity that comes over us occasionally in our weak moments. But usually we shake it off. But still we try to define it and figure it out in a sort of hobby way. But you know.

Occasionally a random drop of it splashes up toward us. And we run to capture it. It is small and weak compared to from where it came and it does not threaten us. It is just the tippy-tippy end of a whip of energy that cracks occasionally within our hearing. And we run to capture it.

It will be dissected and analyzed to death before things are over and we will feel like we accomplished something, something important. It will give its life for our curiosity. In the end 99.44 percent of it will be turned into numbers. This is the language that we understand and that we can slice and dice and compare with what else we know.

But what of the deep and wide river that we have analyzed a drop of? What does it think of our important attempts to explore its scary mysteries? What have we learned today in our few moments that we have allotted to this project?

All good, alperfect really loves, Felipé.

MARCH 27, 2019 / HUMP DAY

Not that Hump Day makes too much difference around here. We are open weekends, holidays, whatever. Here to serve you, pilgrims worldwide, is what we are about.

The middle third of the Camino Francés might be called the dreaded Meseta in the sense that it is hard and demanding. It is skipped by some. I remember hearing all this early on and deciding that I needed to walk that part for sure. It is part of being the guy that does everything the hard way.

But in the end it was my favorite part for I found refuge in its seclusion, in its desolation. I loved its dry land farming, the miles and miles of it. It was all very real to me. Pilgrims looked out for each other in a way that they didn't in easier stretches.

Even though I bussed from Léon to Samos I was still plenty beat up for the last 100 kilometers. This limping, rumpled, dusty look separated us from the clean people at Sarria. We love them too of course but there was an obvious difference in the populations.

OK, off I go. The sun is shining and there is a long list yet. We are together and that is what counts. Thanks for stopping by. Dusty loves, Felipé.

PS—And to think of it, the Meseta is actually the hump or middle section of the Camino, how appropriate. It all fits together nicely in the end.

MARCH 28, 2019 / GRATITUDE AGAIN

I think that it wouldn't be inaccurate to say that gratitude is the gateway to everything. We need to give thanks before asking for our impossible. Before feeding the five thousand Jesus gave thanks for what He started with.

It is not a sin to think big. I don't know exactly where I am going with that but just let it sit there and rest. It is a part in another puzzle.

Almost five years ago now I remember being a part of the miracle of the tiny piece of soap. I got caught without my usual soap that I carried and there on the sink in plain sight was the tiniest piece that someone just before me had left recognizing it's value. I washed with it and there was still plenty left when I was done so I left it where I found it. For all I know it has been there for twelve hundred years. St. Francis may have used it on his pilgrimage before me. Really Felipé?

Here we are halfway to Easter. Time flies here at Caminoheads. We are privileged, we are thankful, we are open, we are ready, we are first and foremost grateful!

Soapy loves, Felipé.

MARCH 31, 2019 / CHURCHY

Today at Mass I was overwhelmed with the thought of how heavily I am invested in living on borrowed time. I easily take all my medical treatment for granted but not that many years ago there would not have been any of that. Or I take my own tenacity for granted and don't give myself credit for coping so well with the ups and downs of treatment for all these years.

What is there about my ability to wrestle with this strong opponent successfully? I must have picked up some clues somewhere in my past. And it just struck me that in my high school wrestling career I leaned heavily on the principles of jujitsu. In Japanese it means gentle skill. As I understand it and as I used it, it is the way of using an adversary's strength against them. In other words, there is always someone who is stronger than you out there. These techniques work on everyone but they work better on those who are stronger. The secret being that through the use of timing and adding energy an opponent can be unbalanced.

The more I think about it the more I see how I have used this against my cancer. Not in a battle of muscle, speed and leverage but with similar mental/spiritual components. One can win battles from positions of weakness is the takeaway.

Walk and tapas later today. Life is good even on borrowed time.

Wishing you the best, Felipé.

April 2, 2019 / A Tale of Two Wheelbarrows

Half of life at the ranch is fixin' stuff. Trying to get one more season out of a mower or a tool. Or finding a broken something that I think I can get back into shape to be useful. Or figuring a piece of gear is close to breaking and getting it fixed while you have time. They are all different variations on the same theme.

Right now I have two wheelbarrows that need repair. Things don't usually gang up on me like that but it is happening today. But then again it's all not rocket surgery.

I used to work for a local construction company run by a farm genius named Robert. The construction business was just part of the whole scene. There was a landscape and a cider effort going on too. I take a lot of my cues from him as to how to make an operation happen. I often thought that his whole thing was held together by will power or hypnosis. It is all about intention really.

And yes, the business is gone and the land sold but the skills and the knowhow live on. Thank you, Robert and Betsy, for the education. And that's where the name of our road comes from, Wax Orchard Road. Wax was Betsy's maiden name.

And today is Day 24 of Lent. We are further down that road. Annie's quote: "If you love it enough, anything will talk with you." —George Washington Carver.

There is a good one. Well, they are all good but some strike you in ways that others don't. And that really did happen on the Camino. I thought that I had made love to the whole thing by the time things were over. Isn't it funny how we develop this personal relationship even though we are just one in a million or millions? Marvelous really.

Well, my time is up for today. Have to run to town to get some parts for my project. This afternoon I am meeting with Henriette, who is working on a book about Cancer and the Camino. A little bit of this and a little bit of that.

Fixin' it loves, Felipé.

April 14, 2019 / Sunday, Complete With Palms

Here it is, the beginning of Holy Week with the commemoration of Christ's triumphant ride into Jerusalem to begin the Passion. Oh, such a heavy-duty time. It doesn't really get any more substantial than this.

As part of the week's activities Catherine and I are doing a pilgrimage on Good Friday. We are walking from Raven Ranch to St. John Vianney's through the trails and backroads. It is about seven miles through the boonies and we are allowing four hours for our walk. If you want to go with us we are leaving here at 1500.

Enough of this loves, Felipé.

April 16, 2019 / Incredibly Sad

My heart breaks with the news of Notre Dame Cathedral's fire. It seems so unreal. Gives a hint of how fast things can change. It seems that "the worst has been avoided" there. It is bad enough as it is but in pics of the interior this morning things looked hopeful. Apparently most or all of the relics and portable art has been saved. Ah, breathe.

Kudos to the four hundred firefighters that got control of the situation. Again, it could have been a lot worse. But the ache is here and for real. It has the feel of September 11th to me. It is an interesting coincidence to have this occur during Holy Week. Ah, breathe.

I hate to be too cheery too soon but perhaps the rebuilding will be a platform for the world to work together on. A nice thought, one can only hope. I would love to go and work on something like that. Your work would have to dovetail with work centuries old. Maybe you would find hidden messages or graffiti from the past. A fun thought finally.

Well, I managed to fall asleep and have used up my time here. Just as well, I need to go and move around to feel better. Off I go.

Charred loves, Felipé.

April 18, 2019 / Thursday Of Holy Week, Soil Temp 60 Degrees

Trying to get the corn started which will be ripe in August for you to enjoy then. Got the field rototilled almost a week ago and it is drying out and warming up. The soil temp yesterday was 60 degrees, which is still short of the minimum of 65. I predict that we will be planting about May 1st, God willing. I am thinking about the final product and how good it is, so fresh, so sweet.

Yea, walking this morning. Have had poor attendance lately, blame it on tax time I guess or Holy Week. Oh, the seven-mile pilgrimage to church is still on for tomorrow. Wish us luck on that as it is more than we are used to lately.

I think I just saw a pair of swallows—nothing swoops like they do. Swooping loves, Felipé.

April 20, 2019 / Felipé's Pilgrim Report

Well, I am happy to say that Catherine, Jessika and I pilgrimmed the heck out of it yesterday with our Good Friday Trek. It was lightly raining and cloudy the whole time of the four hours it took to walk to church. I had torn my jeans and had dried blood on my face but I got there.

It was fun to see some of the trails that Kelly, Rick and I trained on back in the day, back in 2014. It was spring out there with mushrooms, little blue flowers and one random turkey. We were reminded of what a beautiful place we live in.

Holy Saturday here today. It always seems like a strange in-between time. I like to believe that Jesus was visiting the ancestors giving them the Good Word, bringing them to salvation during this veiled time. And now we all live for tomorrow.

Today as I calculate is the fortieth day of Lent, and Annie O'Neil's book *Everyday Camino with Annie* gives us this last quote:

"Recently I shifted from my beginning mentality of worrying about conquering the Camino and have settled into just cruising along being happy I am able to do it." — Phil Volker

Well how about that? I got lucky enough to get into this group with Dalai Lama and Yogi Berra, not to mention the other notables. Well, thoroughly flattered I am. My being in there at all was a result of Annie and my meeting on March 2nd 2014 when Martin Sheen handed me over to her for my further training. Our meeting caused her book to be finished and our film to begin to be, heady times.

Thanks for being here today and see you tomorrow for celebration. Only the best to you fellow pilgrims, love, Felipé.

April 21, 2019 / This Is The Day . . .

"This is the day that the Lord has made; let us rejoice and be glad." That might be from Psalms but from the Bible anyway, close enough. Yea, here we are having moved through Lent. Hope we learned something in all that. It looks like I saved my whole Lenten effort up until Good Friday and the pilgrimage. Cramming last minute, hey Felipé?

Lately I am so thankful for my Christian faith, for its ability to build and maintain resilience in me. I seem to be able to walk my cancer walk without spending time in the dark regions of despair. I can see it from where I am and sometimes I brush up against it, but the ability to remain positive in all situations seems my strong suit. And Easter is the crown jewel of the Church year in terms of the theme of positivity. Here we are!

So, wishing you a big Happy Easter! My Rebecca and I are going to catch some lunch and then take a Sunday drive. Nothing serious. A walk at 1600. Easter loves, Felipé.

APRIL 30, 2019 / SCAN TODAY

Well, this is usually the time cloaked in anxiety and worry, this scan time. The whole process is when I have the worst time, but am feeling strangely peaceful at the moment. I am trying to be as optimistic as possible to hear news of this new treatment that I have been receiving. It has been six weeks now and the doc and research nurses are keeping close tabs on my every move. And this scan is the first look at my insides. Ah, my insides, the place that has been steering my life for eight years now.

I will share the news with you after I learn about it tomorrow at my doctor's appointment. But really enough of that for now. There are other things, other important things, going on. Such as I look out the window and the swallows are swooping once again. There are bunches of them right now, so happy to be back at the ranch after their long trip south. See, that's important!

The walnuts are still bare but they are some of the last to leaf out. And the corn patch is looking mighty fine after six times through with the tiller. Just needs a few more degrees of warmth.

And I need to finish up my prayer for the "sick and infirmed" for National Day of Prayer. I have a good theme; a good beginning and I am working on the body of it. If I can come up with a great wrap-up ending I will have it in the bag.

OK, have to go shower up and get pretty for my nurses. Enjoy your day where you are. Swooping loves, Felipé.

MAY 2, 2019 / HAVE TO ADMIT

I have to admit that I am a little disappointed in the results of the scan from Tuesday. The results were no real change. You could see slight growth depending on how you measure it but nevertheless no turn around. We decided to give it another six weeks as sometimes these drugs need sufficient time to build up to the right level. But in the meantime I feel beat up.

There was also a glitch in the numbers for my kidney function and I am getting a week off while they double check. So, my nerves are somewhat jangled at the moment. I was hoping for some significant dismantling of those tumors equal with the work I have been putting into it the last sixteen months.

Ah, so it goes. Yesterday I saw some of my favorite nurses. I miss those guys since I don't go in as often with this latest drug that I take orally. Anyway they are very supportive. And one of their own is on the Camino right now, ten days into it and blogging. And another is also a pastor at a local church and wants me to come and show the documentary to his congregation. That's all good.

Off to the prayer service at noon and will be offering my prayer for the sick and infirmed. I worked hard on the crafting of it and will be glad to read it here soon.

Off I go. Lots of moving parts here today, have to get started. "sick and infirmed" loves, Felipé.

MAY 3, 2019 / A PRAYER FOR THE SICK AND INFIRMED

As our earthy clothing becomes torn and tattered
in the rough and tumble
so it goes with our bodies.
Why is this Lord? we ask
Some of us, we suffer.
Why us we ask?
Is this fair we ask?
Please Lord open our eyes and our ears.
Some die before others.
And whose turn is next?
Who sets this clock?
Please Lord open us to understanding,
Why are some of us chosen for this journey
of the "The Sick and Infirmed"?
What is our purpose now?
We wrestle to make sense of our suffering, of the uncertainty.
Give us a hint Lord.
We know that you are the Wellspring of Mercy.
This mercy is what ultimately will bring us to peace.
In the shelter of this peace we are hoping
some of the answers will appear.
May the tangles in our minds be loosened, our knots untied.
May the knowing of your bigger picture bridge over
our times of personal smallness.
We are grateful.
We are hopeful.
Give us strength.
Lead us through.
All in the name of our Savior. Amen.

Phil Volker 5/2/19 National Day of Prayer

MAY 5, 2019 / WHAT A BEAUTIFUL DAY!

Mass was very moving today. To start, Father David always finds an excuse to bless the whole congregation with holy water by walking through the whole space sprinkling us with droplets on our heads. I think that is one of his favorite things to do. But his homily was good too, with talk of Christ buoying us up. Over the years we have used that word a lot, "buoying."

But I hadn't thought about buoying within my relationship with Christ although it has certainly to be there. To ask for help I have to surrender to the other. That is why I think off of the Camino we don't usually do it or at least do it so easily.

But there we were in distress on numerous occasions. There would be some Camino angel who would appear to help and you/I would say sure, help me. But it is a thing that we balk at with Christ a lot of times. Oh, I got this. Or oh, I'm fine when we are not. But most of the time I think it is pride, oh I got this, thanks. So the help is maybe always available but our surrender is not.

Well, time to travel on. Jim and Gloria are coming on Wednesday and staying to Sunday as house guests. Have some cleanup to do, sort of streamline the situation and make room. It is good to have a deadline to get this worthwhile work done when we don't seem to be able to always pull it off without.

Beautiful springtime blessings to you. Thanks. Sunny loves, Felipé.

May 6, 2019 / In Preparation

I am planning on planting the corn on Thursday. Jim will be here from Buffalo to help. So, God willing, Thursday it is. The weather is supposed to be fantastic and I am close on having the soil ready, just have to level it and lay out the rows and set up the irrigation. It will be good to have that helping hand for the actual planting.

So, this morning I set the corn seed to soaking in warm water. I'm saying, "Wake up you little guys, it's time!" Have the three varieties in the three coffee cans with the water. The early is Sugar Buns which has a smallish ear that matures quickly so it's there when you are craving. The middle is Bodacious which takes longer and is cornier tasting with a bigger ear. It is a favorite. Then the late is Golden Jubilee which has the biggest ear and takes the longest. It won't happen in a cold summer here at this latitude but it should this year. All of that just means that we will have fresh corn for a month or maybe five weeks at best. It is called succession planting when you have different varieties that come in waves and don't interfere with each other.

So, John Conway, Pilgrim Farmer John, will be here from Iowa later this month to put his blessing on all this. And the real point of this is to help feed the pilgrims who will be here in August. Yum!

Walking in a few moments here. What a beautiful morning too. See you tomorrow. Corny loves, Felipé.

May 8, 2019 / Just A Wednesday In May

Writing from the ferry boat, on my way to the hospital, then airport. It is beautiful again this morning. The sun is breaking through the usual morning marine clouds. The water is very calm as we cruise. The barometric pressure is high with stable weather for us. Looks like corn planting time to me.

The planting project is in high gear with the prep all done and with Jim coming today. Hopefully we will start putting the seeds in tomorrow morning. So, exciting!

There always is that thought rattling around in my brain that this could be the last corn crop for me. Can't be helped really with the state of things, the uncertainty of things. Of course this is true for all of us, young or old, that every darn thing is the last, but we never ever dwell on that naturally.

Coming into the dock, another successful crossing. It is really a miracle that we continually take for granted. No problem, we are good at that. But today I am thinking that my corn could be my last. Maybe this is my last hospital visit. Maybe this and maybe that. I guess the takeaway is to not take things for granted, right?

I am going to sign off for now. The doc is going to call me in momentarily. One thing at a time loves, Felipé.

MAY 11, 2019 / TRYING TO GAIN WEIGHT

During these breaks in the chemotherapy I try my best to put on the pounds that I will need to get me through the next hard spot on the trail. Jim and I went to my Bible class this morning and stopped at the grocery store on the way back. He kindly bought me six cartons of ice cream to help in my effort, saying that this is the fastest easiest way. OK, doctor's orders on this.

The weather continues to be summery and we are off after I get done here with this post to water the corn. My babies, all 1600 of them.

So, I got some more positive feedback on my poem/prayer that I read at National Day of Prayer. I am so happy that it resonated with so many folks. Part of one comment was that yes, inspiration can come from bad things. Yup, that's part of the Camino of it all and a large part of the Cancer Camino.

OK, up, up and away. Saturday sort of loves, Felipé.

MAY 15, 2019 / A BREAK IN THE RAIN

Off to the city this afternoon for a check-in at the hospital. And taking Jessika to the airport for her trip to Rome. In the meantime, the sun is out over Raven Ranch. The corn and the weeds are growing. I can put some energy and time in on weed control since the intermittent rain is watering it just dandy.

Off I go, love, Felipé.

MAY 16, 2019 / HELD UP AGAIN

Oh, not a holdup but I had another obstacle in the clinical trial of my cancer treatment. After my testing yesterday my number that was too high was still just slightly too high so I have another week off. It is coming down to the good range but not quite good enough for the protocol. So, one more week of good energy with no chemicals and the corn will appreciate it I am sure.

Am I seeing everything in terms of the corn, well maybe I am. Well, could be worse, a lot worse. At some point lately I started realizing all the little myths and quests that I would think up to keep myself excited and going. None of it is so-called "real" or "factual"—it is just Philthink. I hope I am making slight sense. Some of my best blog posts are in this category.

So, yea, it's all happening as usual and this and that needs to be contended with but we march on, we walk on, we journey on. If we hear the music in our heads that keeps us sane during all this we are truly blessed.

Love you immensely, alperfect, later, Felipé

May 17, 2019 / Trying To Get Organized, One More Time

Oh look, a little patch of blue sky, a hopeful sign. We could use a little dry out in-between the rains. Well, they have all been light rains, showers really. Don't want to scare anyone away.

I am having a conversation with Karen of Cambridge. We are talking of the importance of inspiration in our ability to keep going on our cancer camino. Spell check doesn't like an "s" on the end of camino to make it plural. And maybe that is better that way, yes? Maybe we share this camino although we have never met in person.

And I realize that in my case the importance of myths and quests in my daily going-forward that serve to organize my life for me. They organize the chaos of cancer and other things. They simplify and streamline the jungle of it to let me pass through on my way. I realize that I am not using earthly logic here with this method of navigation. Somehow I have been able to maneuver outside of the standard thinking and that has given me some sort of advantage in this journey.

There is a "for instance" here that I would like to mention because it is screaming at me presently. When we read the Beatitudes or the Sermon on the Mount in the book of Matthew we quickly run into the difference between earthly logic and heavenly logic. All our standard knowledge and thinking don't seem to fit there anywhere. We are forced to start questioning our normal ways of thinking about things. Standard doesn't work anymore.

And I am not saying that my view of my situation is somehow heavenly logic but it certainly is influenced by it. Or at least I was able to break with standard thinking by understanding that there are possibilities of other ways. Just sort of babbling here. All of a sudden I am self-conscious. Anyway I got that out for the world.

Looking forward in a few moments of getting some time in the corn. Weed control is the name of the game presently. One hour spent here now will be worth ten down the road.

OK, have to leave you, things call. Off we go loves, Felipé.

May 20, 2019 / Ragtag But Enthusiastic, That Be Us!

Wow, what a visit! Pilgrim Farmer John and his gang rode in to Phil's Camino around high noon yesterday. We may never be the same around these parts.

Two trucks pulled up in the yard, one a Suburban with John's guys and another a pickup with a nice sweet couple Richard and Julie. Julie is local and a cousin of one of the guys, Ken. But the guys piling out of the Suburban are Marine and Navy vets, various flavors of officers, mostly flyers. They have experience leaving kisses and destruction in their paths. I think that is fairly accurate. Anyway they left us kissed and exhausted. They still have it. Let's see if I can recall them all: Kent the Elder, Doctor Tom, Ken aka Bruiser, Dapper Dan, Garnett the Swabbie, and of course Pilgrim Farmer John our Caminoheads Heartland Bureau Chief.

Having arrived earlier than expected (thus interrupting my last-minute cleanup attempts) I put them to work in pairs to get things ready. That worked out well and we managed to talk and laugh away a couple of hours before the 1600 hours walk.

Sometime in there, Farmer John walked over to give the blessing to the corn who were all standing proudly at attention for him. I was happy.

As John was the only one in the crowd that had seen the *Phil's Camino* documentary, we piled everyone into the living room and played the DVD for them. They were duly impressed. I hadn't seen it in at least six months so I was reminded how good it is.

The walk went well of course without any falls or animal bites. It all looked great to me after months of cleanup from the winter snows. Of course I'm the only one who saw that. Oh, I need to mention that Jane, one of our pretty regular walkers, showed up to help out the home team. Thank you, Jane.

So, the guys brought a huge pile of food and bottles and a giant frosted cake for the sagging tapas table. We all did a mighty fine job on that and I doubt that supper was needed by anyone after that. Thanks guys! So they are all flying out today to various points on the map: Iowa, Vermont, South Carolina, Oklahoma.

Walking in a minute, later loves, Felipé.

MAY 22, 2019 / VERANDA BLEND

Veranda Blend is a coffee by Starbucks that is offered here at the hospital. I just totally love the way that sounds so I thought that I would keep it going here.

Hooping and hopping and hoping you are having a great day! Come back loves, Felipé.

MAY 23, 2019 / ON THE VERANDA

Veranda, I love the way that rolls off the tongue! It seems to have been around for a while, like old money. It has accumulated a bit of history for better or worse. People have come and enjoyed her and now they are gone. But we are here to start afresh. She seems feminine like a big messy lap. Big enough to hold a group. Maybe there are those wicker chairs that the air can blow through to lend to our comfort. The Veranda has a comfortable hold on us, bringing us together when we have been off on separate adventures and quests. Some of us have been injured, some have won awards, some have created, some destroyed. But the Veranda holds us so that we can reunite and its time provides us with the opportunity to see how we have grown while apart. We are together now and out of the glare that is often taken for reality. The din and the glare, they go together. But that seems far away for all of us now. We loosen our ties and let our hair down, we plan to stay for a while. Air is moving to keep things fresh and to rid us of the unwanted. Maybe it means the weather is up for a change. The Veranda will shelter us in a shower and we are beyond worry. Who has a story for the good of the order? Maybe something about pirates or pyrites or parakeets. We have fun even when we aren't having fun if that is possible. A few of our group go off in search of refreshments. The icebox can't be far. Something light please, vino verde or iced blond coffee perhaps. I have dozed off but the light touch of a napkin on my hand has awakened me. Ah, my wine has arrived. Gracias.

Enjoyed the time with you, love, Felipé.

May 25, 2019 / More On The Veranda

Well, after playing with so many possible names for the August get together, I have settled on The Veranda. Yea, The Caminoheads' Veranda. It will grow on you, I guarantee.

Maybe this came partially from a naming trend that has been happening here on the Island. We have an informal music venue that has been happening for a while called "The Coop." And then recently another popped up called "The Greenhouse." Also small, friendly and informal. So we are right in that zone.

We had a few oysters for dinner last night. Haven't had any in a long time, exotic little units. Maybe we could round some up for the Veranda this summer. We barbecued them on the grill and put them in butter and cocktail sauce. Then eat on a saltine. No fuss, no muss.

Off to work, love Felipé.

May 27, 2019 / Smaller Than A Dime

I just noticed this morning that I am missing a little something. Five years ago, after losing two little Virgin Mary medals on the Camino I found a tiny silver shell in a crack in the sidewalk. It was some little town, big-enough-to-have-a-pharmacy-type town, and I was with Maryka in the last 100 kilometers somewhere. Doesn't matter, a crack is a crack. But I have been wearing it on a chain around my neck along with a silver cross that was my Mother's.

Well, it is somewhere, right? Somewhere safe for the next person to find is the right way or a good way to look at it I suppose. A certain amount of randomness is refreshing and welcome.

We saw the Sam Cooke documentary film last evening on Netflix. My Rebecca heard about it from a friend. That was a good one to catch up on, some important history.

Memorial Day today. The local vets are putting on a ceremony at the Vashon Cemetery. I ran or helped with that for something like twelve years when I was serving in various offices in the American Legion Post. I had to quit that when my cancer hobby got so time and energy consuming. But we remember those on whose shoulders we stand.

OK, have a walk in a few minutes. The day is supposed to be beautiful and maybe eighty degrees. Holiday loves, Felipé.

May 30, 2019 / Leaving The Little Corns Behind

Off to the airport and Orlando tomorrow. It will be another world. Here we are going to weed and water the little corns so they will be happy while I am gone. They are two to four inches tall now, getting on up for the Fourth of July Knee High Test.

Things are shaping up for the Veranda. It is starting to take on a life of its own, which I was hoping for. Getting this many fantastic people together in one place will be enough to start something good happening. The rest is just details.

Thursday loves, Felipé.

JUNE 2, 2019 / GETTING BACK AND LIVIN' THE DREAM

OK, got 'er done. On the plane heading out of Orlando. Our event went well. We had maybe 75 professionals and students involved with different aspects of sports medicine. Not a huge group but an enthusiastic one.

I am looking forward to getting back to the ranch. I want to check out the corn and see what it looks like. Maybe it grew another inch. It is trying to stay ahead of the deer chomping on it. Ah, and there is Mass in the morning.

Well, there you have it. A high day was had by all from one coast to the other. Love you, Felipé.

JUNE 7, 2019 / I FOUND MY CAMINO SHELL

A few weeks ago I discovered that my tiny remembrance of walking in Spain had fallen off of my neck chain. I think that I described it as smaller than a dime. Well, I found the little silver shell on the carpet in the living room last night. I felt like throwing a party! See? it really pays to cut down on vacuuming all the time.

In the corn news, it is supposed to rain today, which we really need badly. I am managing to keep up with the weeds barely. And the deer are letting me know that they are still around.

I am expecting around fifty folks at the Veranda in August and that would be great if we could get that many.

I have a friend Sui who walks here as often as possible and lives and works in Seattle. She has connections with Taiwan. And there is a bishop there that is intent on coming to visit the ranch and walk with us. How about that? We haven't had a bishop yet.

Just a few more minutes, maybe I can squeeze in one more news item. Our Catalina, Kate Barush, the Art Historian for the documentary is coming to the Veranda. We are assembling some heavy hitters.

Just saw an eagle soar by the window, a nice omen for our day loves, Felipé.

JUNE 15, 2019 / HERE WE ARE ON THE VERANDA WITH WISDOM

This morning we had a great Bible Guys meeting and we talked of a lot of things, but one thing that came up was a definition for wisdom. And that was that it is healed suffering. Wisdom, any thoughts on that? Yes, you say that it reminds you of the phrase School of Hard Knocks. Yea, haven't heard that in a long time. That is learning through living life, right?

Well yes, each one of those knocks needs to heal up to garner wisdom out of them. Yes, otherwise we could complain about them and not get any further. Or we could be unforgiving and it wouldn't go beyond just a painful memory to relive and relive. I see that.

How else can we think of this? Yes, we know heart rocks. We like to collect them and have them around, yes, rocks that are in roughly a heart shape. So, you are saying that the cleft in the heart rock is basically an injury. That the rock is rolled and tumbled for a thousand years afterward and it becomes worn smooth or healed but there is still evidence of the injury. That's cool, yes I can see that. In order to have heart as we say we need to have suffering and healing. I will think about that, yes.

All right, there you go! Heart-shaped loves, Felipé.

JUNE 18, 2019 / SOMETHING NEW EVERYDAY

Yesterday was a bit much, speaking of something happening. It was just the most absolutely ordinary day with us puttering around the ranch like a lot of days. It was an all-of-a-sudden realization that my wedding ring wasn't on my left hand anymore. After forty years of traveling with me it was gone, solid gone. I stared at my hand; it didn't even look like my hand.

I exhausted myself searching for it. What a frantic feeling. Oh, it is wearing me out right now just thinking of it. There was one spot where I was convinced it had fallen. I went over the area with a metal detector, put stuff through a half inch mesh to no avail. Had to finally give up and lie down.

A couple of years ago My Rebecca had made a beautiful silver ring, inspired by wind-blown grasses, that she gave to me and that I have been wearing on my right hand ever since. She suggested that I just switch hands, easy-peasy. That made sense and felt good. And then she had a story for me about a young friend of ours, a new Mom, that found a wedding ring while gardening and it wound up being her wedding ring some time later. I feel better. Maybe I am part of some bigger story yet to come together.

Life is like that—I should remember from the Camino where it seemed like daily I was losing and finding things. Of course in the end these things are only things and sharing them with people that we don't know may be important somehow.

Walking later today. Henriette will be here with a bottle of Sangria. That could be the opening line in the great novel that I need to write yet.

OK gang, time to scram loves, Felipé.

JUNE 20, 2019 / SOME BLUE SKY

Last night one of the guys from my Bible Guys group who we haven't seen in a while spoke of his challenges with his wife's cancer. It was very open and moving and brought us all up to date. And other guys shared stuff about what was going on with them and theirs. It all seemed to have a central theme as I listened. And that was getting to the place where one can operate, function and maybe even thrive in that place of dislocation and discomfort. That is what I am calling that state for the moment, dislocation and discomfort. It is the place where we may find ourselves even after we have spent a lot of time and effort trying to avoid it. The place that is the opposite of our best dreams for ourselves and our loved ones. It's, in my own case, dealing with cancer.

But how do we get on top of those obstacles? How do we get to the point where we can work with that and live with that and make it into something positive? Yea, and that is really the bottom line of this blog and five years of blogging. It has been the unfolding of this process for me. It has been a long drawn-out process but worth every penny and minute of it. That's what I am beginning to see anyway.

Hey, time to go find my shoes for the morning walk. So glad I can still ambulate. Thanks for being here loves, Felipé.

June 22, 2019 / Saturday Morn

All checked in at the 2-Day Cutaneous Lymphoma Patient Conference here in Manhattan Beach, California. We go on stage at 2 this afternoon with a screening and Q and A session. So, I got time right now to be with you. I found a semi quiet corner overlooking the golf course and the cement pond.

I've got my name tag on and underneath my name is the title Cancer Commando. I like it.

Drs. Asher and Wertheimer are showing up tomorrow to give their presentation on the GRACE Program, "Growing Resiliency and Courage." Really great to be with this group. Standing up to it loves, Felipé.

June 27, 2019 / A Little Help From Confucius

I saw this quote today: "You have two lives. The second one begins when you realize you only have one." —Confucius.

I have never zeroed in on a quote from this guy before but this one is speaking to me loud and clear. It is taking me back to writing to you about cancer. This diary is supposed to be about Cancer, Catholicism and the Camino. It is more often than not about the Camino in one form or another. But traveling backward to reach the cause of that you quickly find the other two of that trinity.

Catholicism for me could be termed a bridge between the Cancer and the Camino maybe. But the cancer diagnosis was the spark that started the whole thing ablaze. In various talks I have termed it a catalyst and that really is non-judgmental. It can cause a change is all I am saying. And it's usually seen as a big deal so it can easily cause a big change. But that change can be a good change as this quote points to.

That is an amazing phenomenon really. But it makes sense that we need a jarring announcement to shake us awake. It's the old 2X4 to the head that sends us into another dimension.

But it does spell disaster and doom and gloom to people too attached to earthy concerns and earthly logic. It is death come early. It is more though. It is the death of great expectations. And isn't that one of the lessons of the Camino? We learn that our expectations generally get us in trouble. Life just isn't that predictable, it is twists and turns and plan B's over and over again. We know that.

Off to walk. Patches of blue sky and occasional rain drops falling. Traveling together loves, Felipé.

July 1, 2019 / Summer Has Hit

Thinking of the souls on the Camino now with the current heat wave there. I remember crossing the Meseta with Kelly and we would get up a half hour earlier each morning trying to get more of it done in the dark and cool. It was brutal in the afternoons.

But the Pacific Northwest is not Spain. We are in comfortable temps for sure. Walking in a few minutes and conditions are perfect.

Well, time to go round up my hiking shoes. We'll see who comes by this morning. Sometimes the mornings are just me and I tend to work on my rosary then; today is the joyful mysteries. I pray for the whole rock pile here and all the things that you have placed there over the years.

You guys are the best. Buen Camino loves, Felipé.

July 2, 2019 / A Change In The Weather

"Let's review" as Kelly would say.

A thick layer of gray has enveloped us this morning. A little rain is falling now and again. I think that I will put some time in at the woodshop this morning. Maybe we will have some sun breaks this afternoon in time for our walk.

Henriette is coming to the walk and tapas. Kelly may show up also as well as some mystery guests. Rain coming down now. Our plant world needs a good soaking. And Henriette is coming early to talk about Cancer and the Camino, the theme for her new book. A rainy day, we won't be distracted.

The Camino may be a natural solvent for Cancer. I am using a capital C on cancer here just to acknowledge its power. The Camino we always capitalize. But the Camino may be something that has the right properties to loosen the hold of Cancer. It is powerful enough to match it. To believe in The Camino leaves little room for other concerns. I am groping for something here that I am not quite sure of. Sometimes things get interesting when we don't have the proper words.

One needs powerful positive things in one's life to ward off the negative that trolls for us. Old French: *troller*—to wander here and there in search of game. We are being hunted or fished by negativity I sense. The Camino may be a natural repellant to this.

A lot of talk right now as folks get ready for the Fourth of July, one of our big holidays. There will be parties and cookouts everywhere you look. Fireworks overhead. America's birthday party!

Thinking of you loves, Felipé.

July 5, 2019 / Making Sense Of It

I boil it down and I boil it down like maple sap in the spring to finally get to the point where there is something significant left in the pot, something sweet enough to brag about. It's been years now of this process to make some sense of my life with Cancer.

What is it after all this time and all this walking, after all this talking and all this writing that my effort amounts to? What does all that seek to accomplish? I think I have an answer and I want to spring it on you momentarily. It seems the only thing that I have power over. The only thing that is worth the fight. The only thing that I seem to be good at, my gift maybe. What is that?

What if it amounts to waking up each day and figuring out how to kick a little more fear out of this massive mountain called Cancer. That's it finally, in very short form. It appears to me that at this point I have accomplished walking around it, this mountain of my personal Cancer, to say, "Ha, I see you are not infinite and I am putting boundaries on you." That is where I find myself.

And so I am not just going to be on the defensive anymore. It is time to say things will be different from now on. I am reading the Riot Act to Cancer to say I am in charge of this situation. I may very well die in the process but dying is not defeat; not living is defeat.

Feeling feisty on the Fifth of July loves, Felipé.

JULY 6, 2019 / MORE SENSE

Kicking fear out is an important concept and goal. There is way too much of it around. And definitely way too much swirling around cancer the disease. As a matter of fact, cancer the disease should be written with a lower case "c" while that ugly thing which results when all the fear is added to it is another animal altogether and could then be spelled with a capital "C." Yes, how about that?

There is a reason why the Christian Bible (the New Testament) is always saying "Fear not!" Fear is a tool of the darkness and it abounds in our environs now and then. It is a hindrance to us to say the least. It is more like a burden which can overwhelm us.

Anything that we can do to lessen it for ourselves and others is a major step in the right direction. It is necessary to be aware of this continually, day in and day out, minute by minute. Whack-a-Mole it for yourself and for me please. You have my eternal permission, whenever and wherever it appears.

The other "mole" to whack is the idea that death is a defeat. Cancer patients can get wrapped up in hopes of cures to a frenzied degree, only to be finally faced with death and then feeling that cancer defeated them. This is so common. The point to me is to do what one can in the curing department but to balance that with living life. We all have a unique life to live, for ourselves, our family, our neighborhood, for God. This is what I was getting at yesterday. To miss out on our life is tragic and is the real defeat.

Let's not miss the joy loves, Felipé.

JULY 15, 2019 / THE MORNING WALK

I have a few minutes before the regular morning walk at 9 o'clock. Maybe a brave soul or two will show up. It looks like it could sprinkle on our heads. And we are getting down to the final laps of this our third walk across Spain. There are somewhere between forty and fifty laps to go I am recalling. Maybe by mid-August we will be in Santiago!

Any ideas where to go next? I need a map or guidebook from another route maybe. Remembering back to the start of this trip across and I was then looking for another route and nothing came up so we did the Francés again.

Oh, a light rain out. This is going to so help our wild berry crop this year, all this rain lately. I'm predicting they will be super juiced because of it. The king berries are starting to appear. That is the singular blackberry at the very end of the vine that ripens first. So, coming soon.

Out of time for now. That's how things go these days. See you soon! King berry loves, Felipé.

July 16, 2019 / Sometimes A New Perspective Comes About

Years pass sometimes as I trudge through certain aspects of my life. I don't even sense that I am in a rut. Everything seems present and accounted for. Then one day somehow I stumble on a new way to look at it. It was there all the time but it wasn't available to me. How many things are like that?

Last evening I was doing energy work over the phone with my friend Janet from California. I'm the subject, she's the worker. We were having our weekly session Monday evening. It was warm out and I decided to move my end of the operation outside to the deck by the tapas table. You know the place.

I stretched out on a reclining chair and found myself looking upward at the big cherry tree which overhangs the area. It was there before we got there in 1980 and it has turned into quite a presence over the years. And as I was there working with her, I was becoming more and more lost in the structure of this gnarly old tree.

It was like meeting an old friend that I hadn't seen for a long time. Look at that! And look at that! And look at that over there! I enjoyed that immensely. And Janet wove it into the treatment nicely. But that tree has been in my life most every day for decades now and it took a different perspective to see it and enjoy it, to appreciate it anew.

It has a great cantilevered way that is spread out horizontally to cover most of our house. This is totally different from the structure of the conifers growing in the crowded forest here. They are interested in height as they strive for the sun. This guy is out in the open and is intent on growing outward.

So, I scurry around under this magnificent tree in its shade and protection doing our tapas rituals. Our guests enjoy themselves laughing and sharing stories. And I take the tree for granted. So that is what I was awoken to last evening. It was fresh and new remarkably.

I wonder how many other things are lurking around waiting for me to rediscover? And a major part of that is slowing down. So thank you, Janet, for slowing me down for that hour.

Off I go to the day. Unexpected loves, Felipé.

July 18, 2019 / Blast Off

Somehow death has always seemed like it would be a dimming of life. We want to continue onward to another day but our capabilities ultimately fail us as our fire dims. But taking a cue from my cancer, it is possible that a person as they approach death could grow so large, robust and wacky that they outgrow their venue like cancer does to the body. Maybe blast into another dimension!

I am so lucky to have options for my mind and spirit to fly to. There doesn't seem to be a good reason to be small about things. Where does that get us anyway?

It's a blast loving you, Felipé!

July 19, 2019 / The Blackberries

The blackberries, that really are the owners of our property, are starting to strut their stuff. The upcoming crop is looking totally outrageous. This wild and crazy plant is once again going to bring a cascade of abundance down upon us. Maybe we will have some guests here this summer to help us pick them.

But it was in February of this year that we had the big heavy snow and everything was crushed including the blackberry brambles. Things looked bleak for them but hark, look at them now. This plant just screams resilience! Cancer patients need to study this. What do they have that we could learn? It is a gnarly nasty plant by suburban landscape standards, way too unruly for the lot. But out here at the ranch it owns the land in between the forest and the pasture.

I know I curse them continuously, true, true, true. We compete for square footage. I hack and I burn and I sweat and I curse. Maybe some of their orneriness has worn off on me. You think?

Otherwise on Vashon Island there is the annual Strawberry Festival this weekend. There will be a parade and vendors and dances. Thousands of folks from the mainland will descend to partake. I will be hiding out here pondering blackberries and resiliency. None of that wimpy strawberry stuff for me.

None of those wimpy strawberry loves, Felipé.

July 20, 2019 / Remembering Lourdes

I remember how I struggled to try and capture the experience at Lourdes last May. It was hard for me to do that. It was hard to separate my idea of pilgrimage that I had developed from the Camino. I had to put that on hold to consider Lourdes. This took some doing but I did it.

Now more than a year later I see something maybe that I missed in my writing then. Well, basically the Camino is all about action. Walking, walking, showers, tapas, sleep, walking, walking and on for hundreds of miles and many days. If it is not action. it's that you are resting and getting ready for more action. If we have to stop for good you would feel defeated.

Lourdes is all about sitting still, being still and receiving. It is all there for you, all figured out. Good people cart you around, literally, from one religious experience to the next. You are with thousands of other malades, pilgrims with an illness, receiving, receiving and receiving.

Of course I had trouble sitting still, the Camino guy that I am. So this is what I was wrestling with there and after. And what did we receive ultimately, what did we come away with beyond all that? What did I finally find and boil down to put in the blog? Well, in brief it was all about healing. And by healing, I mean beyond curing. I mean we experienced a closeness, a glimpse of the bigger picture. That is beyond suffering. Something that can make it all seem OK or, even better, can see it all make sense. Or even better yet see as something to find joy in. Yea.

Well, just a flashback to last year. And a year can be an eternity when you think about it. A lot can happen and you can get a lot done in a year. Here's to the future!

thinking of you loves, Felipé.

JULY 23, 2019 / REPORT CARD

And you need a report of my foray into Swedish Cancer Institute yesterday. That sounds like a university, I wonder if I can be a college graduate now; Mom would be so proud. Shoot, I've been going for eight years now, I ought to be getting something to hang on the wall, don't you think? Anyway, I passed all my tests, turned in my forms and answered all my questions right. So I am still in the clinical trial! Yea! I really didn't think that I was going to get through all the hoops this time. But voila!

So besides all that, I hope that these little pink pills are beating back the little growies in my lungs. That would be the important thing here. So, I have three weeks back here at the ranch before I have to show up at the Institute. The Institute, that sounds important. Be there for a full meal deal scan, tests and appointment. I am so lucky!

OK, so there is merit and benefit in celebrating small victories I have learned. This here is one of those. At tapas today raise a toast to Felipé's ongoing contribution to medical research. That's only half funny, I really mean that.

Our family is all here now at the ranch. That's why I'm locked in our bedroom where I can talk to you in peace. My Rebecca is having the time of her life playing with the kiddos. We should take a family photo to let you know what this looks like. Yea, good idea.

OK, time to get the day going. Have to go peek at the corn. It is all tasseling now, forming those precious ears of golden delight. All for your eating pleasure!

golden delight loves, Felipé.

JULY 26, 2019 / THE NEIGHBORHOOD

I am the luckiest guy to live in such a neighborhood as I do. This is the Camino brought home. We have found something priceless in a world so topsy-turvy. It seems an opposite, a germ of better times.

And you, too, are with us. The more the merrier is the story. We will all drink to it when we get together.

pay attention loves, Felipé.

JULY 27, 2019 / THE CORN A-COMIN'

The corn is galloping into our future, our enjoyment future. It is making amazing leaps toward maturity.

And the blackberries are starting to ripen, had a few. That is just going to be a cascade once it gets started in earnest. I made four berry picking buckets to help with the harvest. Hope you come to help!

Tonight it's my turn to cook dinner. Thought I would do a whole chicken in the Dutch oven in the campfire. And add some potatoes wrapped in foil. Then marshmallows on sticks afterward, summer fun!

This is absolutely my favorite time of year when everything is in such crazy abundance. Time for Felipé to gain a few more pounds, fatten up for winter. I am coming along on my weight gain program coming in at 178 pounds at my last visit to the Institute (new word for hospital, sounds impressive).

Verandatime is also galloping at us. Hope that you can join us for part or all of it. Preparations are coming along.

let our love ripen, Felipé.

August 7, 2019 / We Had Five

Yesterday was our afternoon walk and tapas and we had five pilgrims partake. We did it up right too. Catherine and Dana, Jim and Jen and Henriette were here. So great to have good weather and be out at the tapas table and comfortable.

We are getting closer to the end of this "walk across Spain." We are slowing down so you all can join us and we can walk in together at the Veranda. So most days I have been doing two laps instead of my usual three, which is OK in this heat.

Things are working out for the Veranda. Folks are checking in and making arrangements. The excitement is building!

getting closer loves, Felipé.

August 8, 2019 / Gosh

I am thinking about all the thoughts and notions about love my Bible class uncovered this last Saturday. The chapter was the 4th chapter of First John. All about how love works. It's about how God loves us and how to return that love and how we need to love one another.

In this blog over the years, I have had numerous posts about how the Camino works and how it works in me and in us. And we all know this. We know because we drank of that wine. We may have a hard time explaining what happened there but we know that something significant did happen there.

John goes a long way in explaining these things. This is his blog from the end of the first century AD. He does a nice job. It is as relevant now as it was then. This is one remarkable thing about the Bible, how it stays current. It's timeless stuff.

John was the last of the Apostles. The only one not to die a martyr's death. He lived out his days on the Greek Island of Patmos, a Roman penal colony. And he wrote these inspired letters for the fledgling church and for us.

Walking here in a few minutes. Time to join the salon of thoughts, ideas and laughs at Phil's Camino.

salon love, Felipé.

August 12, 2019 / The Best News Ever!

Yea, hey, out of this world news! Corn season is officially open here at Raven Ranch! We got into a dozen ears yesterday at tapas to start the season officially.

The Sugar Buns variety is ripening, which is impressive earliness. It is tender and very delicate. It will run about two weeks 'til it peters out. The next variety Bodacious will be ready, of course God willing, for the Veranda party. This is a perfect example of alperfect!

And as long as we are talking corn, the final variety Golden Jubilee, bigger and better than anything, like third gear, will come along. What a show, almost better than the fireworks on the Fourth of July!

OK, preparations proceed for the Veranda party. People are asking how they can help and I am assigning things for them to do. I am going to drop all other duties here pretty quick so I can concentrate on it. Oh boy!

Monday morning walk coming up. Where are my shoes?

bodacious loves, Felipé.

August 13, 2019 / What To Do With All The Beans

This is the time of year when surplus is the word when it comes to the fields and gardens around us. Harvest, harvest, harvest day and night. What to do with the surpluses?

Everywhere you go people are handing you zucchinis. There was a time on Vashon when they would regularly show up in your shopping bag after you got home from the market. The checker had thrown one or more in there for you, spreading the wealth.

Anyway, I was actually thinking of beans here, green beans. In Spain they served them in a broth which I loved. So, that is what I am doing lately. The beans are cut into one-inch pieces maybe at a bias to make them more interesting looking. Then for each serving cook in one cup of bouillon. The amount for two people could be cooked in two cups of broth. Then it is served in the broth in a bowl with a spoon.

Of course you can only eat so much fresh produce and that is where freezing and canning come in. This is a big chore at times, trying not to have waste.

OK, just giving you a snapshot of the time and place. Off I go now to work on preparations for the Veranda.

serve with a spoon loves, Felipé.

August 14, 2019 / A Traveling Post

I have a few moments before I have to leave for the Institute. My day to make an appearance. Once every three weeks seems like luxury. Scan today, a lovely anxiety producing procedure. This must be my way of getting ready to give you the update. It will be a very long day with a rushed drive back to the Island to catch what I can of My Rebecca's book launch starting at 6 PM for her first novel, *That One Day in August*.

It is such a lovely event for her and I hope that she has many more books and launches in her future. This fits her well as a transition from teaching. And I who have not as of yet read her novel will try to get started today with all my "free" time at the hospital.

At the Institute. Such a day outside, I'm staring out the window at it. They could feature drive-through treatment maybe. I know we are always way ahead of the times here at Caminoheads. Waiting on getting my tests started. I am getting way too used to this crazy stuff.

Speaking of My Rebecca, I need to start reading her novel now to see if I can make a dent in it before this evening. The husbands are always the last to know.

staring out the window loves, Felipé.

AUGUST 15, 2019 / ABOUT YESTERDAY

Wow, a big day for us yesterday.

First, I was off early to travel to Seattle to what I call the Institute (Swedish Cancer Institute) for my scan and the doctor's interpretation. Under normal conditions these scans are so incredibly anxiety producing for the scannee. So much seems to ride on this one snapshot. How could any one thing be so important? But it seems so.

My scan showed the cancer in my lungs stable, no growth! That is a win in my world, a "W." And two other parts of the puzzle were good also. One, my side effects were near zero and my numbers from all my tests were in the good zone. This is what a win looks like anymore, no growth and tolerating the drug at the same time. Yay!

And rushed back to the Island to catch most of Rebecca's book launch party. She had a good crowd and a fun reading. So happy that she has this going. A lot of books were sold and signed. And I personally am very close to finishing the book. Somehow actually reading it has escaped me over the last few months. But it's good, quirky and comical.

Afterward we cleaned up the venue and went across the street for a drink and dinner to celebrate. The whole day was something to be celebrated and we tried to do a good job of it!

So, off to the morning walk. We are so close to Santiago. Sort of dragging our feet and not trying too hard lately so you can catch up and we can finish at Veranda time.

celebration loves, Felipé.

AUGUST 16, 2019 / MY FIFTEENTH LIFE

I went to evening Mass yesterday as it was the Feast of the Assumption of Mary. These special services are always interesting to me in that I get to see a lot of people that I don't normally. Our little church has three Sunday services per week and folks tend to get habituated to one or the other, and if that isn't your slot you normally never see them. So it is refreshing to be there.

One of these that I talked with was Catholic Collin, as Wiley calls him. He yells out from a distance, "Phil, hey what are you on, your fifteenth life now?" That's hilarious. I said something about that I was losing track!

But it is something to check in with once in a while or daily. It is easy to take life for granted most times especially on the good days. Yes, but I do feel like I have been given fifteen lives sometimes, crazy as that sounds.

Well, time to jump up and continue on the prep for the Veranda. A hundred little things that I would like to get done before people arrive. Some of those might actually happen. Sometimes I feel like one of the characters in my Rebecca's novel where the quirks of life really rule everything in spite of best intentions.

fifteen loves, Felipé.

August 18, 2019 / The Sunday Before . . .

The Sunday before the very first Caminoheads Veranda. I am asking all other pilgrims to spend a quarter of their time here helping out. That means you are open to help out if something needs doing while you are on duty. Things like serving food, dish washing, or manning the sign-in table for instance. We are just a big loose albergue.

OK, maybe that is it for now. This is just the kind of stuff that is filling my brain during the countdown, lots of nuts and bolts issues. But it is all for our Veranda! Our get together is the important idea, everything else is secondary.

Everything else is secondary loves, Felipé.

August 23, 2019 / Opening Day 2019 Caminoheads Veranda

Here we are: 8:40 AM. Have coffee brewed and stories are coming out in droves just with the few of us present so far. The rain has stopped for good, fingers crossed. Looking like Spain in August here early this morning.

William from Calgary and Rho are here with me starting this out. Will just write a few words in this lull to let you know what we are up to. So, with that I need to get back to scurrying around getting the venue oh so just so.

Oh so just so loves, Felipé.

August 24, 2019 / Veranda Saturday

We walk into Santiago this AM on Phil's Camino. Our 909 laps will be completed, God willing.

Then a few hours' break and then off to the Vashon Theater for the high noon showing of *Phil's Camino: So Far So Good*. *Phil's Camino* is up on the movie house marquee next to *Apocalypse Now*. Maybe it's two for the price of one.

We are experiencing a deep manifestation of God's love here at the Ranch. We had a marvelous first day yesterday and things are ramping up for more shenanigans. I have a feeling that this energy will start to be noticed from space.

Anyway we are merrily pilgriming along here. The best to you there. Know that you are loved.

noticed-from-space loves, Felipé.

PART VII
The Guestbook

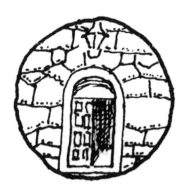

I.

When I came to walk with the pilgrims gathered at the 1st Veranda, I especially needed the attention of our fearless leader, Felipé. In the midst of all who were there, he was willing to give me his whole self for one lap of his Camino walk, sensing my great need. I had felt pastored by this gentle soul all year, in each day's writing of his blog.

At that particular time in August, I was just 2.5 weeks into my recovery from breast cancer mastectomy surgery.

I had not yet told Phil of my cancer diagnosis 4 months prior. I couldn't seem to live it "out loud." I was still reeling from the whole scenario of medical protocol required leading up to surgery.

I had retreated into my inner cave. I felt safe there.

I knew however Felipé would understand and provide the needed consolation I was looking for. He did not disappoint. I felt seen and heard, as if I were the only person on the trail that day.

My spirit felt relief in my confession, the weight of the burden lifted, by sharing my journey with another, had received the balm of healing that follows.

Felipé's Camino has touched us all. His writing, so refreshingly raw, gives one reason to ponder life in perhaps a new way, each and every day.

A community has been created from sheer Divine intervention. And I am grateful.

~ ANONYMOUS

II.

"The universe conspires to support the dream."

If ever I wanted evidence of Paulo Coelho's prophetic lines in my own life, I have only to recall how I met, and came to know Phil Volker.

In the spring of 2014, at the age of 59, I announced to my wife, Dana, that I knew what I wanted to do to celebrate my 60th birthday, walk the Camino de Santiago Compostela," an ancient Christian pilgrimage route that stretches 500 miles across the north of Spain. I only had to voice my nascent idea and it suddenly appeared before me like a very big dream. Immediately, Dana was excited to join. "We need to start walking now," she said enthusiastically. And then, as if considering the personal importance of the idea, she said, "Unless you want to go by yourself." "Are you kidding?" I replied, "There is no one else I would rather walk with than you." And with that, it was decided. But, because we were still more than a year away from making the dream a reality, we moved it to the back burner of our conversations, focusing our attention instead on the more immediate work of planting a garden and taking care of our small farm.

Later that summer, however, on a Sunday morning, our parish Priest asked us to pray for a fellow parishioner who was making a holy pilgrimage across Spain. Coincidence, or the first of many signs that the universe was already conspiring to support the dream?

Every Sunday for a month we prayed for our fellow parishioner and then one Sunday in September we applauded his safe return. Our parish pilgrim, it turned out, was Phil Volker. I told myself that I needed to meet this man and all that fall, as Mass let out, I would start in his direction. But, since I am somewhat shy, I put off our eventual meeting until "next Sunday."

Finally, the new year rolled around—2015. We were at an island party when Dana asked me: "Isn't that Phil Volker?" As I agreed that it was, she already was leading me to him. Phil greeted us warmly and when he heard that we intended to walk the Camino in Spain, in just a few months, he invited us to come and walk his camino here on Vashon. He took out a business card and wrote the days and times that he walked on the back. When we read his address we realized that he was our neighbor, our neighbor! It turned out that Phil lives less than a mile down the road from us.

My first impression of those winter walks with Phil, on his camino, were like dating; slowly getting to know one another while passing the steps across his land together. We got to know his story: the story of his cancer, his conversion to Catholicism and his eventual pilgrimage across Spain. We learned how his camino had come to be, how he had walked to strengthen himself physically, mentally and spiritually in order to better meet the demands of his cancer treatments. We also talked about all manner of things "Camino."

In preparation for our upcoming trip we had many questions most of which were practical in nature: what to expect, what gear we should take, how to adequately train? More than once Phil said, "People focus too much on the little stuff, the Camino will take care of you." His message then, as it remains today, is that the preparation of the open heart and the receptive soul are primary, and the physical and intellectual preparations secondary. So, from February until we left for Spain on April 1st, my wife and I walked and talked, and walked some more with Phil, 2 or 3 times each week.

Before walking the actual Camino, Phil's camino was more about Phil as mentor. The actual trail around his land while beautiful, seemed like only that, a beautiful trail that encircled his land. It starts beneath a blue pop-up tent with a pile of stones at its center, ambles out beneath a large plum tree, through a pasture gate, across open fields, one adjoining another, and then along his corn patch and into the woods. In the woods the path crosses over a little stream that runs clear in winter. Then, it finishes back at the tent. At the streambed we would pick up a rock to add to the pile along with a prayer for someone we had been keeping in mind. After each lap, and there were always three, Phil would record the date, who was present and where we were on the actual Camino in Spain. He used a tattered map, the one he had carried on his pilgrimage, to help him track of our virtual progress. I remember being fascinated by that map, trying to imagine the landscape it traversed and marveling over the names of the towns, names I tried to sound out and pronounce, "Cizur Menor, Castro Jeriz, O'Cebreiro . . . " towns Dana and I would eventually walk through, with shuttered windows at siesta, lively tapas scenes at evening and a holy reverence at dawn.

As Dana and I walked across Spain, we carried Phil with us, often mentioning him to one another, wondering how his health was holding up, sharing his story with our fellow pilgrims. We came to realize that Phil's story was embedded in our own, he had mentored us, he had become a dear friend and he had given us his tattered map as a going away present – nothing could have been simpler, more generous or more profound. The Camino does take care of you. When you are in need, other pilgrims always seem to have just what it is that you are missing; even if it is only a smile or some words of encouragement on a long uphill grind. We too shared what we had whenever we could, a few segments of an orange to an older woman, out of breath, tired and thirsty.

When my wife and I returned home to Vashon from our Camino, the first thing we did was walk over to Phil's and walk with him. It was a celebration that rivaled the one we shared with other pilgrims upon our arrival in Santiago. Phil was so welcoming, "Catherine y Dana" he shouted and we hugged with easy joy. So often in Spain at the end of a day we would enter a town and see our pilgrim friends who had arrived ahead of us, packs dropped, sitting around a café table having tapas. They too would welcome us by shouting our names, pulling up extra chairs and ordering another bottle of wine. Now we knew what Phil knew and now the walk across his land became a way to hold the spirit of the Camino alive in our hearts and our actions. Now, Phil's trail was not only beautiful, but something imbued with meaning and memory.

The Camino taught me that being a pilgrim is a state of mind as well as a way of being. I can see now that Phil tried to share this with us long before we went to Spain. I wonder, if we had never gone but only kept walking here with Phil, would we have learned the lessons he was offering? I like to think we eventually would. Because, Phil embodies the pilgrim spirit, he is an inspiration to so many and his story continues to spread. He lifts me up, by who he is and how he lives his life. Dana and I still walk with Phil at least once a week, and we never fail to fall into that Camino state of heart: easy in conversation, easy in silence, appreciating the beauty of the seasons, the weather, whatever it might be, making small prayers for those we love and often finding ourselves suspended in the peace that *surpasses all understanding.*

When Dana and I arrived in Santiago, we attended a Mass for pilgrims. At its end a Cardinal spoke to us in English. He told us that the real pilgrimage would begin now; the destination - our deaths, the journey - how we would choose to live our lives. He encouraged us to continue to live as true pilgrims, as those who give their selves to something larger, who travel lightly, who rely on the kindness of others and as a result extend kindness whenever and wherever possible. And always, the Cardinal said, walk with gratitude. Then, switching to Spanish he said: "Gracias, Gracias, Gracias." The last "Gracias" he spoke as a whisper. It was a challenge, an acknowledgment, but most of all it was a blessing. And so we continue to walk with Phil on his camino, full of gratitude for the blessings in our mutual lives, for each other. Sometimes I catch myself whispering in prayer and in blessing. "Gracias Phil Volker, gracias."

~CATHERINE JOHNSON

III.

Veranda. Front porch. Unobstructed, comfortable, laid-back view of the outside world. A beckoning place, looked forward to, and back on, as far back as our memories will allow. A place of freedom as a very young youngster, noise and rambunctiousness allowed, maybe even encouraged. Quiet times, too, with loved ones, and soon-to-be-loved ones, welcoming the night and the coolness before the days when we were mechanically cooled.

So, all in all, a word that evokes good memories, and good times, and yet not much used in this modern day and age. Yet, this is the invitation we all received: "Come to the Veranda! Recall and reconnect with all things Camino, meet old friends and make new friends. It matters not that it is to be held on an island off the coast of Washington!" The call is unmistakable, and irrefutable, and eagerly accepted. Time and distance mere details, as we were all taught by our shared Camino experiences. The "want-to-need-to" easily pushing aside the "but, what about————." Phil has invited us, and we will go!

And August, as August is wont to do, rolled quickly into the calendar and plans were put into motion, again so similar to our shared Pilgrim experience of our past Camino, or Caminos; it's here! The time is now. Planes, trains, automobiles, and ferries bring us once more as strangers together. From all over the country, from all over the globe, Pilgrims, and hoping-to-be Pilgrims meet, greet, and reunite. Strangers only in the respect of being friends we haven't yet met.

Bonding, in such short order, and with ties stronger than chemistry could explain. Eating, sleeping, talking, laughing, drinking bond strengthening LIFE for all waking hours, and some hours that weren't meant for being awake. We were all again in the Camino Life. We were all on The Way. Thank you for that, Felipé.

~JOHN CONWAY (AKA PFJ)

IV.

Nowhere else would I have delayed a trip to Southern California than to spend that time instead with Phil at Phil's Veranda in 2019. I needed to go. Going to Phil's for me is like getting spiritually re-centered with many like-minded people. Never in my life would I imagine being in the middle of the woods in the middle of an island in the middle of Puget Sound with Phil at a Monastery with Monks in the summer. But I did and that was an amazing experience and it never fails to spend any sort of time with Phil and Rebecca at that beautiful Raven Ranch.

~Ryck Thompson

V.

To give
To gift
His raison d'être.
His "just one more thing to do."
Empty handed, he gives advice: "There's mushrooms here for you."

In Pilgrim Lourdes, he's naught to give,
save self, to waters deep.
Waters holy
Waters cold
Waters washing, whirling, wishing well,
Profound and blue.
Compliments of Mother Earth.
Compliments of Mother Mary.
Merci beaucoup!

To give
To Gift
His raison d'être.
Himself he gives,
In prayer he lives.

To his tumors he turns,
"Be kind," he pleads.
"Benign, that we both live."

"To give
To gift
Our raison d'être.
Our one last thing . . . .
To Live."

~Fr. Tom Hall (aka the Padre)

VI.

He Never Shakes

Dedicated to Phil Volker

He never shakes
His faith stakes him to the ground
where the earth spills tomatoes and corn,
the cedar and Doug fir cast shadows,
and the shy maples drop their golden gloves vying for a suitor.

He never shakes
his faith stakes him to the saints
who draw pictures of him with carpentered knuckles,
wrapped with a pomegranate-beaded rosary.
He protects what he has,
and what he does,
and what he sees in the dappled light through the apple trees.

He never shakes
he makes shelves, promises,
light of a subject,
and when he hears the soul's whistle,
he stops to walk his Camino trail.

He faith never shakes
he awakens our rude, boastful pride
and limping life stories
to the mysteries of the tomato—
a vibrant red balloon
in the hand, in the salad, in the belly.

He never shakes
the earth quakes because life is now uneasy, unsteady.
When you've gone to as many treatments as he has,
you've earned the angels holding you close,
the sun to warm the weary bones,
and the rain, fragrant with roses, growing sweet gardens of sound.

He never shakes
his faith stakes him to the ground.

~JESSIKA SATORI

Afterword

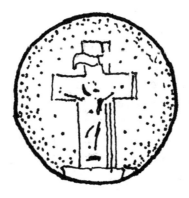

PHIL VOLKER WAS AN ordinary man, and Phil Volker was an extraordinary man. It brought me great joy to recognize how extraordinarily ordinary he was. It's one of the great paradoxes of life: by our own ordinariness we can become extraordinary.

I was lucky to see Phil about once a month when we were bringing the film, *Phil's Camino* to film festivals. Nothing would make me happier than to watch the audience when Phil himself would walk out onto the stage after a screening. We often played around with it, having the moderator ask me "Where is Phil today?" to which I would respond "I think he is in row 7" and have him walk up. The audience would be delighted and erupt into applause as he joined me.

What can I say that Phil himself hasn't already said in this book? Phil would have another thank you, I am certain. That would be to you. You who have opened this book, read the words, and are preparing to move forward in whatever direction you are heading. He would be so grateful to you, so thankful that you shared some time together. If he could, he would invite you all to tapas and a glass of wine, and find out what connections you shared. So on his behalf, let me tell you thank you. Thank you for being here, and thank you for whatever it is you are about to do, about to undertake. I just know it is going to be wonderful!

A month or two before Phil made his transition, I was visiting him. I had planned my visit around one of his chemo sessions because in the past, that had been a way of getting several uninterrupted hours together as we sat in the infusion center while he got his treatment. Catherine and I both sat on chairs by the wall as Phil got his vitals taken. It was during this time that I heard about some of the side effects that he was experiencing, since Phil never complained.

After a while, his oncologist, Dr. Gold came in to speak with him. He sat directly opposite Phil, their knees practically touching, and after looking over his chart, set it aside. "It pains me to say this to you but I don't think we should continue treatment at this point." He went on to talk about the negative side effects, and what exactly each one of them meant, then pulled up his scans to show the growth of the tumors. Somewhere in this I reached out to hold Catherine's hand as we sat silently in our chairs, two loving witnesses to the visit none of us wanted to have happen. Phil listened with a light smile playing across his face as Dr. Gold talked, and when he stopped, he simply said, "Well, we knew this day was coming." And they both agreed that this day had in fact come a lot (a whole lot) later than they could have predicted.

Phil's treatment ended that day, and his journey into home care and hospice had begun.

We left the hospital and got into the car. We were now several hours ahead of schedule since Phil hadn't received treatment. He had arranged to see his old doctor, Dr. David Zucker (AKA Danger Zone) who was no longer caring for Phil professionally, but the two men had forged a strong friendship and Danger Zone had wanted to see Phil when he was at the hospital.

The three of us grabbed some sandwiches at a local supermarket and went to a nearby park where we had a picnic. The conversation was one of three old friends, as many silences as words. After we ate, Catherine had an old blanket in the car and spread it out for Phil to take a nap in the shade while we waited for Danger Zone to be free. Phil had dozed off and I was wandering around the lovely park when Danger Zone called to say that he was unexpectedly free. We rounded ourselves up and got over to the hospital. Phil and Danger Zone had some time to themselves before we all sat and talked together. Then Catherine, Phil and I got into the car and headed out for the ferry. Parked on the ship the three of us dozed as we went across the water. As we drove off the ferry that late afternoon, Phil said "What a beautiful day this has been," and the other two agreed. Later I realized that for Phil, this was a day where he had learned that his life was coming to an end sooner rather than later, and yet, he still had had a beautiful day.

I started the film *Phil's Camino* with something that Phil told me one day as we were driving around in his truck on one of the first days of filming: "I had this practice of giving a gift to everyone I met." This book, like *Phil's Camino*, is Phil's gift to you.

Annie O'Neil
Director and Producer, *Phil's Camino*
New Year's Day, 2022

The Last Lap

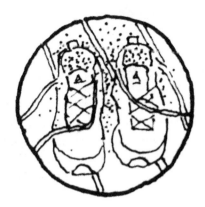

A COOL BREEZE RUNS through the General's tent[1] between hail storms. It brings a patch of sunlight, dappled by the great cherry tree overhead, like a vast umbrella. Resident Raven's wings above that. Heaven just above that.

I sit with Phil, my hand on his shoulder while Will calmly reads a lullaby from the Bible. We are playing a game of telepathic charades. Pulling blankets off, then on again, trying to bring tidbits of relief where we can. It's tough. Communication is at a minimum. Consciousness is hardly here, spanning many distant planes at once. A moan, a groan. Sometimes a word, repeated if urgent.

Currently, the word is leg as he reaches down to his left one and is obviously trying to change something. I gather that he wants a stretch and help him bend it toward his chest, gently swaying back and forth. "Leg. Oh, leg. Ah. Leg, leg . . . " It's not enough. Just trying to get some blood moving, I continue. Bending, rocking. "Other leg" he says, wincing. Will sets the good book down and uncovers his right leg.

"More. More. Ugh. Mas, mas" Felipe at the helm. "Move" he groans. Will and I catch eyes in a joint effort. We sense that he wants them moved closer to the edge of the bed and slowly, we oblige. As his right leg nears the edge, I chuckle and try to explain that we can't move him any more without his leg falling off the bed. "Yeah" he says "fall off." Ok.

---

1. While in hospice, Phil had a vision of dying like a Civil War general. True to his life-long D.I.Y. mentality, he and Wiley pitched their old hunting tent ("Elk Hotel") in the backyard and friends brought over furnishings.

I'm worried that what he wants is to get out of bed, but this doesn't seem to be the case. As his knee bends over the edge and Will lifts and lowers his foot, he breathes a sigh of relief. I'm bending, he's bending, but it's still not quite right. He's still groaning, knees creaking. We lift both legs so that they are in front of him and bending in sync, as if he's pumping on a swing. Getting warmer.

Finally, in an Aha moment, I delay the rhythm by half a beat and we-as a team-fall into stride, literally. That unmistakable motion that most of us do every day . . . the one that saved his life. His face relaxes, maybe even tries to smile. With the tent flap open, breeze still gently rustling through the Hawthorne beyond the decaying garden, it's a perfect vision of autumn in the northwest, a beautiful day for a walk.

Will and I lock teary eyes now. We can feel his muscles and tendons flexing beneath our grasp. Yes, we are helping him, but he's walking and he knows it. One foot in front of the other- one in the spirit world, one in ours. Content to stroll, we carry on. To Burgos or Léon, I suppose, or maybe to the next albergue or bird feeder. Not sure, just happy to be on our way there. On the road to awe. This was a defining moment. One of those ones where time melts away, ceases to exist. Only love. Simple, boundless. Will and I loved him and we knew he loved us back.

It wasn't a full lap. Perhaps only to the corn and back. But it was his last lap. And I was glad to be with him. I write this now on his 74th birthday and trust that he's walking still, walking with God. Walking will never be a meaningless activity to me, I'm sure many of you feel the same way. Keep on walking.

WILEY VOLKER
December 21, 2021

Eulogy for My Dad

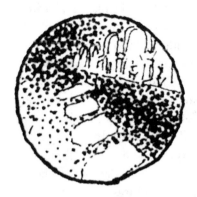

THE SPIRIT THAT SETTLED in and took up residence in my parents' home in the last few years was the spirit of hospitality. I am struck over and over again by the camaraderie, and the raucous laughter that fills that house, or that spills into the house from the back porch. It is remarkable and beautiful to me.

In my memory, in his earlier years dad was a more withdrawn person. I think many of us remember those times when his heart was not out on his sleeve . . . it is worth mentioning because it is evidence of a great transformation. I've tried to thank many of you for the "support" you provided to dad, and over and over again you mention his generosity of spirit, the enjoyment and deep companionship that you felt a part of. Dad was transformed by this spirit of hospitality that he found in Spain, as well as on his own camino, and home with him it traveled. In my home, with my children, Osian and Freya, we read a lot of fairy tales. Our favorite ones have the moral, God favors the fool. The fool of course ends up a hero, and he is a person with a simple outlook. He leaves home with some idea like he is going to build a flying ship and go marry the Tzar's daughter. He doesn't overthink it, he doesn't talk himself out of it because it is impractical, he just simply leaves home and sets out on his way. Of course he meets a magical old man who tells him, "here's what you do. You take this axe, you go up to an old oak tree. You take one huge swing at the tree, and then fall back on the ground, and fall asleep. When you wake up, you will have the flying ship. The fool/hero doesn't overthink this improbable idea, he just says "okay! I'll do it, that sounds great!" He follows the directions exactly, and he is indeed rewarded with the flying ship.

Well, in this real-life fairy tale that we are in now, It occurs to me, God favors the Phil in a similar way. It's not a direct comparison . . . but I think dad also had a fairly simple outlook. Dad had a simple idea. A couple of simple ideas. He would walk the camino in Spain, and in the meantime, that he would create his own. And if this is a fairy tale, there are many magical creatures and fairy godmothers who came in, and you know who you are. But anyway, my point is the simplicity of the camino idea. It is just a path! And he did not overthink it, in the sense that did not talk himself out of it. If it had been me, I would have said "well, that was really fun to have that cool idea. If I act on it, here's what will happen: I'll wake up on many mornings, and it will be raining. I won't want to walk. I'll have so many other things to do. Or, it won't feel like God is walking with me. The idea will lose its magic . . . it won't feel like the platonic ideal, it will be corrupted by all manner of things in reality. But in this tale, God rewards the Phil who has the simple idea, and with a simple outlook says, I have this idea, and so that is what I am going to do. I'll do my part every day. God might intervene, my doctors might intervene, but I'll do my simple part every day.

And then, I think also in this tale, God favors the Phil who constructs a method, which he always did. It's not overthinking exactly . . . but it is a thoughtful structure, a process by which to proceed. He never did anything without a method. Every day was organized with a set of instructions on a single three by five card. I am also reminded of the "corn-o-matic," a sort of jig that dad built to help him plant the corn last year. And here's another example: when I was 16, dad bought me a $50 car and once it was generally in working order, he came up with a monthly maintenance plan that we would do and it would teach me about how to maintain a car.

So here's where we get to do an interactive activity. I want you to think: if you had to come up with a list of all the car maintenance activities one should do on a monthly basis . . . yes, monthly car maintenance activities . . . I'll give you part of a minute . . . Okay tally up the number, turn to the person next to you, and tell them how many you have on your list.

Okay . . . so dad came up with a list that was a whole page long . . . I want to say there were 18 items. It included such things as checking the battery fluid. Yes, there is fluid in the battery. It was more exhaustive than a yearly inspection . . . But I'll tell you, that car did live for another 5 years. So God favors the Phil who has his method and sticks to it with fidelity, day after day, month after month. As you all know, dad certainly had a method for his camino . . . the calculation of the mileage, the mapping out of all of the landmarks and towns . . . The journal to record exactly who walked . . . the predictable schedule of his walking times. People knew where and when to find him. Every day, or according to the schedule, he did his part. By the way, when he walked and no one was there walking with him, he would write in the journal "not alone." It was simple, and methodical at the same time . . . it was a structure that could be built upon and that people could join in with. And you did. He was a carpenter after all, and he knew how to build a sound structure.

As much as it was completely unpredictable that my dad became a Catholic pilgrim, it makes perfect sense, in retrospect, knowing him, knowing those inner traits . . . the stamina . . . fidelity, his simple delight in a plodding kind of progress.

Each step was as important as the last step. He never expected any destination to be near at hand . . . He always expected gratification to be delayed . . . but he did learn to pop open a bottle of wine with you and enjoy the journey immensely.

Tesia Elani
Eulogy delivered at Phil Volker's funeral Mass
October 30, 2021
St. John Vianney Church, Vashon WA

Glossary

Albergueing: a cozy gathering of friends, as in an albergue (pilgrim hostel) along the Camino de Santiago (see also "tapassing")

Alperfect: better than all good, an appreciation; example, 'I am going to go and make a big lunch. See you, Alperfect love, Felipé'

Althankful: being thankful for all manner of things

Bureau Chiefs: Folks that Phil has appointed to write guest entries for his blog and to brainstorm, dream, and scheme with. The idea was that they would take over his daily blog after his death.

Camino dust: there is no denying that the ultimate way or The Way is following the path that Jesus has taught us. That is the twelve-hundred-year-old draw to that trail. That is the reason why the whole thing is so saturated with the Holy Spirit's magic dust. You can't go ten feet on the Camino without some getting on you. And the pilgrim walking next to you is dusted with it. And then a whole group of you walking together gets covered with it and it starts working on you and them. And the whole trail is covered with it. If you could see it, it probably is drifted up like snow in places as the wind blows it.

Caminohead: a person with the state of mind that makes a walk of their life following the possibilities that the Camino de Santiago teaches (see pp. 64–67).

Caminothink: thinking like a Caminohead

Danger Zone: Dr. David Zucker, Phil's recovery oncologist

Dilly Dally: aimless wandering with a little indecision as we relate outside of time

Goulash: a mix of things

Growies: tumors

Heartship: Having heart or fortitude or toughness or resilience

Maryness: the essence of the Virgin Mary; the epicenter of peace.

Nugget: Dr. Gold

Pancho: Phil's portable chemo pump

Perfectest: In Camino terms perfectest would mean what? It would mean that one is moving forward, experiencing things so to speak. Or if not moving forward, at least healing up or regrouping so one could get going soon, just a temporary state. Perfect is another word for whatever comes up on the trail next. Deal with it gracefully and that's it, we have bigger fish to fry down the road.

PFJ: Pilgrim Farmer John

Philthink: the little myths and quests that Phil thinks up to keep himself excited and going.

SJA – St. James Again or St. James Afoot: refers to the influence and movement of St. James in our lives.

Tapassing (also "tapa-ing"): the act of gathering for tapas with a pilgrim community (see also "albergueing")

Togethernessing: the ability to stick together and have a neighborhood

Uberperfect: "if we can have alperfect it is not too much of a jump to uberperfect"

Veranda: A gathering in August 2019 to celebrate Phil's life; he once called it a "living wake." He lived for two more years after the Veranda and had a second gathering in 2021: the Oasis. For a description of how the name came to be, see May 23, 2019: On The Veranda.

We can't help ourselves: being always connected with each other and things Camino we tend to run into ourselves and each other everywhere.

CPSIA information can be obtained
at www.ICGtesting.com
Printed in the USA
BVHW012345240722
642836BV00001B/3

9 781666 719536